YOGA

From the Ganges to Wall Street

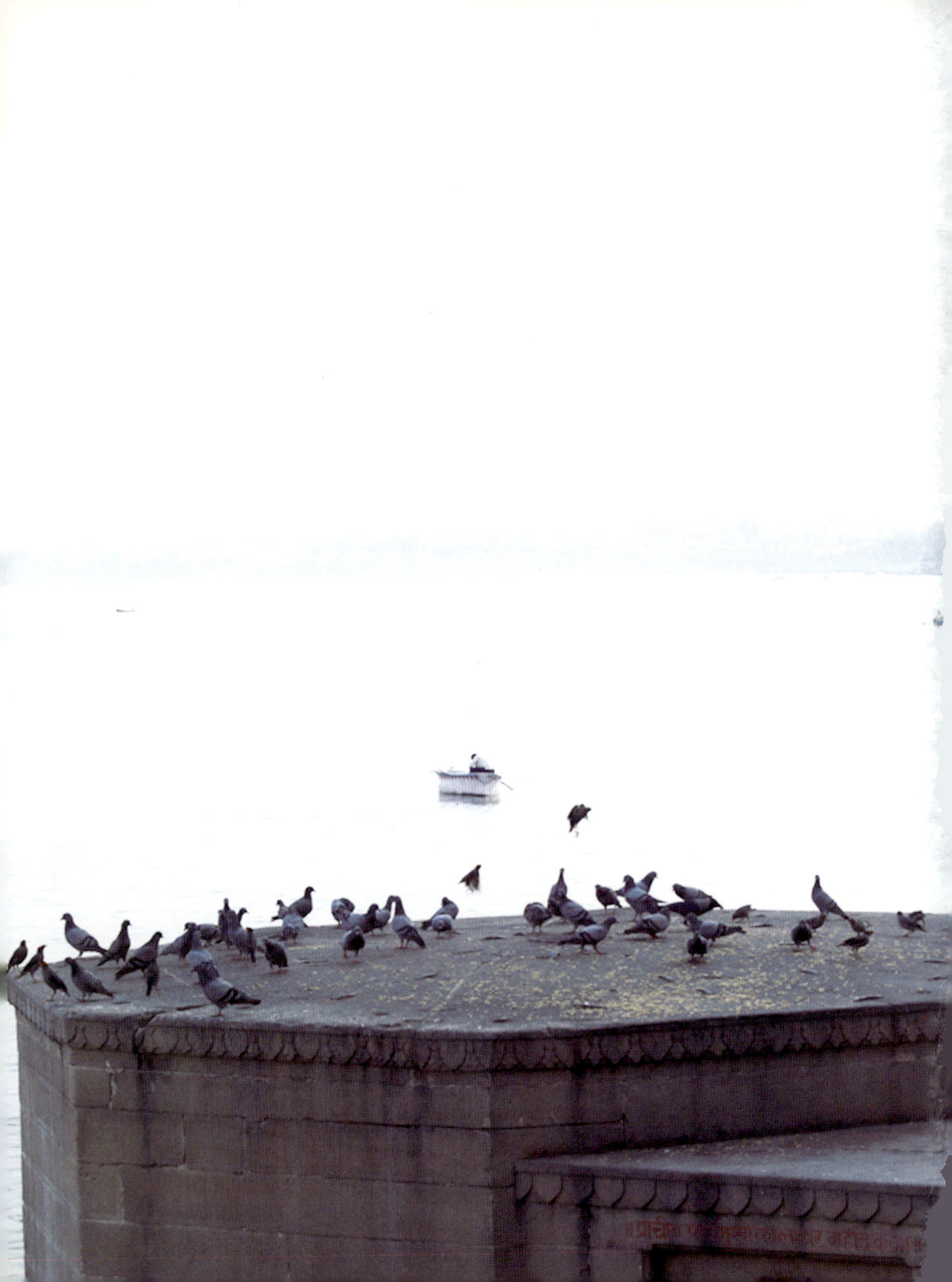

Radhika Khanna

YOGA

FROM THE GANGES TO WALL STREET

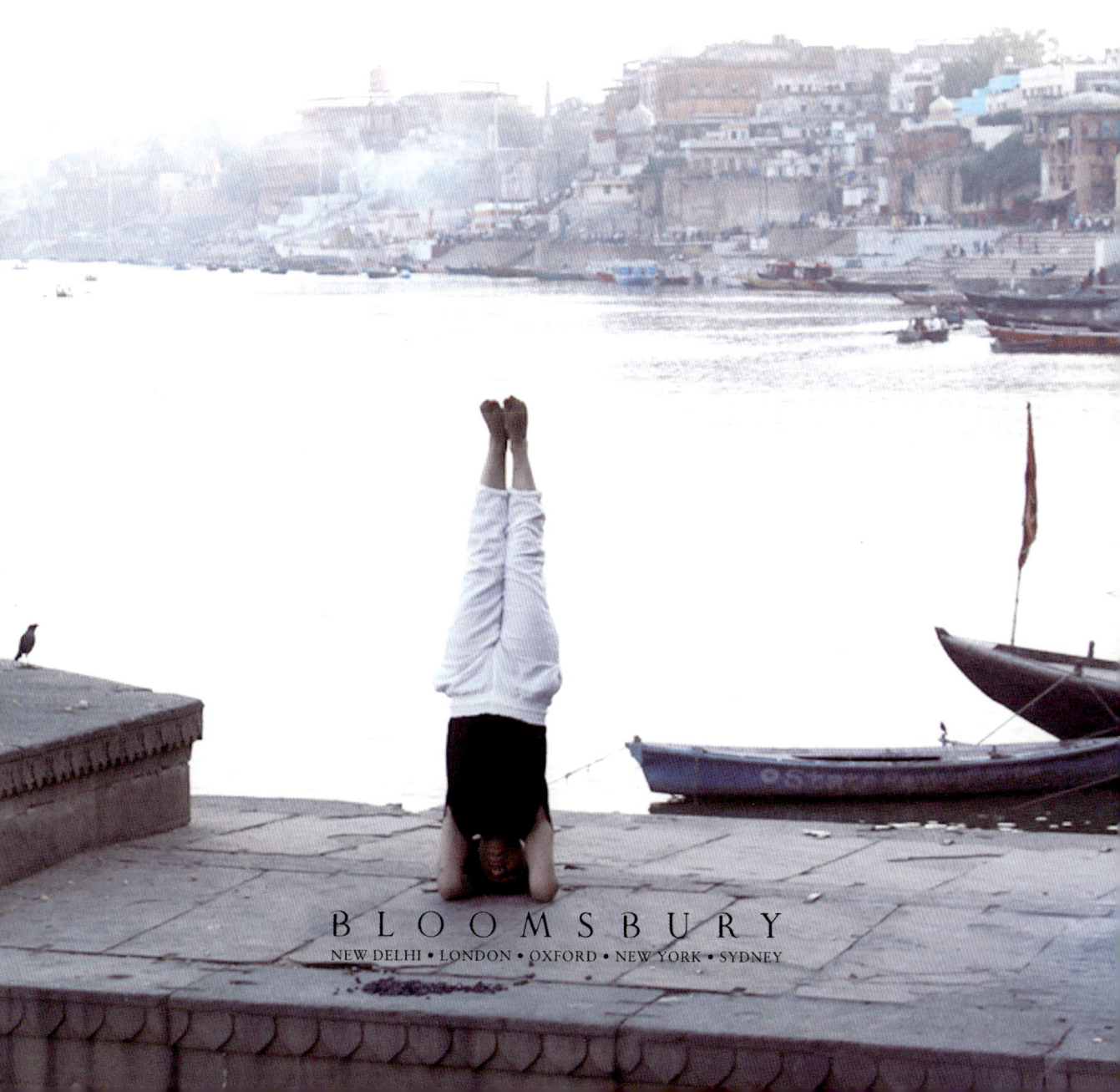

BLOOMSBURY
NEW DELHI · LONDON · OXFORD · NEW YORK · SYDNEY

BLOOMSBURY PUBLISHING INDIA PVT. LTD.
New Delhi London Oxford New York Sydney

ISBN: 978-93-84898-96-0

10 9 8 7 6 5 4 3 2 1

Published by Bloomsbury Publishing India Pvt. Ltd.
DDA Complex LSC, Building No. 4, 2nd Floor
Pocket 6 & 7, Sector – C
Vasant Kunj, New Delhi 110070

Printed and bound in India at EIH Ltd. Unit-Printing Press, Manesar (Haryana)

Safety Note
This book is not intended to diagnose, treat, cure, or prevent any disease or condition. If you have a health concern or condition, consult your doctor or health care provider. Always consult your doctor before starting any new exercise program.

Contents

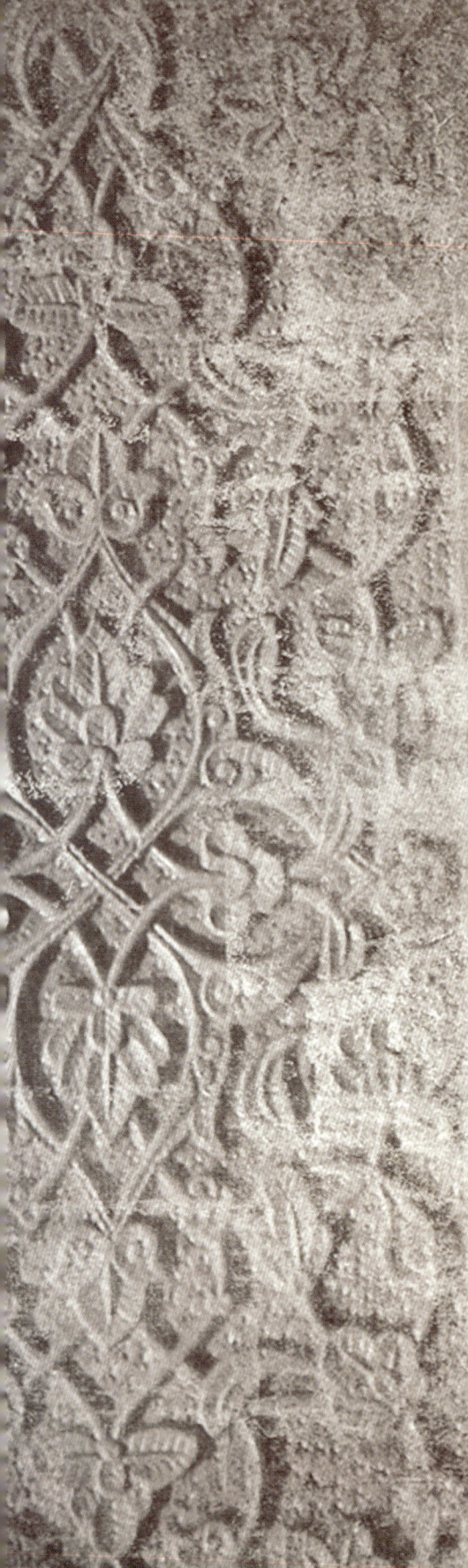

Dedicated to
All My Gurus
All Over the world

Acknowledgements

Thanks to the late Suresh Gopal, Publisher at Bloomsbury, for encouraging me to undertake this project, and to Paul Vinay Kumar and Jyoti Mehrotra for giving it a new vision and seeing it through.

I'd like to thank both Mr Vivek Srivastava and Dr Ashish Singh for the excellent photographs that appear in the book.

I'd like to also thank Vikas Khanna for his chapter on yogic food.

Special thanks are due to the Ministry of External Affairs, Government of India, and to Parmarth Niketan Ashram for their unstinting support.

All proceeds from the sale of this book will be donated to the Clean Ganga Fund. Registered as a society, The National Mission for Clean Ganga is part of the Ministry of Water Resources, River Development and Ganga Rejuvenation initiated by the Prime Minister of India, Narendra Modi.

Introduction

Yoga: From the Ganges to Wall Street is a global journey of yoga, with Radhika Khanna.

The practice of yoga began more than 10,000 years ago, in India. As part of ancient Hindu culture, yoga came before the world's major religions—Christianity, Judaism, and Islam—by thousands of years. Today, yoga is practiced across the world, from side-streets in India and remote caves in the Himalayas to sophisticated western capitals and mountain tops in the Andes. Yoga is shared by India's neighbors in Asia, Africa, and the Middle East as well. It draws people of all faiths, and from diverse backgrounds—economic as well as social. Yoga is not a religion; it provides deep spiritual fulfillment for some, while for some others it is another way to practice good health and well-being. This book seeks to guide the reader on what may become a lifetime's personal path of discovery through yoga. Special attention has been given to yoga's often unanticipated benefits and ways through which it enhances lifestyles of individuals and of societies.

Yoga can be practiced anywhere, at any time. There is no need for a quiet room, perfumed scented candles and soft music. Yogic poses and breathing techniques can be practiced anywhere for a few minutes during the day to bring about peace, calmness, reflection and satisfaction. Yoga can become part of our daily lives, and one can pursue the wisdom of the texts of the *Yoga Sutra* and the *Bhagavad Gita* to deepen one's relationship with one's own self, body and mind. Finding an experienced teacher can also help one discover deep spiritual facets that yoga can bring about in everyday life.

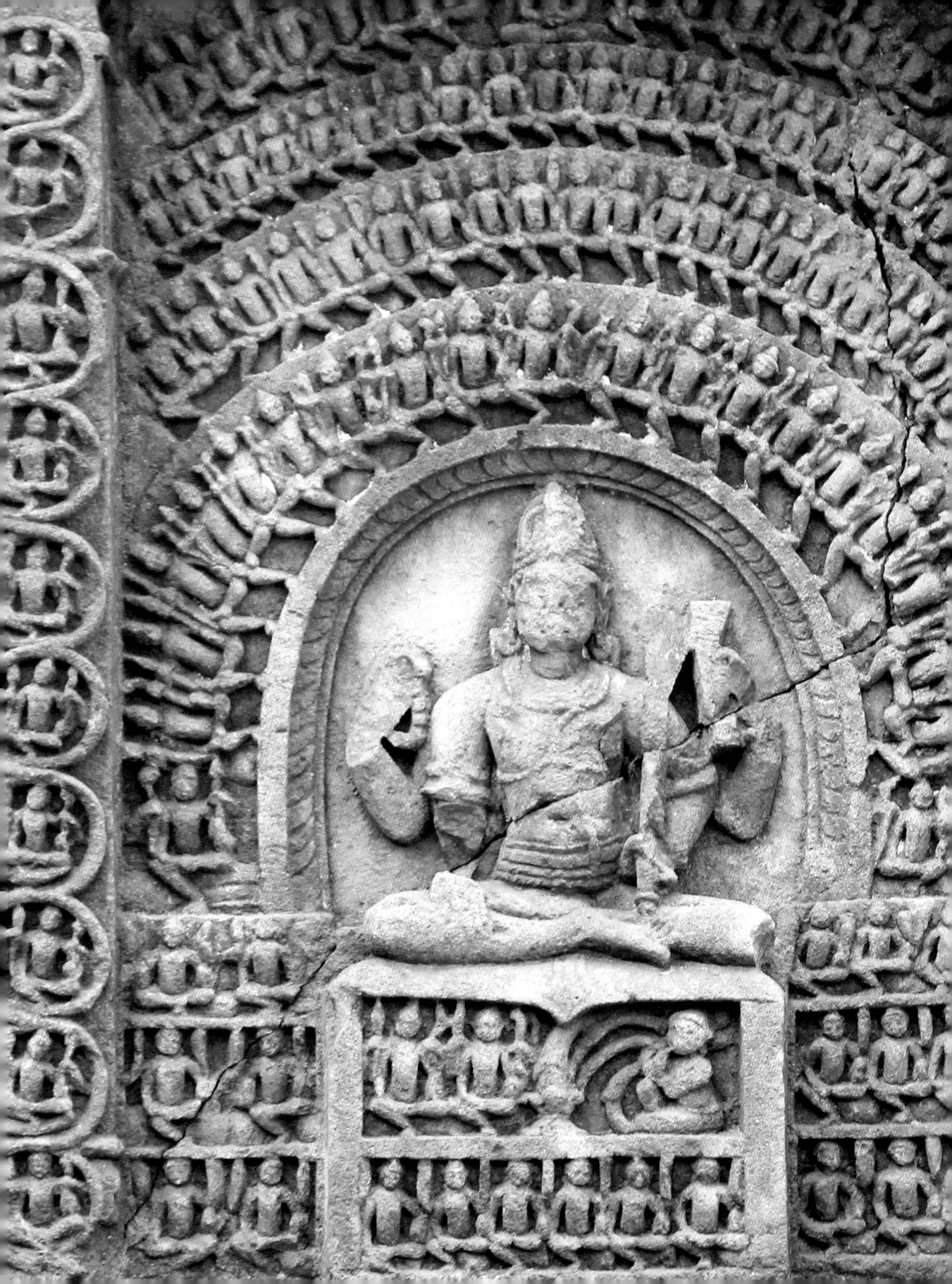

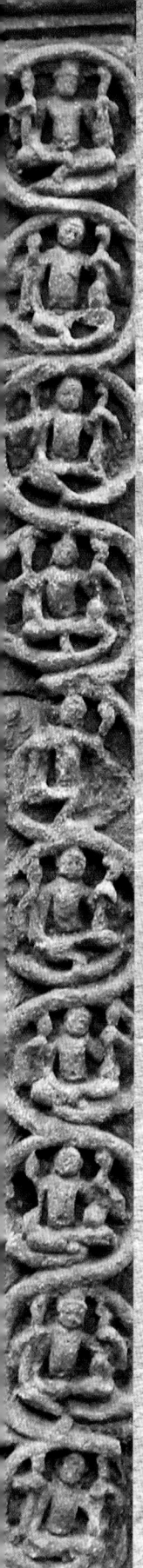

Yoga and Its History

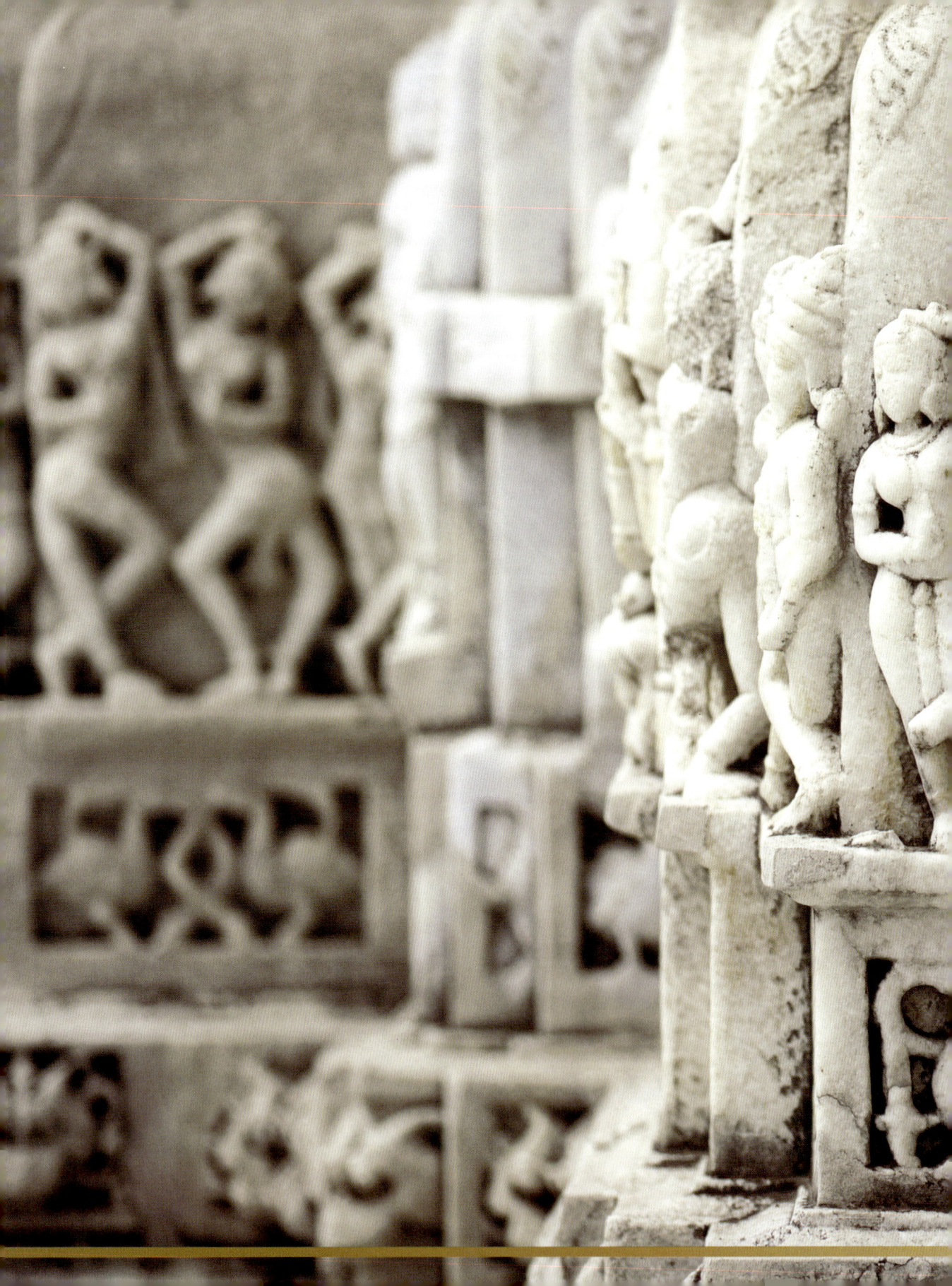

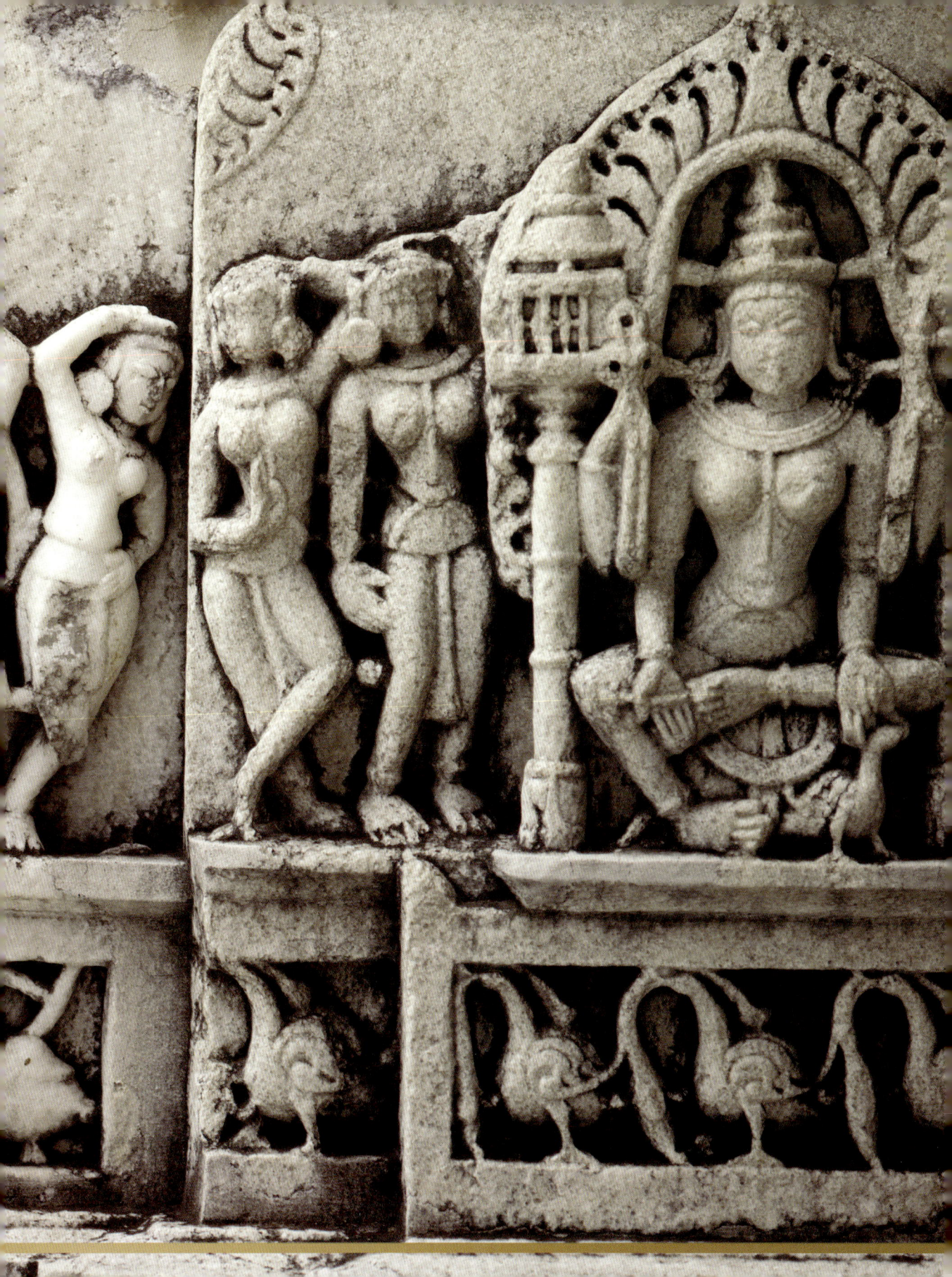

HISTORY OF YOGA IN INDIA

Yoga has existed in India for over 3,500 years. In 1,500 BC, nomads from Central Asia (Aryans) began to move further into the Indian subcontinent, bringing with them their class, or caste system, and an intellectual discipline they referred to as 'yoga'. This included ways of using the mind to retain the senses and control the body. This concept envisioned the intellect as a charioteer holding the reigns to his five horses, or senses, which in turn pull the chariot, or the body, working together and led by the intellectual power or will, of the charioteer.

The *Upanishads* contained volumes of discourses from over the centuries. Around this developed the central philosophical idea that everything is One and consequently, God is in everything and everything is in God. This world view meant that the sacrificial rituals once influenced by religion became superfluous; the self was now interpreted as the Divine. The focal point of practical yoga also shifted during this time, concentrating on recognizing the true self, or *Atman*, through meditation.

TERMS THAT DEFINE SPIRITUAL SELF-DISCOVERY

Let us take a look at the terms that define the journey to spiritual self-discovery as well as physical benefits of yoga.

Asana, meaning seat, defines the myriad postures developed and evolved over centuries of practicing yoga. Asanas are generally understood as poses practiced to expand, stretch, and twist the muscles in our arms, legs, fingers and toes, and even our eyes, ears, jaw and abdomen. A carefully followed daily asana routine provides strength, flexibility, and calmness. Some well known seating postures are over 2,000 years old – the *Padamasana* and *Siddhasana* (explained in later pages in the book).

Bhagavad Gita, which literally means 'The Song of God' is considered a source of wisdom by the Hindus, and has special significance in terms of yoga. It is made up of eighteen verses from the epic *Mahabharata*, which, along with the *Ramayana*, came into being around 500 BC. This great collection of texts represents the historical knowledge about yoga. In the *Mahabharata*, which is a war saga, Krishna, a reincarnation of Lord Vishnu, explains to one of the Pandava brothers, who is also the war hero, Arjuna, that anyone, irrespective of the caste they are born into, can follow the path of yoga to find Atman, the true self and the divine being within.

Brahmins are also known as the priests and sages of ancient Hindu culture. Yoga was practiced as part of religious, mystical and ecstasy related rituals. The Brahmins passed down wisdom and knowledge to their disciples, through oral recitations, and delivering the divine revelations of the *Vedas,* or the ancient texts.

Hatha Yoga is perhaps the most familiar practice in the West today. It is part of the *Tantric* civilization that existed in India more than 10,000 years ago. It comes to us from the *Pradipika*, a Hindu sacred text composed between 800 and 1,200 AD.

Prana is the vital force that enters the body with each breath. All yogic exercises focus on breathing. From prana we draw strength and vitality, and the life energy that keeps us alive and bestows a profound sense of health and well-being: mentally, emotionally, physically and spiritually.

Pranayama is the process of controlled breathing through yogic exercises aimed at creating awareness about breathing.

Sutras literally mean 'threads'. These are the fundamental texts of classical-philosophical yoga, drawn on Patanjali's yoga dating between 200 BC and 200 AD. The *Sutras* describe how the intellect works to offer insight on how to calm the mind and experience awareness of oneself and the world.

Vedas are ancient Hindu writings on religion and philosophy. Although yoga is not a religion per se, it forms the core of Hindu wisdom and philosophy.

Upanishads, a collection of texts from around 800 BC, are the basis for religious yoga.

Yoga, taken from Sanskrit, means 'to join or yoke together'. Yoga, as a form, brings together the body and mind into one harmonious experience. It combines the three key components of exercise, breathing, and meditation. Exercise and breathing first prepare the body and mind for meditation. Meditation prepares a quiet mind, offering healing and a sense of calm from everyday stress. The practice of yoga is based on at least 10,000 years of collective knowledge of the body and mind, and seeks to draw those elements into unity.

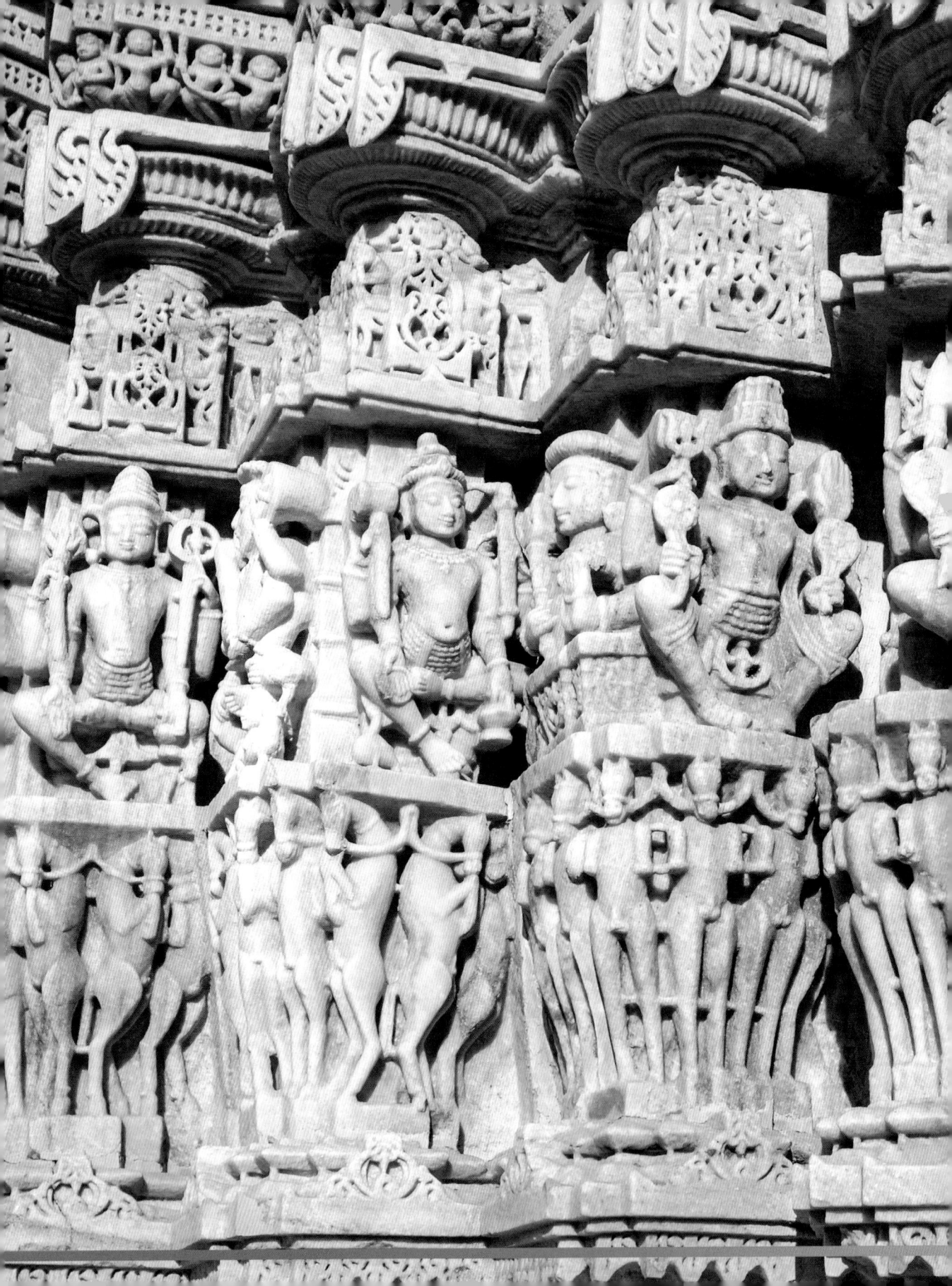

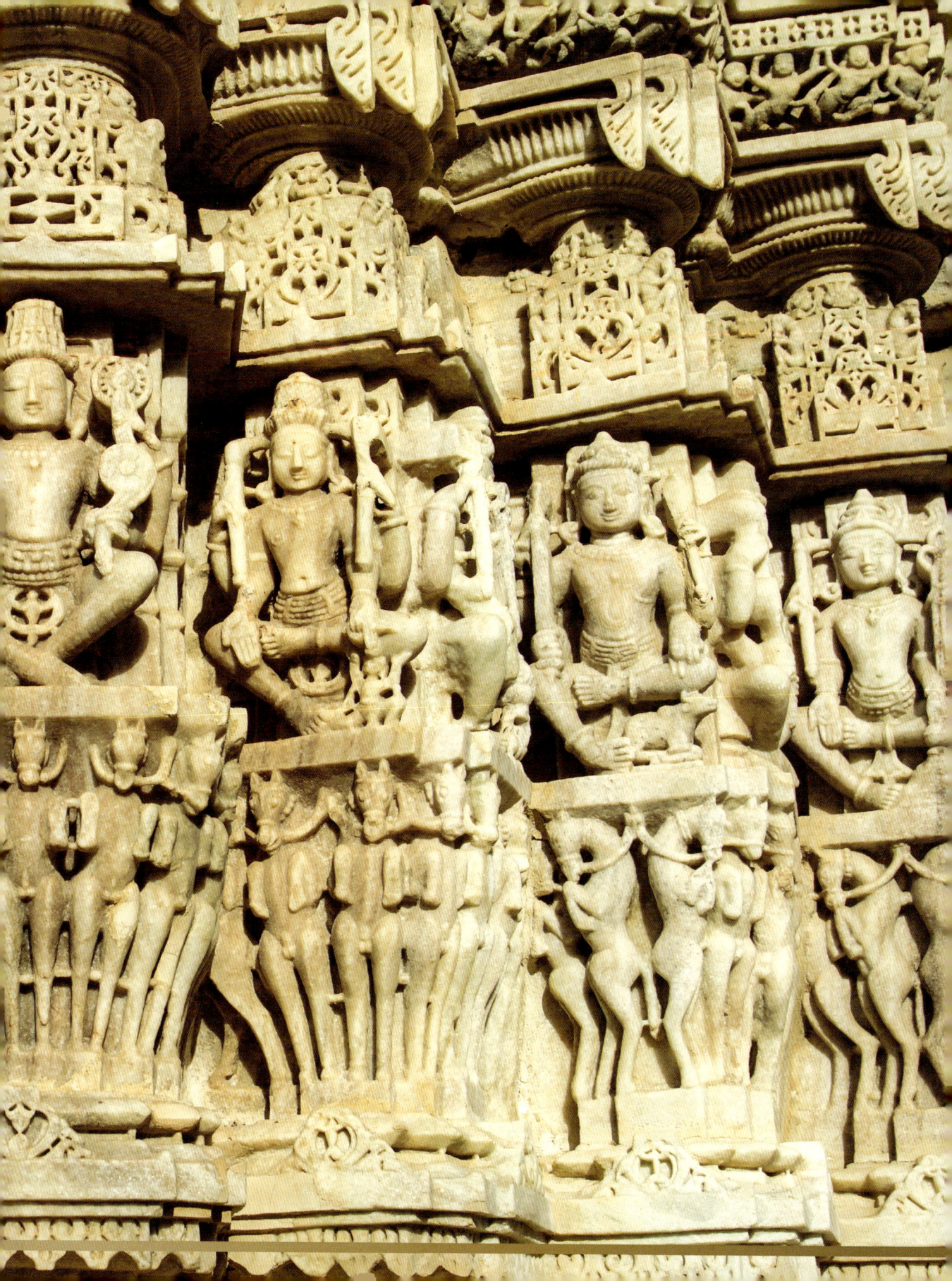

YOGA AND THE ANCIENT HINDU GODS

In ancient times, the Hindu pantheon hosted hundreds of Gods, each with a clearly defined responsibility. Gods ruled the sun, the moon, the wind, the heavens at night, lightning and thunder, air, water and rain. From around 1,000 BC, religious beliefs focused increasingly on the so-called *trimurti*, or trinity of Brahma, Vishnu and Shiva.

Brahma, the God of creation: Brahma, creator of the universe, is usually depicted as the paternal figure. Yet it is Vishnu who is more often worshipped as he protects the faith of all that has been created.

Vishnu, the preserver of life: Vishnu, the world's custodian, is full of sympathy and cares primarily about people. He is worshipped devotedly by many Hindus. He is often depicted with his snake Adishesha, which protects both him and the world with its thousand heads and is the keeper of all treasures. In order to help all creatures, Vishnu has left his comfortable position nine times and returned to this world. Rama, Krishna and Buddha are probably his best known incarnations. Legend has it that Vishnu ordered his snake, Adishesha, to be reincarnated as Patanjali, so that he could bring a practical form of yoga to man.

Shiva, the God of yogis: Shiva, the destroyer, symbolizes death and change. He destroys everything that Brahma has created, including illusions, ideas, models and customs. This makes him the God of yogis. He makes space for new creation and enables transformation to take place. He is frequently depicted either with a trident and blazing hair or as a dancer.

YOGA AS AN ESCAPE FROM THE ETERNAL WHEEL OF REINCARNATION

The folklore and legends collected in the *Mahabharata* and *Ramayana* gave members of all castes, once permitted to learn to read, who were

Yogi in Kukkutasana 1510 BC.

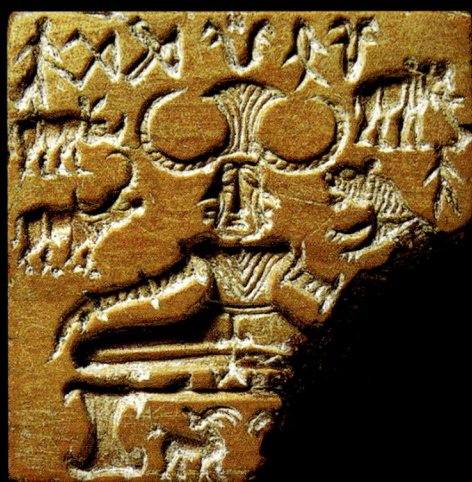

The earliest evidence of yoga was found in artifacts dating back to 3000 BC. A team of archeologists led by Sir Mortimer Wheeler found several objects depicting advanced yoga poses in the Indus valley region

previously denied the knowledge and practice of religious rituals, access to acquiring spiritual knowledge. In earlier times, this knowledge remained available only to men of the highest caste. Since the Brahmins could read, they were revered and well paid for passing on their knowledge of the epics, and of God.

The path of yoga offered each individual a system of techniques and methods of achieving self-awareness and connecting the Divine with their own being. In this way, everyone's blind faith was replaced by an individual's self-acquired knowledge to take responsibility for their own lives, so that they were no longer dependent on the Brahmins to escape the eternal wheel of reincarnation.

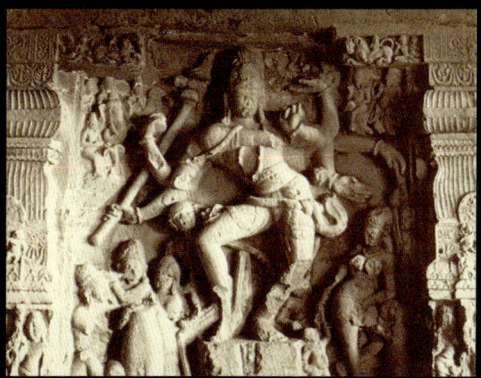

A yogic sculpture from 800 BC.

YOGA AND UNIVERSAL CONSCIOUSNESS

The teachings of the *Upanishads* first introduced the concept of universal consciousness. Early yoga had many names for this state: Brahmin, Purusha, *Ishvara* and Atman are just a few. They were used to signify the state of awareness of the divine consciousness. Universal consciousness embraced the seeing, the seen and the act of seeing in equal measure, and manifested itself both in the external world and in the soul. Atman, for example, refers to the divine consciousness within each individual being.

WHAT DOES YOGA DO FOR OUR PHYSICAL HEALTH?

We largely live our lives based on how our mind or our emotions guide us. Love may be the strongest emotion, but it is our body, our physical being, that allows us to be of this world. Yoga is a series of exercises designed to put pressure on the glandular system of the body, for overall health and well-being. Breathing techniques in yoga focus on inspiration, or the 'drawing in of God'. A yogi treats his/her body with great care and respect.

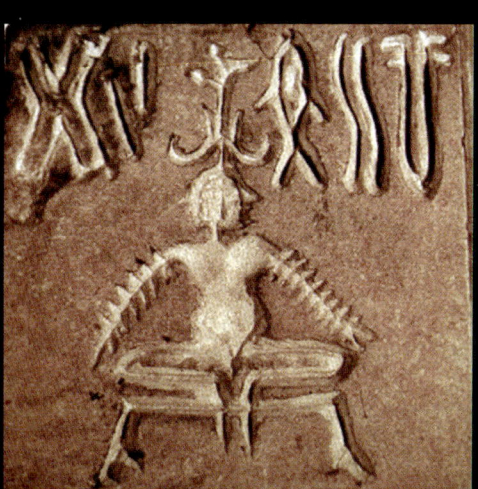

A steatite seal of a yogi seated in meditation, from the Mohenjo-Daro region of ancient India, from 1500 BC.

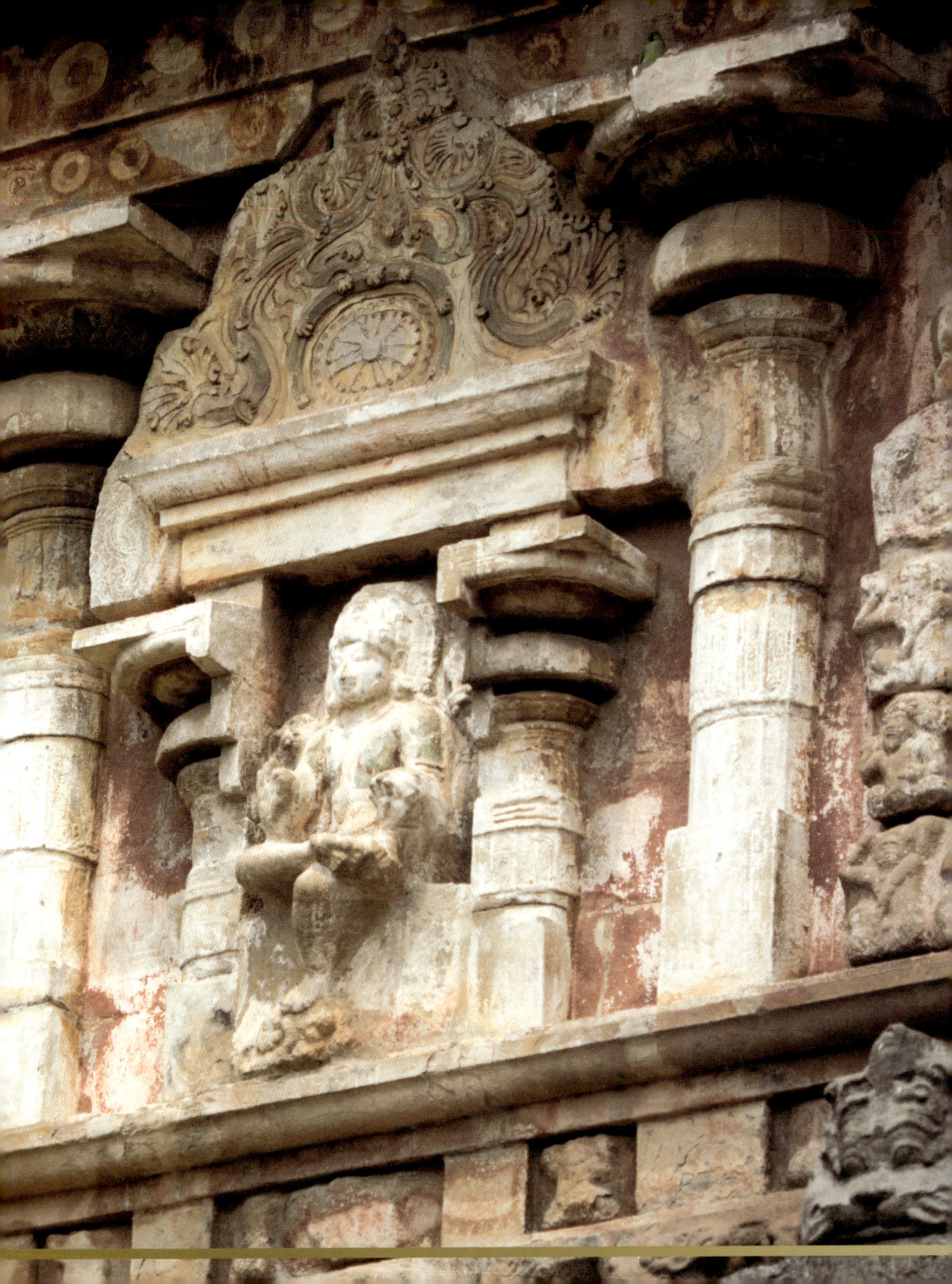

WHAT DOES YOGA DO FOR OUR PEACE OF MIND?

Yoga assumes that each individual is prevented from acting in a clear and conscious manner by physical and mental conditioning. The aim of yoga is to be liberated from those afflictions and to achieve inner peace – the basic pre-requisite for freedom from internal and external constraints. Freedom can mean different things to different people. For many, it is a feeling of happiness, an inner peace and independence from external demands, of self-awareness and enlightenment. For others, freedom means feeling at one with nature, connecting to the oneness, the cosmos or the Divine. Yet others see freedom as being a mixture of all these things. Yoga has a term for this: *samadhi*, meaning the Absolute.

Truth and Illusion

In around 400 BC, an Indian school of philosophy called *Samkya* developed a new way of looking at universal consciousness: this is reality and it has existed forever. Everything else – referred to as *Maya* – is simply an illusion concealing reality. Consequently, the world as it is perceived is simply a reflection of the illusion that is created in the mind and not a manifestation of divine consciousness. According to these teachings, nature, all living beings, bodies, intellect and emotions are separate from the Divine. They do not require any special attention, because they are part of an illusion and are constantly changing.

Purusha and Prakriti – The Two Views of the World

The philosophical view of the world was not entirely shared by subsequent generations of yogis who practiced yoga on the basis of Patanjali's *Yoga Sutras*. They look at the more global view, which corresponded to the dualist view of the world. According to this, the world is divided into universal consciousness – *Purusha* – and individual consciousness – *Prakriti*. *Purusha* is the divine entity that sees the truth and has a cosmic consciousness of immortality. It is enduring, timeless, real and unchanging, somehow representing the primordial state, which itself is Atman, the divine essence of each person. In contrast, *Prakriti* is the changeable nature, the outer shell, which consists of everything that can be seen and experienced. This manifests itself in three forms, referred to as *Gunas*.

Gunas – The Quality of Nature

Everything that constitutes Prakriti has three fundamental forms, or Gunas:

Sattva is characterized by lightness, purity, balance and clarity.

Rajas is characterized by activity, impulsiveness, restlessness, passion, growth, evolution and change.

Tamas is described as darkness, heaviness, resistance, ignorance, sluggishness and inertia.

Prakriti is therefore always a combination these three qualities, with one or the other prevailing. A yogi seeks to achieve sattva in all his thoughts, deeds and feelings. Pure sattva cannot be achieved in the material world, but yoga techniques can be used to mitigate the negative influences of tamas and rajas on the body and mind. Tamas is overcome by rajas and rajas by sattva. Identification with Prakriti is a constant source of distress, due to its erratic nature. Yoga seeks to explore everything material, but without becoming a prisoner of it, with a view to penetrate the essence of universal consciousness or, in other words, to achieve unity between Purusha and Prakriti.

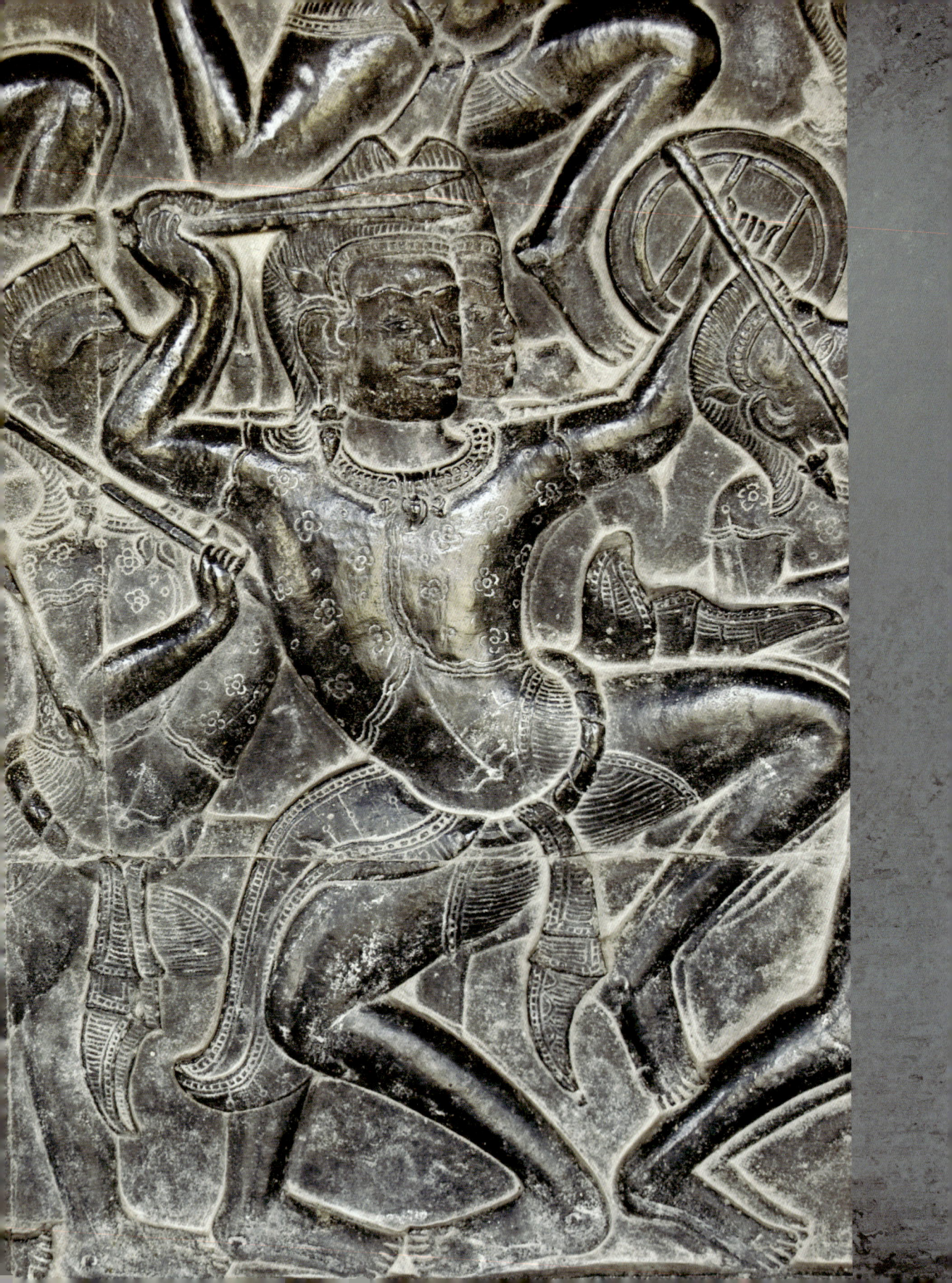

The Vedic and
Pre-classical Period

Yoga and the
Post-classical Period

The earliest written evidence of yogic practice emerged at a time known as the Vedic period (4,500-2,500 BC). The earliest archaeological evidence — that of sculptures — can be traced back to about 4,500 years, to two sites in the Indus Valley. The most significant of the many statues excavated by archaeologists in 1921 at the two sites — Harappa and Mohenjodaro (both in modern Pakistan) — was a horned figure, seated in the cross-legged lotus position and surrounded by wild animals. The *Pashupati seal*, as it came to be known, is thought to be a prototype of Shiva, lord of the beasts.

Harappan culture existed during what is referred to as the pre-Vedic age (6,500-4,500 BC), before the Aryan civilization began to emerge in the Indus subcontinent. As the Indus Valley civilization died, so did its language, and we can only now speculate that these findings denote yogic postures rather than habitual sitting positions of that time.

This chapter looks at the three distinct forms of yogic wisdom, literature and development. The Vedic, denoting the earliest threads of Indian culture, when teachings were recited orally by a wise man, or Brahmin, to groups of students who sat down surrounding him to listen. Towards the end of the Vedic period emerged a new intellectual tradition, known in history as the *Upanishads*. It continued to bring students to 'sit near' — *upani* — the wise man, or Brahmin, to listen to contemplations about the universe, and of being fully alive in a divine consciousness. The greatest text bequeathed in the Upanishad era is the *Bhagavad Gita*, the song of God. Modern yoga practices incorporate teachings from the *Bhagavad Gita*.

Yoga can be said to be a two-fold quest for knowledge in all ways seen, unseen, felt, breathed and thought.

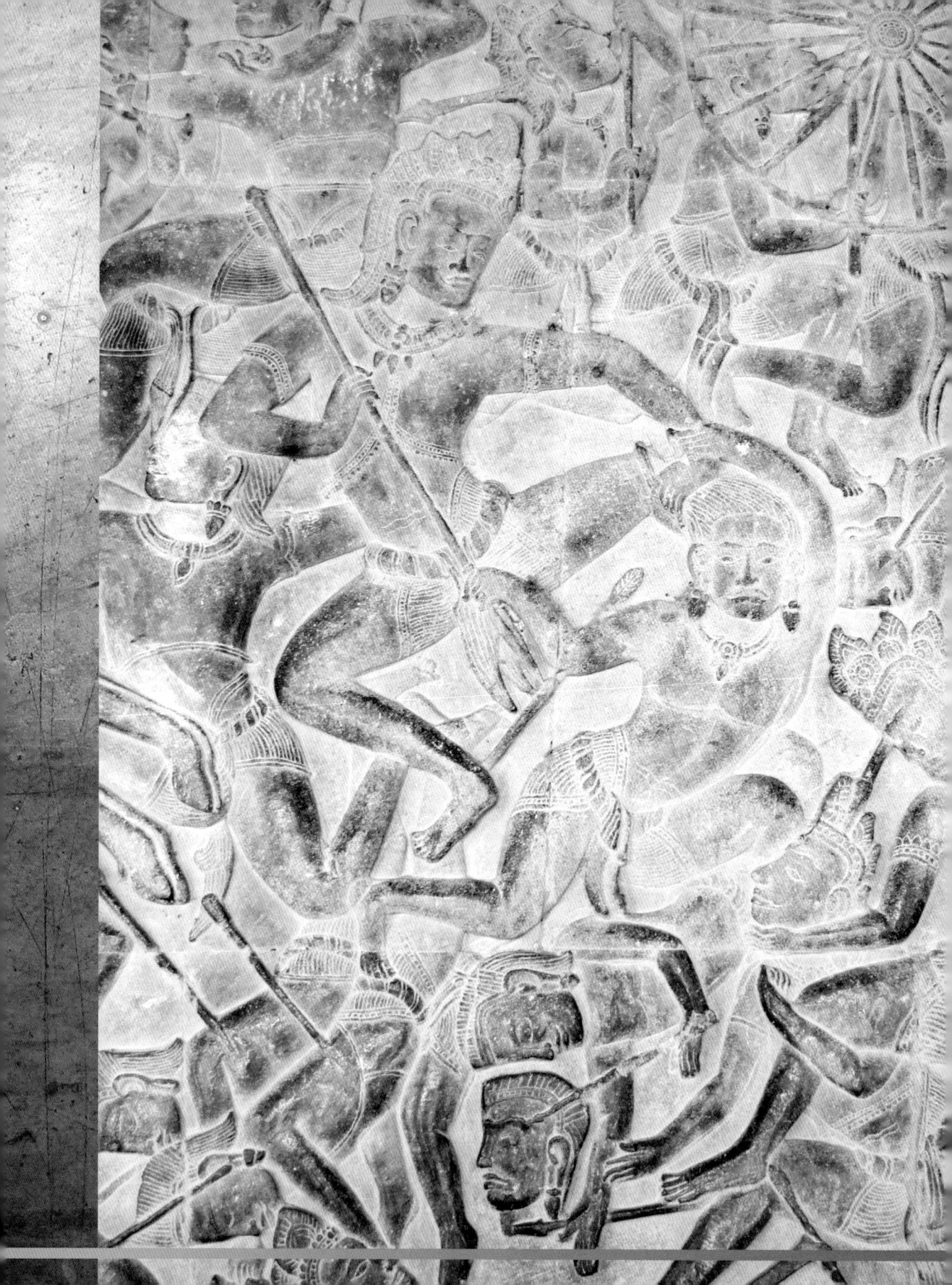

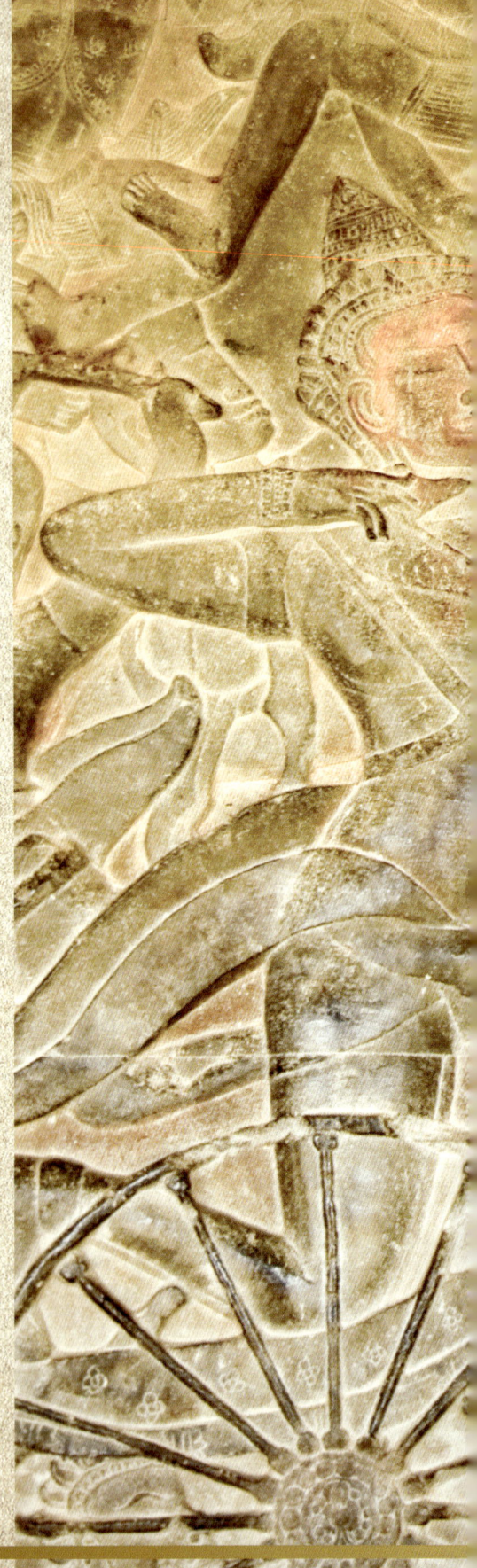

THE VEDIC PERIOD

The Vedic or pre-classical period is the period within which the *Vedas*, the oldest record of Indian culture that also contained the first textual references to yoga emerged. It is also the period from which later religions and spiritual expressions evolved. The *Vedas* are described as *sruti*, which means that their wisdom was only recited orally; it is therefore difficult to ascertain their date, as it was some time before any textual evidence appeared. But most scholars agree that they date back to at least 1,500-1,200 BC. Veda means knowledge, and the *Vedas* were among the first works to speculate on the interconnection between all things in the known and unknown universe. They are said to have been revealed by God to ancient masters of Vedic yoga, who were called *rishis* or *seers*. The main religion of that time was *Brahmanism*, wherein offerings were made to Gods as a means of joining the material and spirit world. Those performing the rituals had to be able to focus their minds for prolonged periods of time. The inner focus, in order to transcend the limitations of the ordinary mind, is at the heart of yoga. The significant Vedic texts still studied today are the *Rig Veda*, *Yajur Veda*, *Sama Veda* and *Atharva Veda*. They help us understand how spirituality developed into physical exercises and how yoga became a part of spiritual living.

THE UPANISHADS

Upanishad refers to the inner or mystical teaching. The term 'Upanishad' is derived from 'upani', which means to sit near, referring to the time when students would learn the truth hidden in mystic revelations by sitting near and listening to the discourses given by their gurus. Deep within forest hermitages, scholars of the *Upanishads* contemplated the mysteries of the world and communicated their knowledge to their pupils. 'Upanishad' also means *brahma*, knowledge through which ignorance is destroyed. As the concluding portion of the *Vedas*, the *Upanishads* are also called the *Vedanata* or the 'end of the

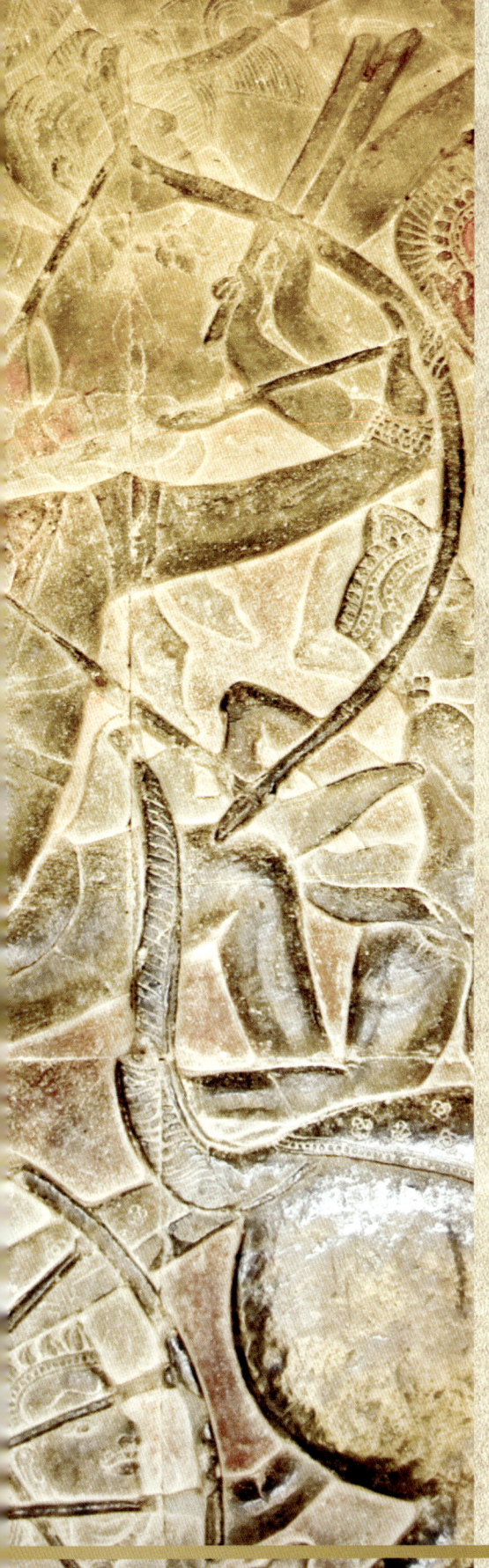

Vedas'. And like the *Vedas*, the *Upanishads*, too, help us understand how spirituality developed into physical exercises and how yoga became a part of spiritual living.

THE BHAGAVAD GITA

The most famous of all texts related to yoga is the *Bhagavad Gita*, which originated from the *Upanishads*, in the fourth century BC. It is part of the *Mahabharata*, one of the longest epic poems in history, generally attributed to the Vedic sage Vyasa. The *Bhagavad Gita* narrates the story of a civil war in ancient India between the sons of Kuru—the *Kauravas*—and the sons of Pandu—the *Pandavas*. It is conveyed as a dialogue between Lord Krishna and prince Arjuna on the battlefield of Kurukshetra. Prince Yudhishthira, one of the son's of king Pandu, loses the Pandavas 'share' in the kingdom, in a rigged game of dice. He and his four brothers, including Prince Arjuna, are banished for thirteen years. At the end of their exile, they try to reclaim their share in the kingdom, which is now ruled by their uncle Kuru and his 100 sons. When their lawful claim is dismissed, the Pandavas declare war on the Kauravas. On the side of the Pandavas is God's incarnate Krishna. Though a non-combatant, Krishna employs divine tactics to help Pandu's sons to victory. The Kauravas, although far more in number, are defeated.

Krishna and Arjuna are friends and companions, but in a deeper sense, they are one soul with two bodies, each one incomplete without the other. Arjuna represents the individual soul and Krishna the supreme soul that dwells in every heart. Arjuna's chariot represents the body, and the blind king stands for a mind under the spell of ignorance. His many sons represent man's evil tendencies. The battle is the perennial battle between good and evil. The overriding metaphor is of God and man, face-to-face, and fully engaged in man's process of discovery which lies hidden in the innermost parts of his heart.

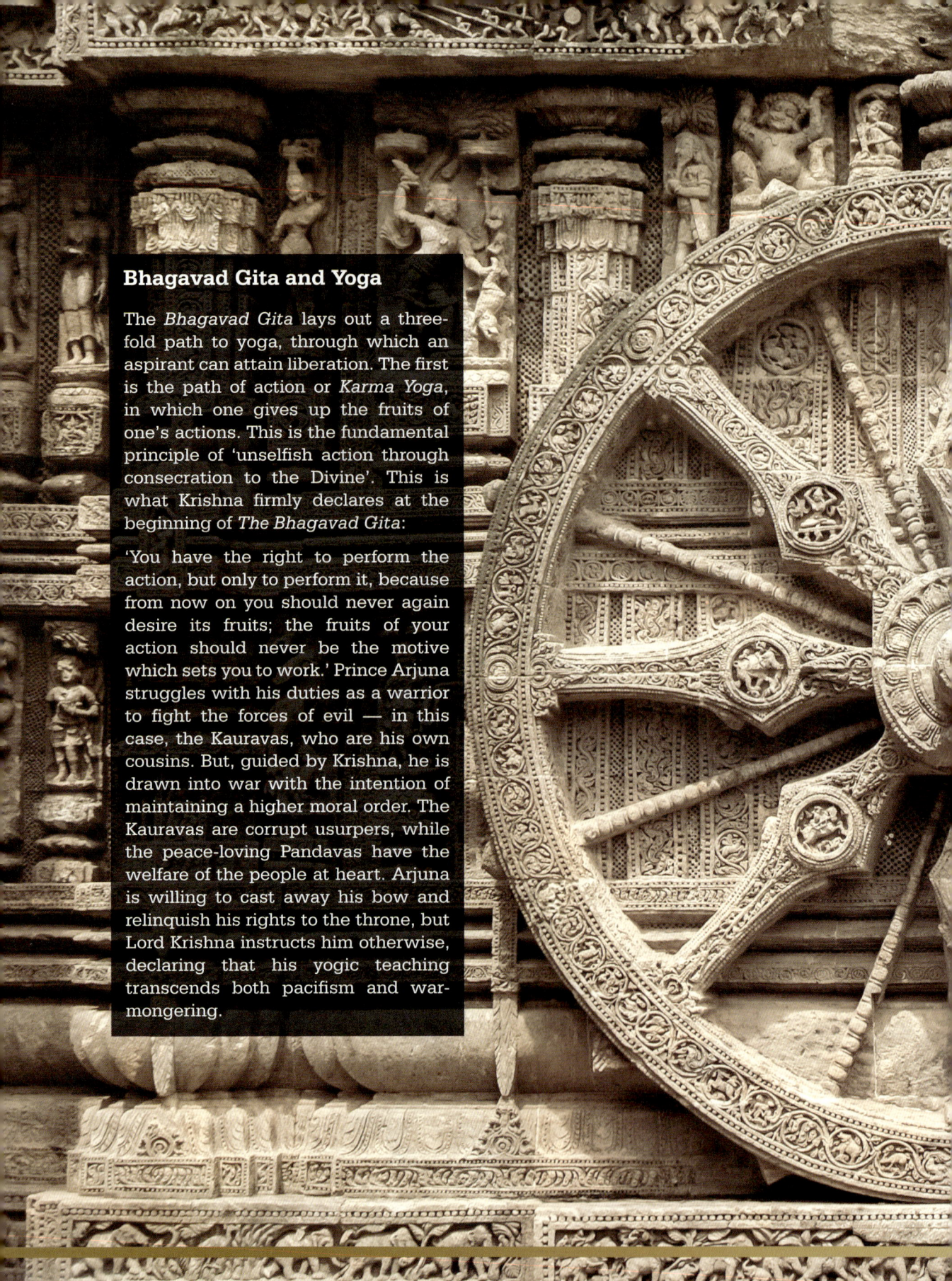

Bhagavad Gita and Yoga

The *Bhagavad Gita* lays out a three-fold path to yoga, through which an aspirant can attain liberation. The first is the path of action or *Karma Yoga*, in which one gives up the fruits of one's actions. This is the fundamental principle of 'unselfish action through consecration to the Divine'. This is what Krishna firmly declares at the beginning of *The Bhagavad Gita*:

'You have the right to perform the action, but only to perform it, because from now on you should never again desire its fruits; the fruits of your action should never be the motive which sets you to work.' Prince Arjuna struggles with his duties as a warrior to fight the forces of evil — in this case, the Kauravas, who are his own cousins. But, guided by Krishna, he is drawn into war with the intention of maintaining a higher moral order. The Kauravas are corrupt usurpers, while the peace-loving Pandavas have the welfare of the people at heart. Arjuna is willing to cast away his bow and relinquish his rights to the throne, but Lord Krishna instructs him otherwise, declaring that his yogic teaching transcends both pacifism and war-mongering.

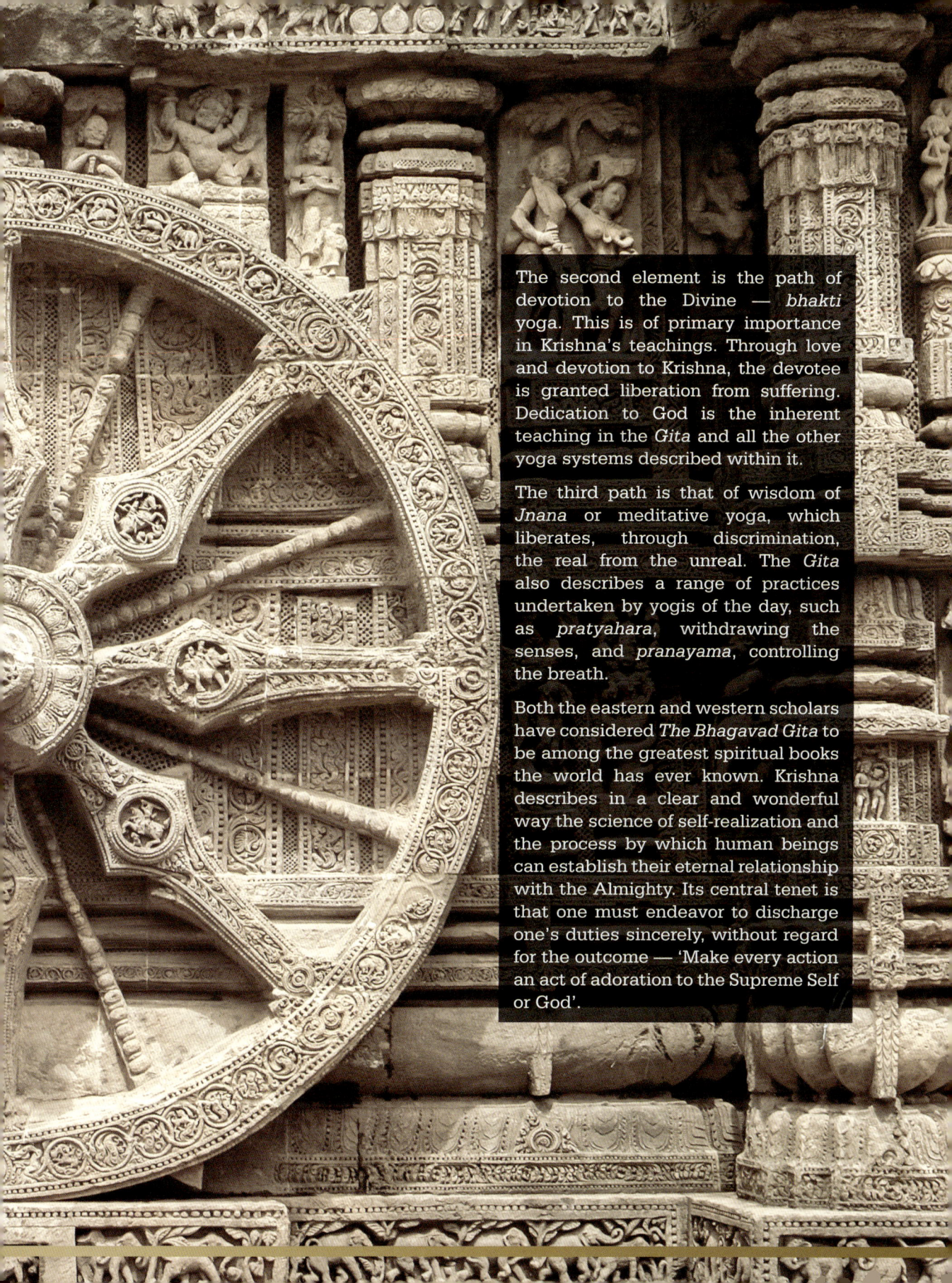

The second element is the path of devotion to the Divine — *bhakti* yoga. This is of primary importance in Krishna's teachings. Through love and devotion to Krishna, the devotee is granted liberation from suffering. Dedication to God is the inherent teaching in the *Gita* and all the other yoga systems described within it.

The third path is that of wisdom of *Jnana* or meditative yoga, which liberates, through discrimination, the real from the unreal. The *Gita* also describes a range of practices undertaken by yogis of the day, such as *pratyahara*, withdrawing the senses, and *pranayama*, controlling the breath.

Both the eastern and western scholars have considered *The Bhagavad Gita* to be among the greatest spiritual books the world has ever known. Krishna describes in a clear and wonderful way the science of self-realization and the process by which human beings can establish their eternal relationship with the Almighty. Its central tenet is that one must endeavor to discharge one's duties sincerely, without regard for the outcome — 'Make every action an act of adoration to the Supreme Self or God'.

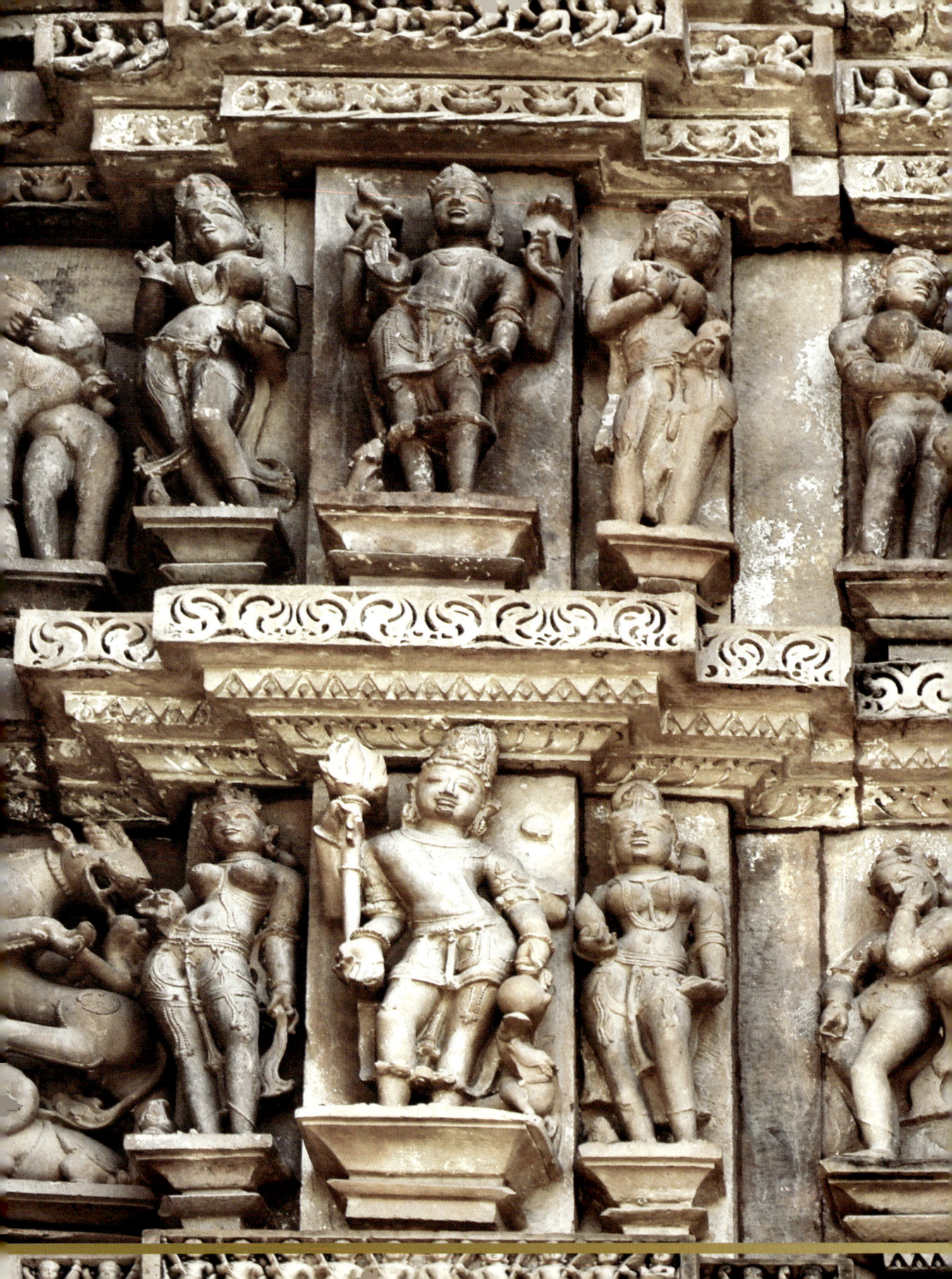

YOGA AND THE POST-CLASSICAL PERIOD

This period follows the journey of yoga traditions and practice to all around the world. Post-classical yoga differs from all the previous periods. The *Bhagavad Gita* says: 'Its goal is no longer a matter of liberation. It does not strive to liberate a person from reality but rather to teach one to accept it and live in the moment.' The boundaries separating various schools of yogic thought are not clearly defined and are impossible to date precisely, but post-classical yoga can be regarded as a reaction to the dualism expounded in Patanjali's *Yoga Sutras* and his eight-limbed path.

Vedanta and its Influence on Yoga

Vedanta was one of the main schools of the post-classical period. One of its most influential sub-schools was *Advaita Vedanta*.

Tantra Yoga

Tantra rejected the *Vedas* and the belief that liberation could only be achieved by ascetic practices such as mediation and renunciation. Instead, it turned to the path of devotion and bhakti yoga, in this case, the worship of the Goddess. 'In Tantra one worships *Sakti* (Power), that is, God in Mother-form as the Supreme Power, which creates, sustains and withdraws the Universe. God is Mother to the Tantrika who worships Her Lotus Feet'.

Hatha Yoga

The physical postures practiced today came from hatha yoga. The term 'hatha' is the combination of two *bija* or seed mantras: 'ha' symbolizing the sun or prana, the vital force, and 'tha' representing the moon or the mind and mental energy. This system of yoga signifies the union of pranic and mental forces. Hatha yoga is the most empowering way to achieve self-transformation. Its techniques are to bring attention to our breath, which helps us to still the mind from any fluctuations and be in the present.

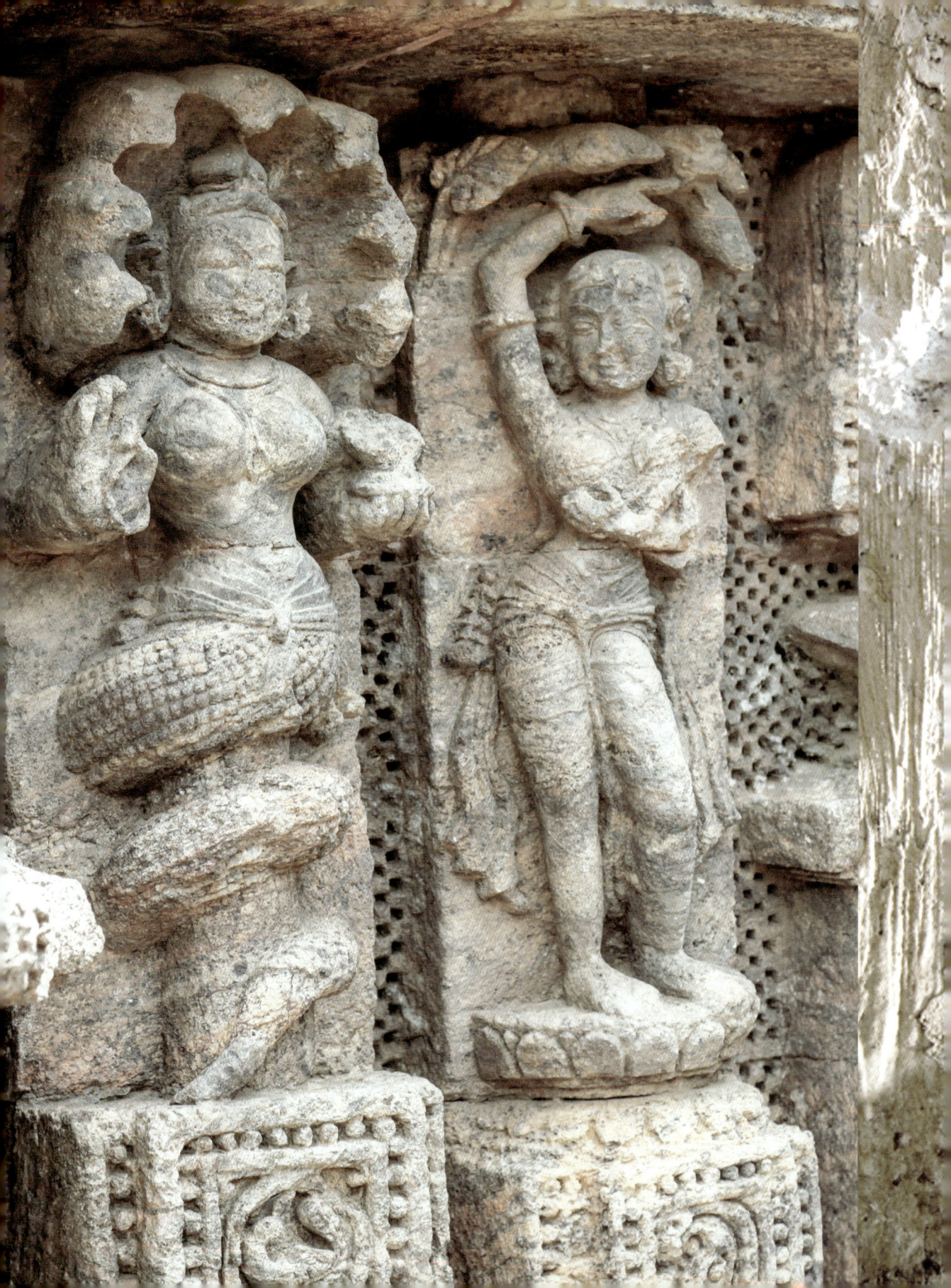

Classical Yoga and Patanjali's Yoga Sutras

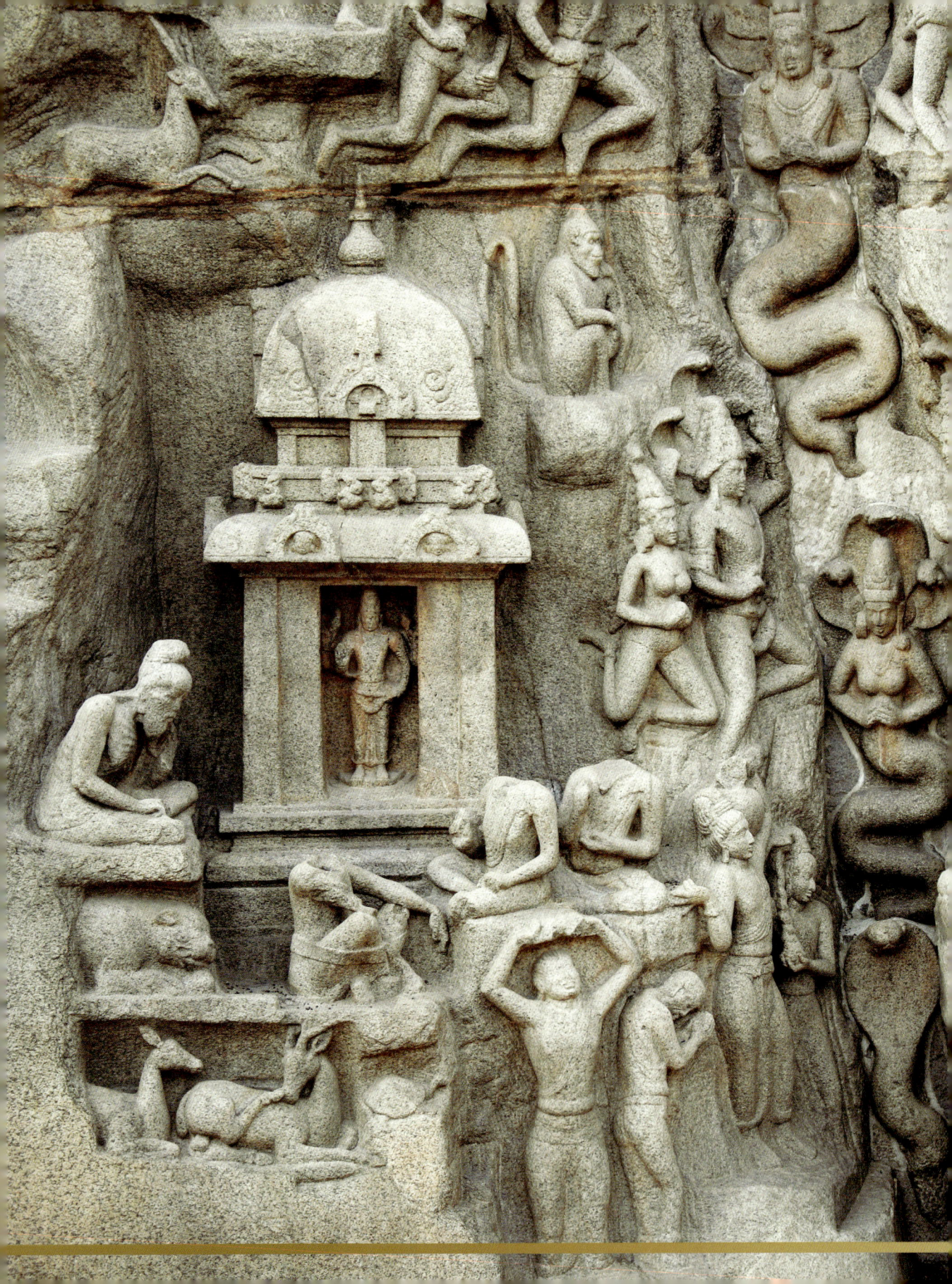

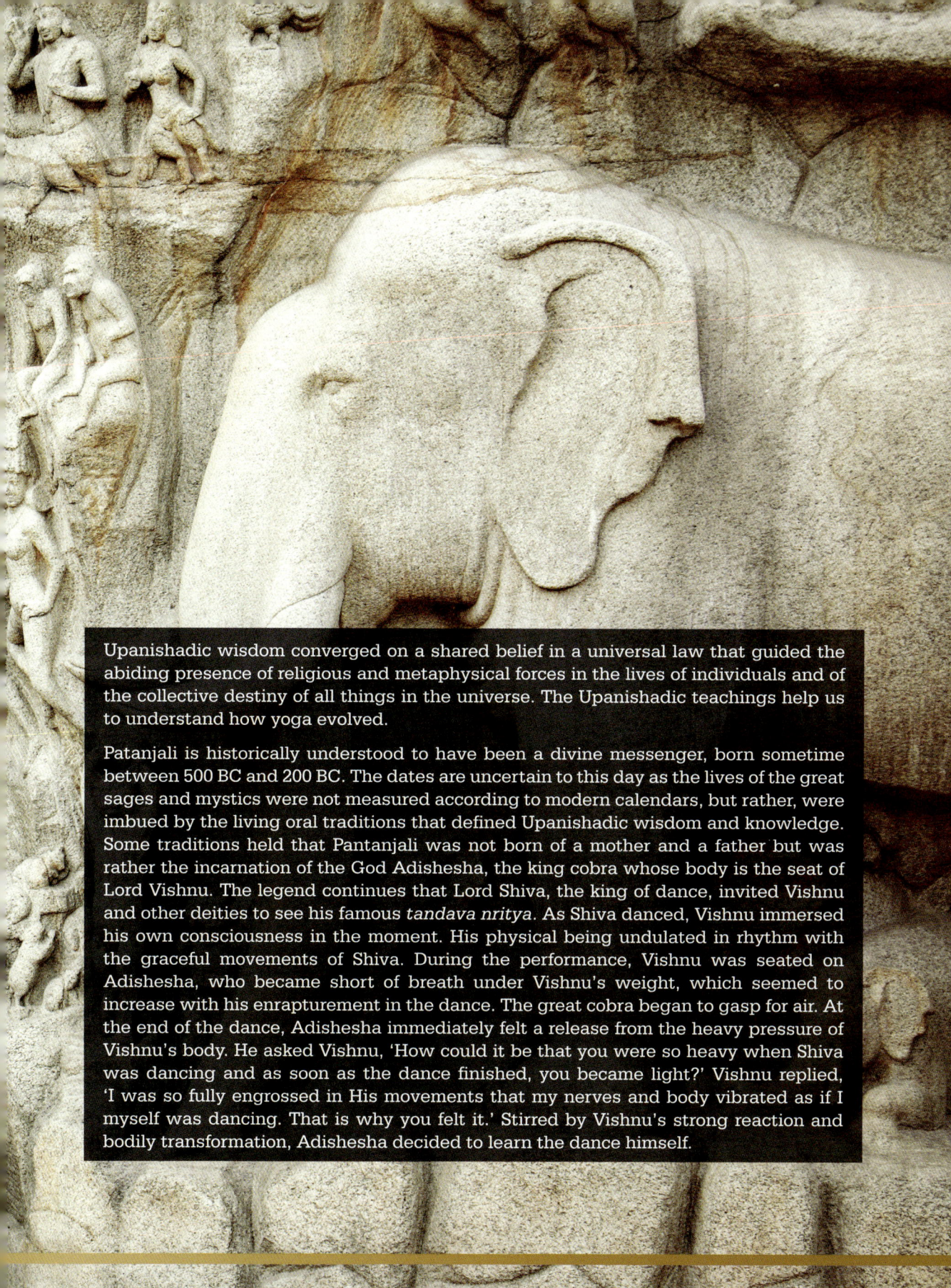

Upanishadic wisdom converged on a shared belief in a universal law that guided the abiding presence of religious and metaphysical forces in the lives of individuals and of the collective destiny of all things in the universe. The Upanishadic teachings help us to understand how yoga evolved.

Patanjali is historically understood to have been a divine messenger, born sometime between 500 BC and 200 BC. The dates are uncertain to this day as the lives of the great sages and mystics were not measured according to modern calendars, but rather, were imbued by the living oral traditions that defined Upanishadic wisdom and knowledge. Some traditions held that Pantanjali was not born of a mother and a father but was rather the incarnation of the God Adishesha, the king cobra whose body is the seat of Lord Vishnu. The legend continues that Lord Shiva, the king of dance, invited Vishnu and other deities to see his famous *tandava nritya*. As Shiva danced, Vishnu immersed his own consciousness in the moment. His physical being undulated in rhythm with the graceful movements of Shiva. During the performance, Vishnu was seated on Adishesha, who became short of breath under Vishnu's weight, which seemed to increase with his enrapturement in the dance. The great cobra began to gasp for air. At the end of the dance, Adishesha immediately felt a release from the heavy pressure of Vishnu's body. He asked Vishnu, 'How could it be that you were so heavy when Shiva was dancing and as soon as the dance finished, you became light?' Vishnu replied, 'I was so fully engrossed in His movements that my nerves and body vibrated as if I myself was dancing. That is why you felt it.' Stirred by Vishnu's strong reaction and bodily transformation, Adishesha decided to learn the dance himself.

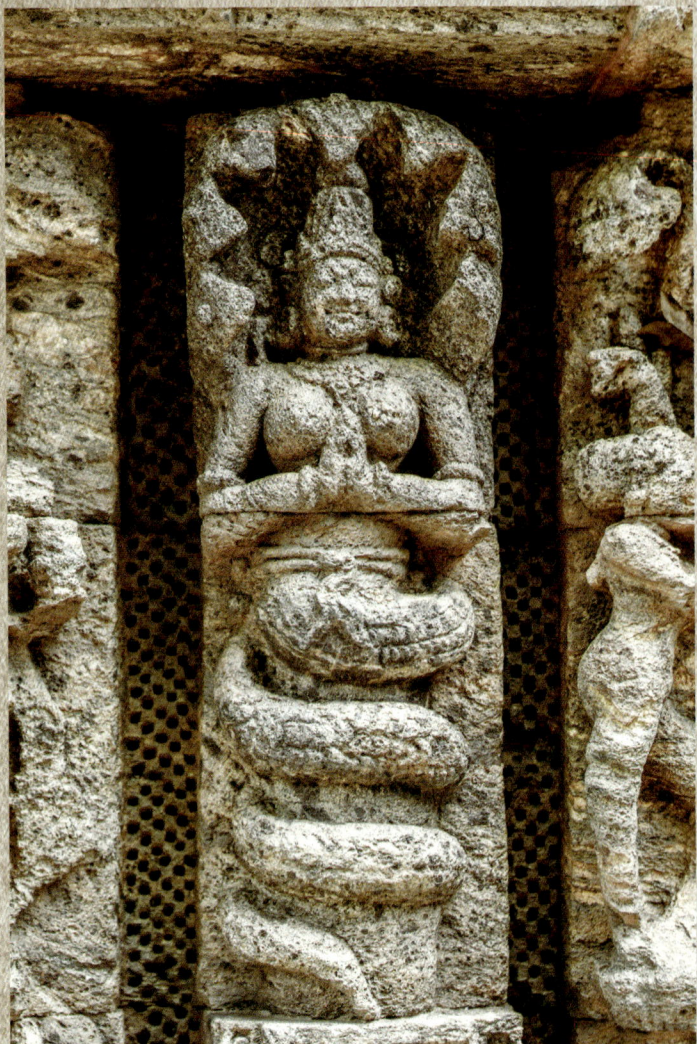

He began looking for a mother who was both a *yogini* and a *tapasvini* – a woman who had done much yoga and fervent penance. After some time, Adishesha found Gaunika, who had no children and who had done penance for several years. She was praying to the rising sun. She took some water to offer, closed her eyes and prayed. As she opened her eyes to offer the water to the Sun God, she saw a very tiny snake moving in the water that she was holding in her palms. At first she was terrified and said, 'What polluted water I have taken!' As she was saying this, the tiny snake at once assumed a human form, prostrated and begged her to accept him as her son. She accepted him as her son and named him Patanjali – *pata* meaning to fall and *anjali* meaning the folding of one's hands during prayer. He is also known as Gaunika *putra* – son of Gaunika. Thus, Patanjali means 'fallen into the palms at the time of prayer'. Eventually, Patanjali completed his first duty – the commentary on grammar. Patanjali took the Indian tradition of language to a definite form. He intuited that movements of the body could be used for understanding the functions of the body. He studied the system of the body, using the knowledge of matter, the elements and their qualities. Through the study of the outer and inner body, he developed a system called *Ayurveda*. *Ayuh* means life and *Veda* means knowledge. So, Ayurveda is the knowledge of life. Finally, he composed the aphorisms on yoga, known as the *Yoga Sutra*.

Much of our modern yoga practice is based on Patanjali's *Yoga Sutras*, but it must be made clear that there were earlier traditions in India which had adopted various yoga practices as a means of attaining liberation. Patanjali articulated in a codified literature of instruction these many threads of understanding in the literature we know today as Patanjali's *Sutras*. This formal body of learning is widely understood to be the foundation of modern yoga. Yoga techniques were systematically summarized for the first time by Patanjali in the *Yoga Sutras* between 200 BC and AD 200.

Yet, much of our modern understanding of the earliest articulation of a yoga system must remain in the realms of myth, legend and human yearning. As a mythic being, it is not known whether Patanjali represented a single individual, a family or a tradition of magis. Legend has it that Vishnu commanded Adishesha to be reincarnated as Patanjali so that he could bring a practical form of yoga to people.

THE PSYCHOLOGY AND THE PHILOSOPHY OF THE *SUTRAS*

The *Sutras*, 195 of them in total, were written in short, concise but meaningful sentences. As in modern psychology, they describe how the mind works and the difficulties, obstacles and emotional disturbances that can affect it and stand in the way of reflective action and self-knowledge. Patanjali's *Yoga Sutras* recommend the so-called 'Eight-limb Path' as the way to changing the mind positively. Following this path leads to recognition of the causes of suffering and provides the means of avoiding them in future, leaving the way open to self-knowledge.

PATANJALI'S THEORY ON 'MONKEY MIND'

According to Patanjali, one of the fundamental characteristics of the mind is that it normally refuses to remain in the here and now. Instead, it jumps about like a monkey from one branch of thought to the next. It is constantly and relentlessly on the move, never focusing on the moment, but instead dealing with all the things at the same time – with past, future and all the incidents it has to process in the meantime.

At the same time, the human mind generally interprets all the things that are seen, perceived and experienced. It is led by its thoughts, habits, patterns, perceptions and conditioning – referred to as *samskara* in Sanskrit. These are learned in the course of a person's life and become habits through repetition – irrespective of whether they are right or wrong, good or bad. So it is little wonder that the mind is usually agitated amid all these activities, with the result that human actions are often also blind and unfocused. On the other hand, conscious actions require a clear mind, a mind that has been stilled. Against this background, Patanjali developed the Eight-limb Path with the aim of stilling the mind.

A STILL MIND IN THE PRESENT

The function of the mind will always be to think and interpret all the time – after all, that is why it is there. Consequently, the aim of yoga is not to shut the mind down, but rather to enable it to be unaffected by its turnings and instead focus exclusively on a single object or thought. The result of this will be a clear perception that is not clouded by the excessive workings of the mind. If this is achieved – a conscious and concentrated action in the here and now – a truly ambitious goal is made possible. However, the mind permanently places obstacles in the way on the journey towards this goal, and these obstacles are referred to as *kleshas*.

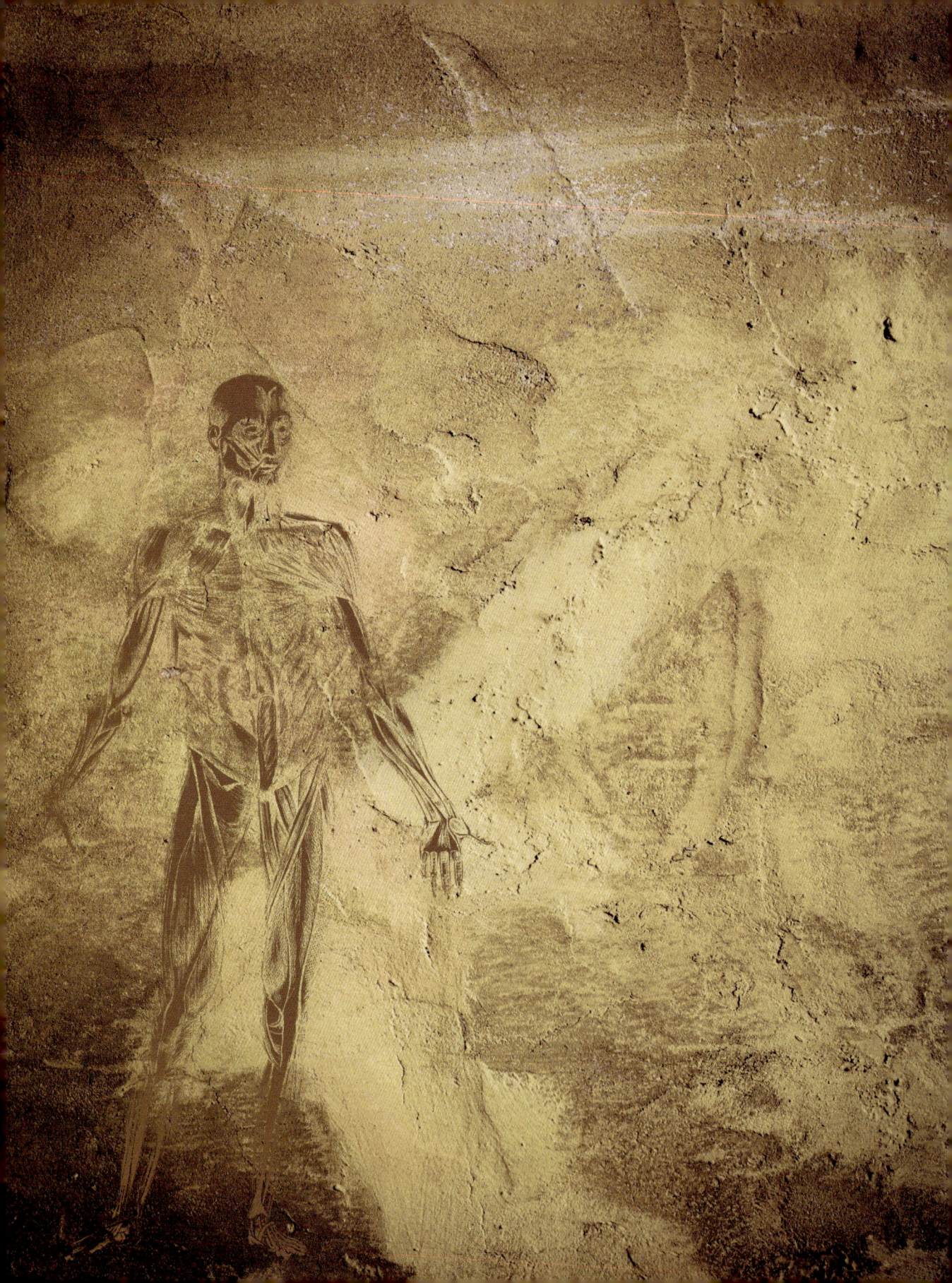

The Anatomical Focus of Hatha Yoga

WHAT IS HATHA YOGA?

Hatha yoga is a series of postures, over 100 in all, that are intended to stretch the muscles, limbs, and organs of our bodies, performed together with careful controlled breathing through the duration and repetition of each pose. Hatha calls into play a combination of postures and breathing that unite our skeletal frame, our muscles, nervous system, vital organs and mind. It is perhaps hatha's main benefit that in performing these poses we become aware, consciously and unconsciously so, of the interplay of mind and body in giving us our sense of self.

THE CORPSE: HATHA YOGA'S MAIN POSTURE

The most important point of reference to which hatha yoga returns throughout our practice is the corpse position. This pose should serve as a resting and reflection point for one to two minutes after each bending and twisting posture that we cycle through; it is held and repeated during the practice. The corpse posture, in which we make ourselves utterly still in a supine position on the floor or some other flat surface, teaches us much about releasing the obstacles we create for ourselves when trying to attain that state of being we might think is simplest: relaxation.

To begin, lie down on a flat surface, the floor covered by a mat or towel is best. Unfold oneself, no bent knees, no crooked elbows, hips loose and symmetrical, spine loosely straight and aligned, arms full length at your sides, feet comfortably apart, hands facing upwards and without tension. Take a full moment to feel the energy of motion slow and cease. Bodily movement is created by the combined working of our neuromuscular and skeletal systems. Feel the force of gravity holding you in place.

The most important point of reference to which hatha yoga returns throughout our practice is the corpse position. This pose should serve as a resting and reflection point for one to two minutes after each bending and twisting posture that we cycle through; it is held and repeated during the practice. The corpse posture, in which we remain absolutely still in a supine position on the floor or some other flat surface, teaches us about overcoming or letting go of the obstacles we create for ourselves when trying to attain that state of being which we often take for granted: relaxation.

To begin, lie down on a flat surface, and make sure that the floor is covered by a mat or towel. Unfold yourself, avoid bending your knees or elbows, the hips should be loose and symmetrical, and the spine straight and aligned, the arms stretched out by your sides, feet comfortably apart, and hands facing upwards and relaxed. Take a few moments to feel the energy of motion slow, and gradually cease. Bodily movement is created by the combined working of our neuromuscular and skeletal systems. Feel the force of gravity holding you in place.

The body is actually a self-contained electrical system in which the motor neurons send signals to the nerves causing little electrical pulses to trigger movement. Your brain controls much of this electrical activity – think of when you pick up a pen or a fork, or stand to stretch your legs after an hour at the computer. Your wonderful, intelligent brain is actually running a very complicated piece of electrical machinery: You! Let your mind listen to what your body is telling you, while you are in the corpse pose. Feel your breathing become slower and deeper. Feel the pulse of movement ebb away from the limbs and organs as the nerve impulses that create movement slow and fade. Just like the gentle pumping sensation that you feel in your thighs for several moments after you finish a bicycle sprint, it's not just your heart pumping slower after you come to rest, but the motion pulses are slowing too. Your brain has the ability to focus on each part of the body as these changes take place. Focused, rhythmic breathing draws you further into relation as the muscles and nerves come to rest. Your elbows, knees, and shoulders are not holding you in place. You do not feel pain in any part of your body. You are comfortably in a state of deep relaxation.

That so much of hatha yoga is practiced in poses on the floor teaches us about the gravitational field that shapes our bodily existence. Hatha works with gravity to strengthen our bodies. Without gravity, as we know from all the studies of the effects of weightlessness on astronauts on long voyages in space, our muscles and bones will atrophy. There can be no walking, running or lifting. Hatha postures such as the cobra, the locust and the bow postures work against the force of gravity as we lift parts of the body off the floor. Gravity holds us to the ground and places all our weight vertically in the shoulder stand. We use a myriad muscles and joints to remain erect when standing. Hatha floor exercises also make use of gravity, as we will see in the following pages when we focus on three floor postures most instructive on bodily awareness in hatha. But first we will have a brief anatomy lesson, to go over the roles in hatha for the nerves, muscles and skeletal system.

HATHA YOGA AND THE NEURO-MUSCULOSKELETAL SYSTEM

The musculoskeletal system is a seamlessly integrated machine of solid moving parts driving our will of mind and our physical movement, with signals sent from the brain and transmitted into electrical impulses that trigger activity in the muscles which in turn activate the joints and the limbs. This action is both consciously directed by ourselves and unconsciously directed by the most primitive part of our brain that controls breathing and swallowing. Speech is the most interesting combination of the mind's will to create thought and the physical instinct to make that thought oral and spoken (the jaw, the lungs, and the throat all working together to create sound, utterance and voice!). In practicing hatha yoga, the musculoskeletal system works to create balance, flexibility and detoxification through movement and breathing.

To illustrate the fact that the nervous system manages posture, let's consider the response of your body when you attempt to sit. First your worried system commands the flexor muscles (muscles which fold the limbs and bend the spine forward) to help pull the upper area of the trunk forward and simultaneously initiate bending with the hips and knees along with ankles. A bare moment after you initiate that mobility, gravity takes centre stage and starts to pull people towards the relaxing position. And concurrently – accompanying this action of gravity – the worried system commands the extensor muscles (those which resist folding the limbs) to combat gravity and hold you from falling in the heap. Finally, once you are settled in the secure seated, the nervous system permits the extensor muscles and the body in general to relax.

The musculoskeletal system serves as a movable container for the internal organs. Just like a robot houses and protects it's hidden supporting elements (power plant, built-in circuits, programmable desktops, self-repairing components, and enough fuel to function for a reasonable time), the musculoskeletal system also holds and protects the delicate areas. Hatha yoga postures teach us to manage both the muscle tissues that operate the extremities, the muscles that run the extremities, and the muscles that are in the container.

OUR MUSCLES

Muscles are made of flesh, tendons and the belly. The belly is made up of individual muscle fibers (muscle cells) surrounded by connective muscle fibers that together form the tendon. The tendon in turn connects the belly in the muscle to the bone. Directed by nerve impulses, those short electrical signals sent by our central nervous system, muscles prepare for movement by contracting, or shortening and lengthening in the opposing muscles (our biceps and triceps for example, are opposing muscles), thus pulling the skeletal elements into motion, much like a pulley system which pivots movable joints such as the hips, knees, shoulders, elbows and wrists. The joints carry the signal to the bones of the arms and legs, and to the spine, to create motion.

The attachments and movements of a muscle can be functionally reversed. When the latissimus dosri muscle pulls the arm down and back in a swimming stroke, its textbook origin is from the lower back and pelvis, and its insertion is on the humerus in the arm. But when we do a chin-up, the arm is the relatively stable origin, and the lower back and pelvis become the insertion for lifting the body as a whole.

Our Agonist and Antagonist Muscles

The actual muscles surrounding a joint act in harmony with each other, but one of them – the agonist – serves as the main moving muscle, assisted by muscles called synergists. While the agonist and its synergists are on one side of the joint, muscles on the opposite side act as antagonists. As suggested by the name, antagonists monitor, smooth, and even retard the movement in question. For example, when the biceps brachii and the brachialis in the arm (the agonist and one of its synergists) shorten to flex the elbow, the triceps brachii (on the opposite side of the arm) resists flexion antagonistically while incidentally holding the joint surfaces in correct apposition.

Muscles also act in relation to the force of gravity. In the lower extremities, extensor muscles act as antigravity muscles to keep you upright and resist crumpling to the floor. They often aid gravity, as you settle into a standing forward bend and then pull yourself down with your hip flexors – the iliopsoas muscles.

The upper extremities differ from the others, because unless you are carrying out something unusual like walking on your hands with slightly bent elbows (which necessitates a string commitment from the triceps brachii muscles), the extensor muscles do not support the weight of the body. In most practical circumstances, it is likely to be the flexors rather than extensors that act as antigravity muscles in the upper extremities, as when you flex an elbow to lift a package or complete a chin-up.

Concentric Shortening and Eccentric Lengthening

To be aware of how the musculoskeletal system operates in hatha yoga, we must look at the way individual muscles help with whole-body activity. The easiest situation, concentric contraction, or even 'concentric shortening', is one by which muscle fiber tend to be stimulated by nerve impulses and the entire muscle responds by shortening, as when biceps brachii muscle within the arm shortens concentrically to help lift a book.

When we wish to put the book down, the picture is harder. We do not ordinarily drop an object we've just lifted – all of us set it down carefully by gradually extending the knee, and we accomplish that by letting the muscle in general become longer while keeping a few of its muscle fibers in a state of contraction. Whenever this happens – every time a muscle increases in length under tension though resisting gravity – the movement is known as 'eccentric lengthening'.

We see concentric shortening along with eccentric lengthening in many natural activities. When you walk up a flight of stairs, the muscles which are lifting you upward are shortening concentrically; and when you walk down the stairs, the same muscles are lengthening eccentrically to manage your descent. When hauling yourself up a climbing rope, muscles in the upper extremities shorten concentrically when you pull yourself up; as you come back down, the exact same muscles lengthen eccentrically.

In hatha yoga, we see concentric shortening along with eccentric lengthening in hundreds of situations. The simplest example of this is every time a single muscle or even muscle group opposes gravity, as when the rear muscles shorten concentrically to help lift the body up from the fold. Then as you slowly bend down along the spine, the back muscle tissue resists the power of gravity that is pulling you forward, lengthening eccentrically to help smoothen your symmetry.

ISOTONIC VS. ISOMETRIC ACTIVITY DURING EXERCISE

Muscles can develop tension while exercising. Concentric contraction is also known as muscle shortening, which influences a joint angle to decrease. Eccentric contraction is muscle lengthening which causes a joint angle to increase. When there is tension in the muscle but the length does not change, the joint is immobile, and this contraction is called isometric.

Most sports are isotonic exercise because they involve movement. Japanese sumo wrestling between equally matched, tightly gripped, and momentarily immobile opponents is one obvious exception. Isometric exercise is also exemplified by almost every hatha yoga posture which you hold steadily with muscular effort.

Movement, Stretching and Relaxation

If few or no nerve impulses are impinging on muscle fibers, the muscle tissue will be relaxed, as when you are in the corpse posture. But if a relaxed muscle is stretched, the situation becomes more complex. Working with a partner can make this work better. If you lie down and lift your hands straight overhead, and then ask someone to stretch you gently by pulling on your wrists, you will notice that you can easily go with the stretch provided you have good flexibility. But if your partner pulls too suddenly or if there is any appreciable pain, the nervous system will resist relaxation up to resist the stretch.

OUR NERVOUS SYSTEM

The agency of specialized, irreplaceable cells called neurons, 100 billion of them in the brain alone, channelizes information throughout the body and within the vast supportive cellular milieu of the central nervous system – the brain and spinal cord. This is all accomplished by only three kinds of neurons: sensory neurons, which carry the flow of sensation from the peripheral nervous system (by definition all parts of the nervous system except the brain and spinal cord) into the central nervous system and consciousness; motor neurons, which carry instructions from the brain and spinal cord into the peripheral nervous system, and from there to muscles and glands; and interneurons, or association neurons, which are interposed between the sensory neurons and the motor neurons, and which transmit our will and volition to the motor neurons. The sensory information is carried into the dorsal horn of the spinal cord by way of dorsal roots, and the motor information is carried out of the ventral horn of the spinal cord by way of ventral roots. The dorsal and ventral roots join to form mixed (motor sensory) spinal nerves that in turn innervate structures throughout the body.

Neurons

A neuron is the basic functional unit of the nervous system. Even though there are other cell types in the nervous system, yet, the neuron is the only one that aids in transmitting information from place to place.

So the neuron is our main interest. It has several components: a nucleated cell body that supports growth and development, and cellular extensions, or processes, some of them very long, that receive and transmit information. Cellular processes are of two types: dendrites and axons. Picture an octopus hooked on a fishing line. Its eight arms are the dendrites, and the fishing line is the axon. A typical motor neuron contains many dendrites that branch off the cell body. Its single axon – the fishing line – may extend anywhere from a fraction of an inch away from the cell body to four feet in the case of a motor neuron whose cell body is in the spinal cord and whose terminal ends in a muscle of the foot, or even fifteen feet long in the case of similar neurons on a giraffe. The axon may have branches that come off the main trunk of the axon near cell body (axon collaterals), and all branches, including the main trunk, subdivide profusely as they near the targets.

Interneurons put it all together. You sense and ultimately do, and between sensing and doing are the integrating activities of the interneurons. It's true, as the first-grade reader suggests, that you can think and do, but more often you sense, think and do.

To sum it up, sensory input to the brain and the power of will both ultimately influence the motor neurons, which in turn preside over the actions of the musculoskeletal system. The reflexes are in the background and out of your immediate awareness, but without them we would be in dire straits. Without the stretch reflexes, our movements would be uncertain, and without pain receptors and flexion reflexes, we would soon be a battleground of burns and injuries. Without the reflexes from our vestibular system, we would teeter about, uncertain of our balance and orientation. Without sensation from touch and pressure pathways, we would lose most of the sensory input that gives us pleasure – and along with its loss, its guidance too. In the end, the nervous system drives the musculoskeletal system, and these two in combination maintain and sculpt connective tissues, which in turn passively restrict movement and posture. All of this takes place within the field of gravity and creates the practice of hatha yoga.

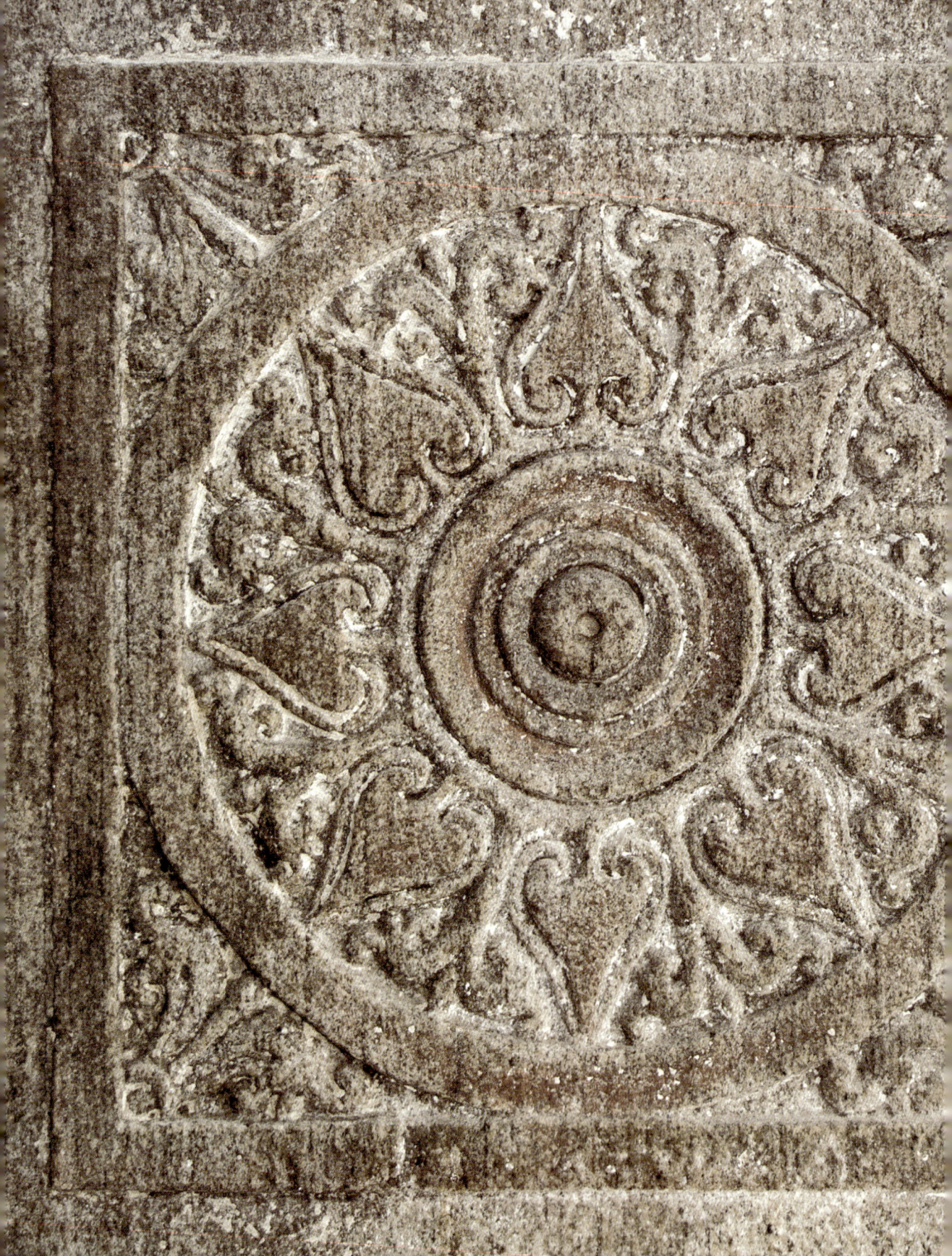

Mantras and Chanting

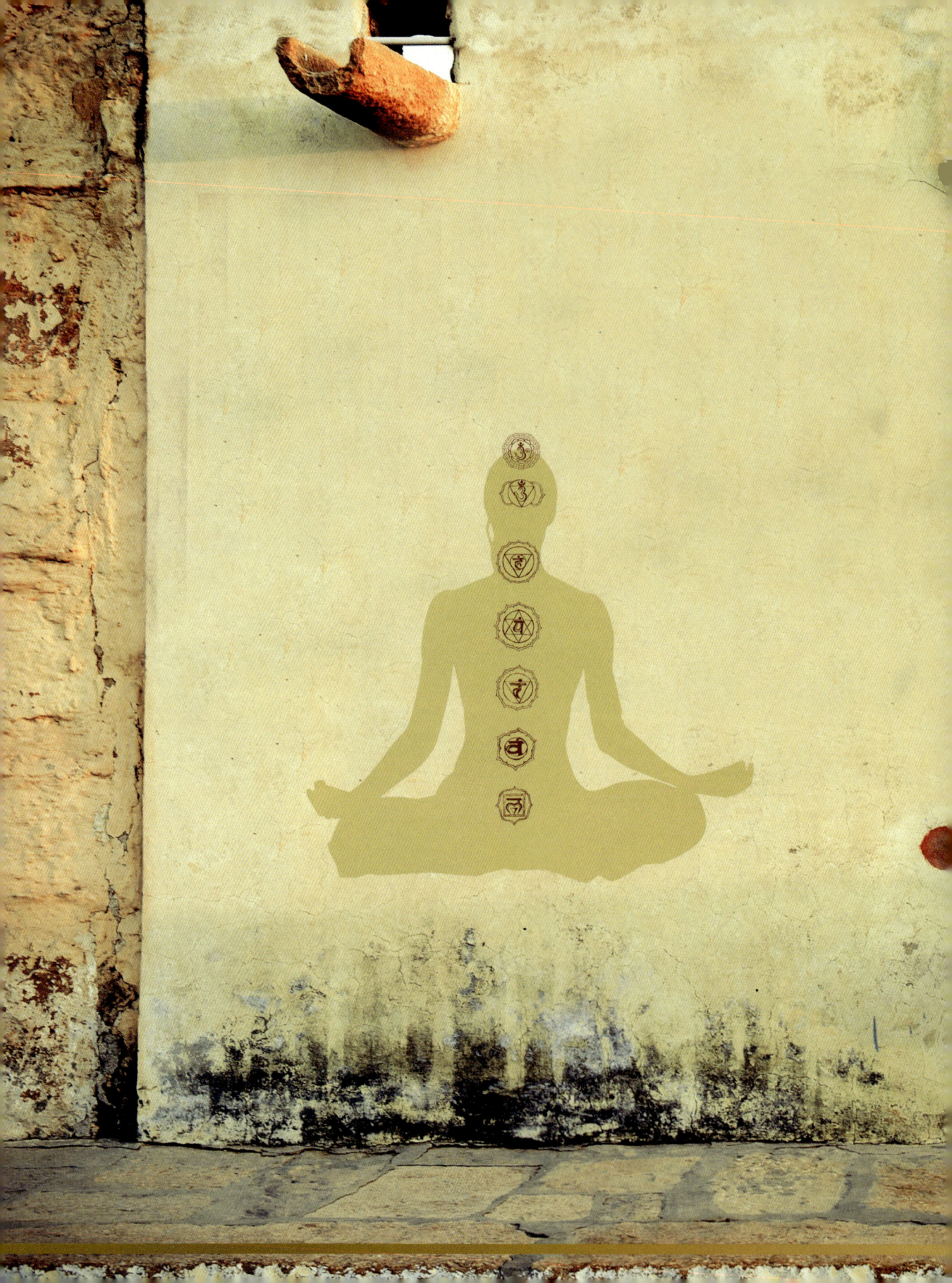

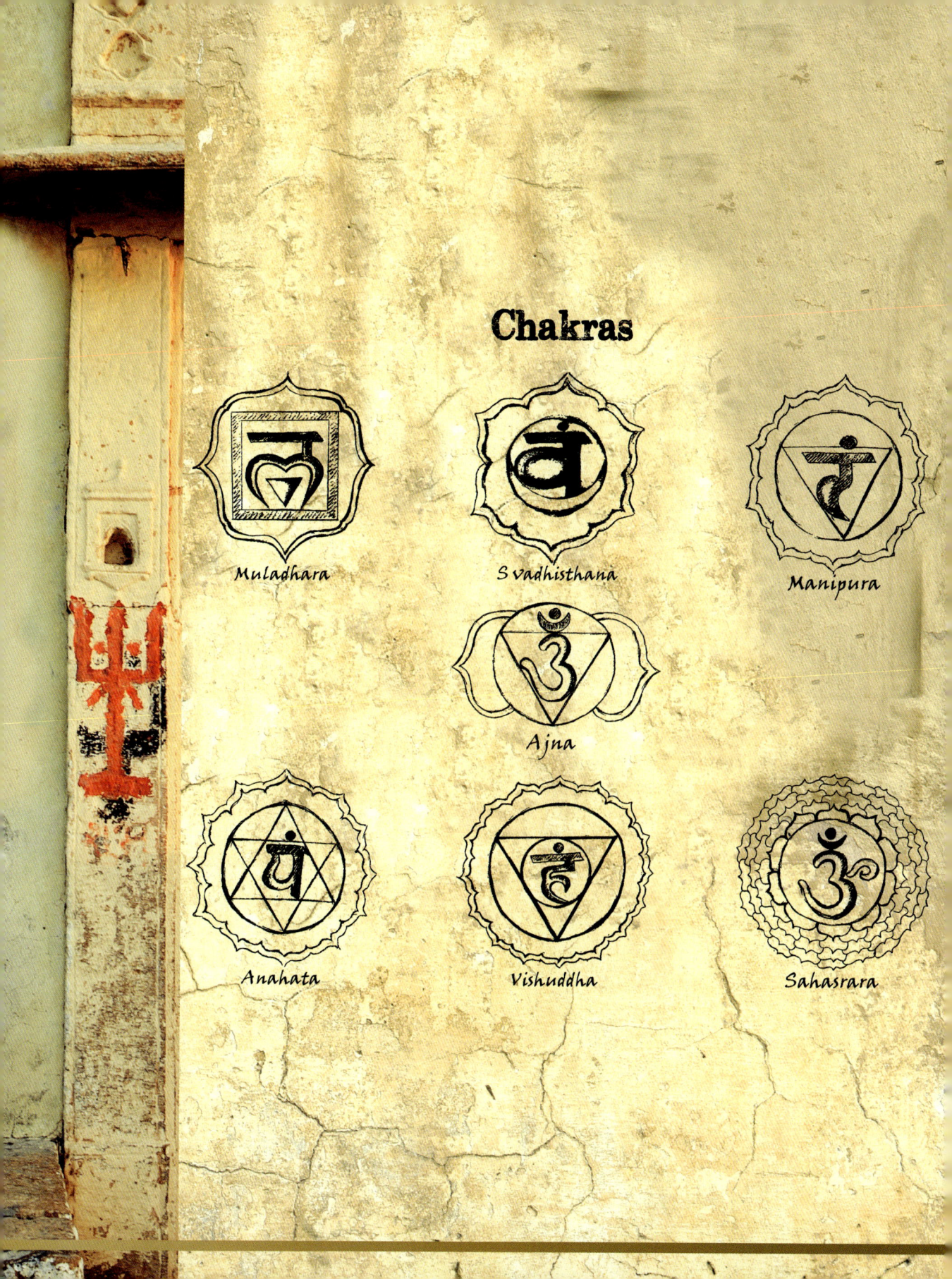

Chakras

Muladhara

Svadhisthana

Manipura

Ajna

Anahata

Vishuddha

Sahasrara

A 'mantra' is a word or sound that is repeated over and over. Mantras offer points of focus for the mind. They serve as positive affirmation and are an effective way of bringing yourself back to your base. Repeating a mantra is an exercise in *dharana* – concentration – that can become *dhyana* – meditation. A vital part of yogic living includes mantras and meditation.

Numerous mantras are in Sanskrit, the ancient language, which is composed of primordial sounds, with each syllable creating a certain resonance inside the body. A Sanskrit mantra is a specific combination of sound vibrations that, when chanted or used in meditation, affects the body, mind and psyche in a particular way. The resonance aids with healing and spiritual elevation. Each repetition of the mantra sends out a certain energetic vibration into the world. The desired effect can only be achieved with correct pronunciation, so if you are not sure, ask a yoga teacher about the right pronunciation for the mantra in question.

Though mantras are traditionally given by a guru, you certainly have the option of choosing your own mantra. Having an exotic-sounding mantra is not necessary. You may feel more inclined to select a mantra in your native language.

To use a mantra for meditation, you can start off by chanting the mantra aloud and allowing the resonance to flow throughout your body. Then, maintaining the reverberation, take your volume down to a whisper. Finally, close out your meditation by repeating the mantra mentally.

Chanting a mantra is commonly used as a method of focusing at the beginning and end of a yoga class. The use of mantras can be as basic as chanting *Om* a few times with the yoga teacher. You can use your mantra practice in a way that works with certain areas of the body and the *chakras* or energy centers of the body. For many people, using a mantra is helpful during stressful times. They can be used in public places since the repetition of a mantra can be silent. Like an affirmation, mantras serve as helpful reminders to bring you back to base.

SOME COMMON MANTRAS

Om is a sacred syllable that is widely considered the mother of all sounds. As with other Sanskrit mantras, it is believed that this syllable sends out a special vibration in your body and mind, which then spreads out into the world. This syllable is used by Hindus and Buddhists alike. Om is composed of three sounds – A-U-Mmmm – running together. The first sound 'A' resonates in the stomach, the 'U' transports the vibration up to the chest cavity, and the long 'M' sound resonates in the head.

Om Namah Shivaya – This mantra is a salutation to the Hindu deity Shiva. Non-Hindus use this mantra as well to honor the Divine.

Soham – This mantra, too, is used to honor the Divine within. It is pronounced as so-hum, and it means 'I am the universal self'.

Shanti – This mantra means 'peace' in Sanskrit.

Om Namoh Bhagavate Vasudevaya – This mantra means salutations to the divine source, the in-dweller of all.

CHANTING

Some people may feel shy about making loud sounds, but chanting is perfectly natural. Let go of any concerns you have about how good or bad you think you sound to others. Chanting is not like singing; rather, it is more like reciting. The purpose of chanting is not to have the most beautiful voice, but to feel the sounds you are making resonate throughout your body.

In the devotional path of yoga, known as Bhakti yoga, God or God's representative – the spiritual teacher – is worshipped. Bhakti yoga is practiced by chanting spiritual verses with great devotion, and it allows one to feel a sense of connection to something greater than the self, known as the universal consciousness. Practicing Bhakti yoga allows the heart center to open up to a crescendo of universal love. Then the emotions settle down and become stabilized once more. This climax and stabilization of the emotions is similar to the way a heart works when a broken-hearted person cries out a song about lost love. It is very healing to experience relief of the emotions before they are left to settle.

Even if you are not a religious person, you may find chanting to be a worthwhile and fulfilling experience. A chanting session is soothing, and feels much like a balm for the brain. It helps wipe away the usual preoccupations, serving as an instant mental holiday. In addition, chanting offers clarity and uplifts your heart. It allows you to find the light you carry within. If you do not feel comfortable practicing alone, you might want to find a chanting group in your area that you can join.

CHAKRAS

In yogic tradition, thousands of *nadis* or energy meridians exist in our body. The largest nadi is known as the *sushumna* nadi. It is not a feature of the Western anatomy, but it follows a nervous pathway and runs from the perineum up the length of the vertebral column.

Yogic tradition speaks of a reservoir of energy called the *kundalini* residing in the body. The word 'kundalini' translates to 'she who is coiled'. The kundalini force is akin to a serpent lying dormant at the base of the spine. Yoga exercises are designed to make the energy path clear by reversing any energy blockages of the spine and purifying the body and mind to allow for the rise of cosmic power. Another method of clearing the kundalini path is working with the chakras.

The word 'chakra' means 'wheel' in Sanskrit. A chakra is like a wheel or vortex in that it is an area of increased energy or prana. A chakra is a center of energy that is able to exist anywhere in the body. We recognize seven main chakras located at various points up the spine. The chakras, which have related nerves and endocrine plexuses, are said to act as transformers. Pranic energy is channeled into the physical body at the points of the chakras. It is commonly believed that when the chakras are fully functional, the kundalini power can travel unhindered up the body's central energy channel from the base of the spine to the crown of the head. As the kundalini 'serpent' rises, it brings each chakra to life in turn. When the kundalini reaches the top chakra, a change of consciousness occurs. As a result, special psychic powers are obtained and the soul is liberated, which is the ultimate goal of yoga.

Each of the seven main chakras has unique physical, emotional and spiritual effect. The lower chakras, which are located from the base of the spine to the solar plexus, have a tendency to be more physical than the chakras that are located from the heart to the crown of the head. Many people focus on the chakras located higher up because they believe that these chakras are more spiritual than the lower ones. However, it is important that each level is supported by a solid base below it. The lower chakras have grounding forces that establish a steady foundation for balanced spiritual exploration. If a chakra is out of balance, you can balance the whole system by stimulating the less active chakras and redistributing energy. Knowledge of the chakras is a way of understanding our mind and body better. Yoga poses offer us the tools we need to create a transformation.

THE SEVEN CHAKRAS

1. *Muladhara* Chakra or Root Chakra

This first chakra, known as the root chakra, is located at the base of the spine. The related organs are the organs of elimination and excretion, which are the lungs, kidneys, large intestine and rectum, and also the skin.

This chakra, which governs your connection to the earth, relates to how 'rooted' you feel. It is concerned with your material and monetary existence. It is involved with getting your basic needs met, such as food, shelter and love. This chakra deals with your emotional stability and your physical setup and is outwardly expressed in your strength and stamina. It gives you the motivation to wake up in the morning. It makes it easier for you to focus, stay disciplined, live a healthy lifestyle, and be aware of your limits.

The balancing of the root chakra is critical; without it, you will lack stability. When this chakra is out of balance, lower abdomen problems such as constipation, diarrhea, hemorrhoids, kidney problems, sciatica and back pain may occur.

Since the base chakra possesses a grounding force, the psychological impact of an imbalance here will lie somewhere on the spectrum between feeling too grounded and not being grounded enough. A lack of grounding may make you feel off-center, like you're living in a fantasy world. You may have difficulty focusing or may go out of control easily.

You may also find it challenging to control your feelings and hold on to your emotions too much. An imbalance at the base chakra may manifest itself in a way that causes you to act as someone who likes to control things.

The muladhara chakra drives the energy related to work. When this chakra is not in balance, you may become a workaholic. You may also experience diminished creative power, which will make it harder for you to enjoy life and experience joy and happiness.

Aggressiveness and stubbornness are other indicators of root chakra imbalance. A tendency towards selfishness, fostering material and emotional possessiveness, are also signs of the same. When there is a threat to your survival, you feel afraid. This fear can immobilize you and ultimately stop you from achieving your goals. Confronting your fears allows the root chakra to awaken.

A balanced root chakra results in general health for the related organs, such as the kidneys and bowel. The adrenal glands, which play a role in the response to stress, will be healthy as opposed to exhausted from chronic overstimulation. You will have a cheerful, fearless and courageous attitude because a balanced base chakra results in heightened self-confidence, enthusiasm, will to live, and sense of identity. In this state, you are more prone to trusting others.

You will have a positive outlook on life and be able to look at the grand scheme of things. You will not over-emphasize the importance of material possessions. You will have a healthy attitude towards work, i.e. being focused while not being so attached to work that you ignore other parts of your life. You will bring an enthusiastic approach to your work and challenges. With this attitude, material success will be easier to come by.

2. *Svadhisthana* Chakra or Sacral Chakra

The second chakra, which is located at the lower abdomen between the navel and the genitals, governs the organs of this area. These organs include those of the urinary and reproductive systems.

This chakra deals with sexuality, relationships and creativity, and governs our ability to nurture, as well as our sensation and pleasure focus. It is concerned with relationships, including our relationship with ourselves. The svadhisthana chakra controls how we adapt to any change regarding growth, movement or life, and helps us go with the flow.

If there is an imbalance in the sacral chakra, it could negatively impact the urinary, reproductive and circulatory system. Impotence, sexually transmitted diseases and bladder problems are signs that the second chakra is not in balance.

People who have an unbalanced second chakra struggle to give and receive either materially or emotionally. Physically, obesity can be a manifestation of a lack of balance between giving and receiving. An overweight person who is eating more calories than they are burning is an example of someone taking more than they are giving. The second chakra also aids with the assimilation of knowledge. The integration of knowledge is a form of receiving.

Feelings of guilt, anxiety, unpredictability and clinging on can result from an unbalanced second chakra. Some people may struggle to separate their own feelings from the feelings of others. General low energy or lack of creativity can also be a result of an imbalance in this chakra. Sex drive can either be too high or too low. Over-the-top flirting or using sex to get attention are other indicators that the sacral chakra is off balance.

A person with a well-balanced second chakra will have healthy lower abdominal, urinary and reproductive system. If the chakra is balanced, you will be outgoing and patient, and will possess a good sense of humor. You will feel comfortable with yourself, including your sexuality. You will have a more positive attitude and greater enjoyment of life.

A main force of the second chakra governs the attraction of opposites, creating a dance between dualities. At the same time, you harbor your own intellectual ideas about the world and where your desires and emotions fit in it.

Problem solving, including the ability to work with others in a creative capacity, will come easily when this chakra is balanced. Even if other people don't share the same ideas as you, you will be able to carve out a complementary path. You will view the different approaches and attitudes of others in a way that enriches your life and allows you to develop and grow.

3. *Manipura* Chakra or Solar Plexus

The third chakra is located between the bottom of the breastbone and the naval. It controls the digestive system and related organs such as the liver, stomach, gall bladder, pancreas, spleen and the organs of excretion.

Because of its closeness to the digestive system, the third chakra deals with the production and the storage of energy that allows us to live our lives in an effective manner. The *manipura* chakra is concerned with emotions, actions, power and will. It helps us to realize that, with effort and action, we are capable of achieving what we want.

The solar plexus center links our comfort level with power, including our sense of personal power. Power originates from the ability to bring things together as opposed to viewing things as separate and unrelated. A balanced third chakra aids with the development of a healthy will and autonomy. When the solar plexus is not in balance, one may experience a feeling of powerlessness, have lower self-esteem, and be more easily swayed by the opinions of others.

Also, if this chakra is imbalanced, one may experience extreme emotions such as violent passions, jealousies, anger and frustration. These emotions can transform into troubling doubts, fear and confusion. One may also feel the need to try and manipulate others. Obsessive characteristics or addictive tendencies might also manifest themselves due to an imbalance.

Without asserting your own autonomy, you may feel powerless or victimized. With an unbalanced third chakra, you run the risk of draining yourself of emotional strength. Apathy and lethargy will result in a loss of energy that makes you want to withdraw from life. You may become overly critical of yourself, and as a result you will not connect with or be nourished by your surroundings. Low self-esteem leads to excessive self-doubt.

You may also experience an imbalance of fiery energy. This imbalance may manifest itself as feeling scorching hot, avoiding spicy food, craving cold drinks, sweating easily, or being quick-tempered. On the other hand, too little fire can make you feel cold, crave spicy foods and hot drinks, or feel lethargic. Any or all of the related organs might show symptoms of an imbalance, like ulcers, upset stomach, diabetes, hypoglycemia, alcoholism, a tight and hard belly, a large pot belly, or a sunken diaphragm.

A well-balanced manipura chakra infuses you with high energy levels, which can result in a warm body and fast metabolism. High energy levels give you an enthusiasm for work and play, as well as an inclination towards development and transformation in your life.

You will use power constructively, directing it inwards, towards the self, instead of wielding it over others. Internal will power will foster proactive, assertive and confident qualities. Your self-esteem will be at a healthy level, and you will be driven towards positive change, instead of passively waiting or wishing for something great to happen. You will be self-motivated and self-accepting. You will have an awareness of your social responsibilities and will approach life from a social perspective. You will feel a temptation to abuse your power to manipulate others. You will use your power to bring people and things together instead of driving them apart. A balanced manipura chakra gives you the inner strength to act with ease and grace.

4. *Anahata* Chakra or Heart Chakra

The anahata chakra is located at the center of the chest, corresponding to love in the pure, unconditional sense. It encompasses both the love of nature and of humanity.

Physically, the anahata chakra is connected to the heart, the circulatory and respiratory systems, the breasts, the chest and the shoulders. This fourth chakra combines the forces of the first three chakras. The first chakra fosters solidity and stability, the second controls change and movement, while the third deals with acceptance and will. When these forces are combined, they can then channelize energy that allows you to achieve higher goals. The heart chakra is a transitional point between the grounding lower chakras and the higher, spiritual chakras.

It is concerned with social awareness, love, openness, devotion, peace, forgiveness, acceptance, kindness and joy. While the svadhisthana chakra has a unifying force that is directed toward objects or people, the unifying force of the heart chakra relates to the state of being. It is less involved with sexuality and materialism. It is involved with the union and harmonious integration of the self into larger social groups in a way that doesn't result in the loss of a sense of the self. The force of the anahata chakra keeps you from being circumscribed by the limitations of the ego. In transcending the ego, we can grow towards true strength. Our boundaries are loosened as we experience the joy of love.

Physically, an imbalance in the fourth chakra can cause heart conditions, including high blood pressure and respiratory problems, asthma and arthritis of the arms. Emotionally, you might experience a conditional type of love. You also may confuse love and sex. You may find yourself imposing your will on others and becoming manipulative. On the other hand, you might become overly selfless and often play the role of martyr. An imbalance in the fourth chakra can result in a lack of sensitivity, making you arrogant and selfish, and harboring feelings of sadness and depression.

When the heart chakra is balanced, the related organs and systems will be in good health. You will experience a sense of connection with life, and in turn feel peace, joy and a feeling of unconditional love for all beings. Your relationships will be more balanced and harmonious. Your emotions will be free and stable, and you will be able to clearly and spontaneously express them. You will be open, willing and able to live your life without fearing vulnerability. You will have a good balance between material things and your emotions because of the heart chakra's integrative force, which allows you to overcome dualities. Furthermore, love is the ultimate healing energy, and the heart chakra is the center for healing.

5. *Visuddha* Chakra or Throat Chakra

The fifth chakra is located at the base of the throat and is linked to communication and expression.

The *visuddha* chakra is related to the neck and organs of the neck, including the voice box and air passage in the throat. The related glands are the thyroid and parathyroid glands, so the fifth chakra affects the metabolism of the whole body.

The throat chakra is concerned with the verbal expression of everything encompassed by the lower chakras. It affects our speech and our ability to express ourselves. It is closely related to truth and honesty. It connects our feelings with our thoughts, allowing them to enter our consciousness and letting us act on them. The throat chakra helps in the formation of our future. In general, needs and desires are more easily met once expressed, therefore verbal communication allows us to shape our own future. Like the sacral chakra, the throat chakra, too, is closely connected to creativity since the formation of speech, communication and expression is a process that is inherently creative. The throat chakra is a deviation from the physicality of the chakras below it. It has more fluid boundaries and is less physical in nature because of its involvement in things such as the sharing of information and ideas.

Physical symptoms of a throat chakra imbalance are sore throats, loss of voice and neck or throat conditions. An over- or under- active thyroid, headaches from neck muscle tension, insomnia, flu and even cancer are also possible manifestations of an unbalanced throat chakra. Any difficulty in expression is an indicator of imbalance, too. You may find yourself holding back, either in voicing your opinion or in expressing your thoughts or feelings. On the other hand, you may be overly dominant in conservation and discussion. You may be critical, tactless, deceitful, judgmental or harsh. You also might suffer from false pride.

When the throat chakra is balanced, the throat area will be in good health. You will effectively communicate your feelings and ideas, which can show in your voice, making it clearer and more pleasant to the ear. You will feel more creative, mature and inspired, which will allow you to deal with yourself and others in an honest, compassionate and tactful way. You can make clear assessments without being overly judgmental of others. This fifth chakra is related to the rhythm and the pace at which we lead our lives, and our verbal expressions because of vibrational rhythms, thereby equipping us with a sense of serenity and devotion.

6. *Ajna* Chakra or Third Eye Chakra

This sixth chakra is located between and just above the eyebrows. It is like a third eye and is considered to be the seat of wisdom.

The *ajna* chakra is closely connected to the brain and nervous system. The ears, nose, eyes and sinuses are all linked to this sixth chakra. The hormonal system is impacted by it because of the wide reaching effect of the pituitary gland in the brain. Our sense of sight has a powerful information gathering capability. With a single glance, we can consume an enormous amount of information. Taking our ability to see further, the sixth chakra deals with the capacity for intuition, imagination, visualization and clairvoyance. This intuition serves as the link between our intellectual and psychic abilities, guiding us from within. Intuition allows us to harness a force greater than ourselves. An imbalance in the ajna chakra may result in headaches or eye, ear, nose and sinus conditions. Hormonal imbalances, insomnia and nervous disorders may manifest themselves, too. Depression is a possible manifestation because the third eye chakra is connected to the hormonal glands of the brain, and therefore to levels of the neurotransmitter serotonin. An imbalance in this neurotransmitter can cause depression.

On a different level, depression might result from losing touch with your creative side. When the sixth chakra is imbalanced, you may experience difficulty focusing and concentrating, and consequently feeling confused and negative. A lack of direction and intellectual stagnation are also indicators of an unbalanced sixth chakra. Many people spend many hours a week in a job that fails to enhance their lives in any way. We should feel enriched by what we do for work. Make sure your work aligns with your beliefs. The sixth chakra can help you determine what will fulfill you. Your yoga asana practice is incredibly helpful as it takes you on an emotional and intellectual journey, which allows you to listen to your intuitive self and the special language of your body related to posture, holding patterns, disease and well-being.

When the third eye chakra is properly balanced, you will be able to observe your thoughts and feelings without getting overly attached to them. You will be able to have a good sense of direction, devotion and ideas. You will feel imaginative, and will have the ability to carry within yourself a sense of unity. This sense of integration will prevent anxiety. When the ajna chakra is fully awakened, you will experience a mastery over the self, which is known as self-realization.

7. *Sahasrara* Chakra or Crown Chakra

The crown chakra is located at the top of the head, at the 'soft spot' that is called the anterior fontanel.

The brain, the whole nervous system and the pineal gland are all related to the crown chakra. The root chakra and the crown chakra have opposing forces. While the root chakra is the entry point of human life, the crown is an exit point. The crown chakra is concerned with transcending materialistic tendencies and letting go of physical attachments. The search for meaning and the understanding that all things are part of a bigger picture brings us closer to unity. The seventh chakra equips you with a coherent sense of meaning. It deals with the highest state of consciousness — spiritual enlightenment, self-realization and consciousness about 'God'. The crown chakra is significant because it is the point where the liberation of the soul occurs. When the sahasrara chakra is fully awakened, the seven chakras fuse together and you experience spiritual boundlessness. At this level of consciousness, you are aware of a higher or deeper order that integrates and unifies everything, including you. It reminds us that although the body is finite, the soul is not.

Physically, cerebral tumors and increased pressure in the skull are possible manifestations of an imbalance in the crown chakra. Psychological symptoms such as psychoses, neuroses and depression may appear. You may experience insomnia because of the crown chakra's connection to the pineal gland. This gland is responsible for producing melatonin, which is essential to healthy sleep and is related to Seasonal Affective Disorder Syndrome (SADS). Emotionally, you may also feel isolated from the world. You may experience a loss of direction, low energy levels, fatigue and closed-mindedness. When your crown chakra is balanced, you will have a sense of unity with others that does not compromise your individuality. You will pay well-focused attention to those around you. You will not have a distorted view of the world, but instead will have a knowledge born of wisdom and enlightenment. You will have the will to follow your own ethical ideals instead of being overly influenced by the opinions of others.

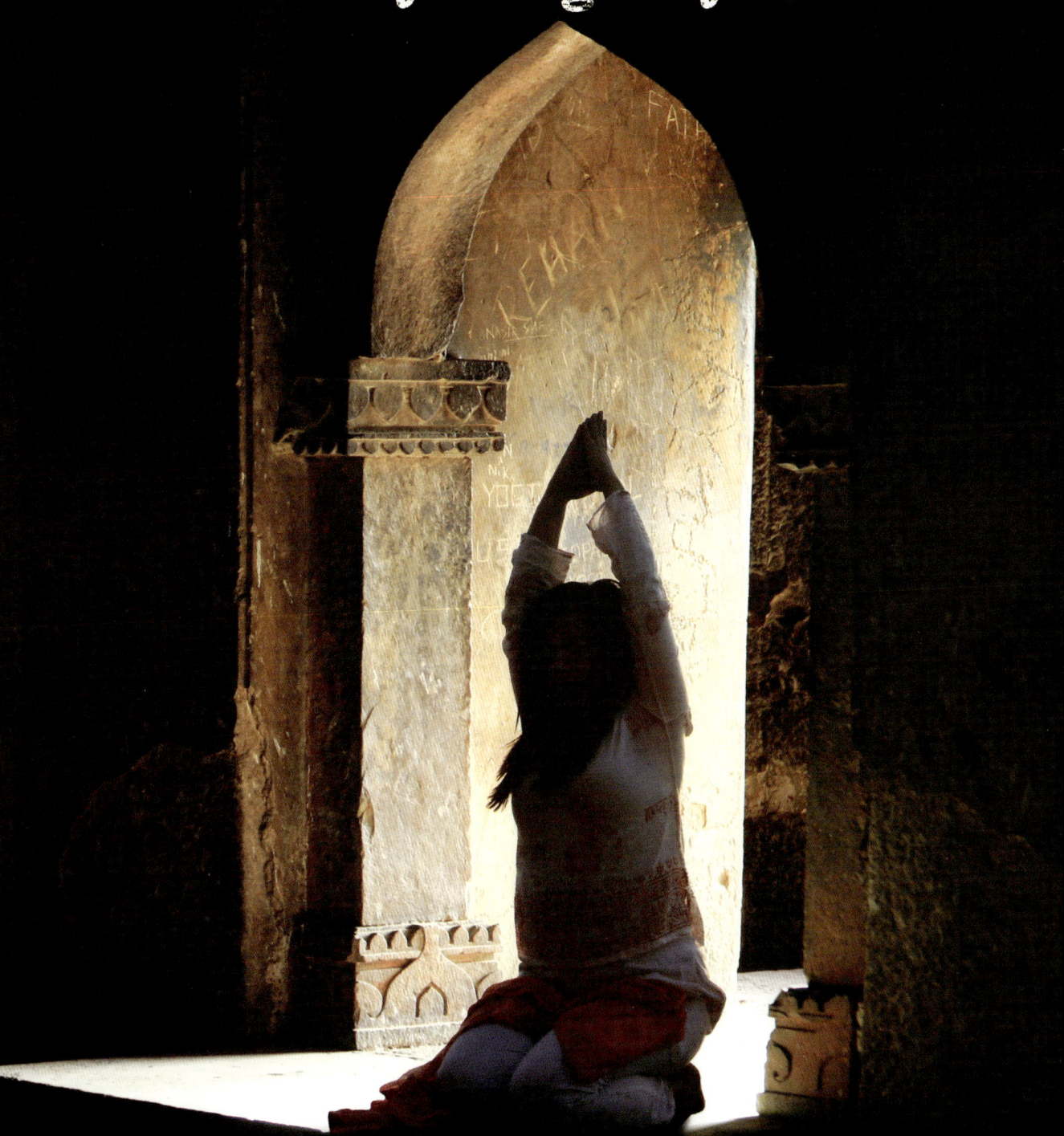

Today's Yoga Styles

The concept of modern yoga is like a maze; many people find it confusing, to begin with. However, all styles of yoga practiced today can be traced back to three historical basis:

1. Religious yoga

2. Yoga based on Patanjali's *Yoga Sutras*

3. Hatha yoga

Here are some varieties of yoga. They all ultimately stem from the same source, differing only in their form.

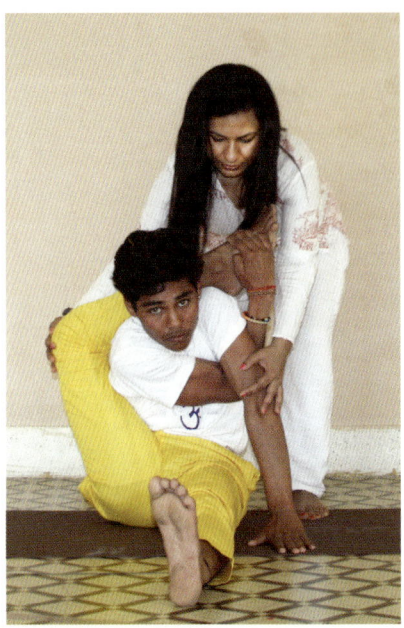

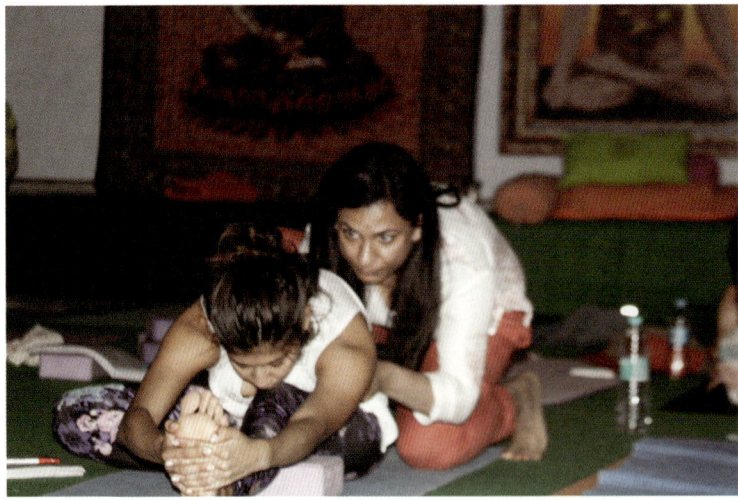

The author assisting her pupils in Rishikesh, India

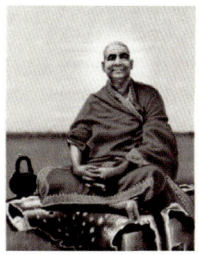

SIVANANDA YOGA

Sivananda yoga started when, at the end of the 1950s, Swami Vishnudevananda (1927-93, India) was instructed by his teacher, Swami Sivananda Saraswati, to introduce yoga to the West. He opened the Sivananda Yoga Vedanta Center in Montreal, Canada, which still exists today. Sivananda centers can now be found all over the world, but predominantly in Europe and North America, where the five pillars of the Sivananda method are taught: asana practice (often referred to as the classical hatha yoga style) combined with breathing exercises, deep relaxation techniques, vegetarianism, meditation and positive thinking.

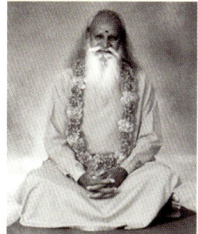

INTEGRAL YOGA

Swami Satchindanada (1914-2002, India) was also a pupil of Swami Sivananda Saraswati. He became famous at the end of the 1960s when he encouraged thousands of spectators at the world renowned Woodstock Music Festival to chant the holy mantra 'Om'. He started the Integral Yoga Institute in Virginia, USA, which spread worldwide. The cornerstone of his style was inherited from his teacher and involved gentle asana practice, breathing exercises and deep relaxation.

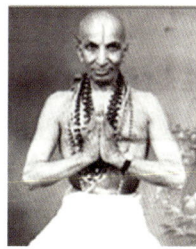

YOGA IN THE TRADITION OF TIRUMALAI KRISHNAMACHARYA

T.K.V. Desikachar (born 1938, India), son and pupil of Krishnamacharya, who founded the Krishnamacharya Yoga Mandiram (KYM) in Chennai (formerly Madras), India. This is a nationally renowned institution where Indian and Western pupils are trained. The yoga taught at KYM draws on the therapeutic background of Krishnamacharya, in that it concentrates on the needs of the individual, and the asana and breathing exercises are adjusted to suit the requirements and conditions of the person concerned. As a result, the teaching is usually on a one-to-one basis.

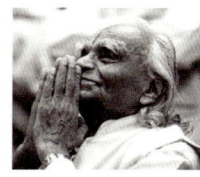

IYENGAR YOGA

B.K.S. Iyengar (1918-2014, India), a pupil of Krishnamacharya and the uncle of Desikachar, was the founder of the Iyengar Memorial Yoga Institute in Pune (formerly Puna), India. Iyengar yoga is one the most famous styles of yoga practiced worldwide. It draws on elements of the therapeutic approach. Instead of focusing on absolute precision of the asanas, it places emphasis on the individual.

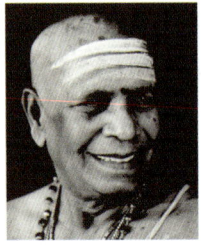

PATTABHI JOIS' *ASTHANGA* YOGA

Pattabhi Jois (1915-2009, India), also a pupil of Krishnamacharya, founded the Ashtanga Yoga Research Institute in Karnataka (formerly Mysore), India. He mainly adopted the elements of *vinyasa* yoga, and refined it. The distinctive feature of ashtanga yoga is the precise sequence of physical exercises developed by Pattabhi Jois, which has remained unchanged. In this exercise cycle or series, each physical posture leads to the next. There is a progression of series, although few pupils go beyond the first series. The asanas, which are physically challenging, are practiced energetically, dynamically and fluently, and are combined with breathing exercises.

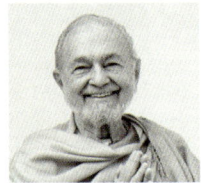

ANANDA YOGA

Swami Kriyananda (1926–2013, Romania) developed this style, which is also known as *kriya* yoga and is based on physical and breathing exercises developed by his teacher, Yogananda (1893–1952, USA), in 1917. This yoga directs the energy flow to particular parts or organs of the body, and prepares the pupil for meditation and spiritual training.

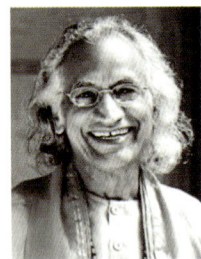

KRIPALU YOGA

Amrit Desai (born 1932, India) is the creator of *kripula* yoga. which is based on asana practice, breathing exercises and the flowing style of Krishnamacharya. It challenges the pupil to recognise his or her own strengths and weaknesses. First, the asanas are practiced, to ensure they are correctly performed, and movement and breathing are coordinated. Then individual positions are held over a prolonged period of time in order to learn how to remain calm in one position. In the third and final stage, pupils develop their own routine in which the sequence and holding of the positions depends on their individual needs.

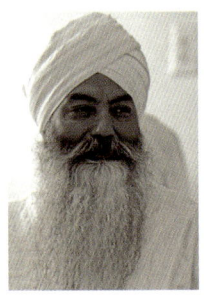

KUNDALINI YOGA

Yogi Bhajan (1929-2004, Pakistan) developed this style of yoga in the religious tradition of Sikhism – a religion practised in India since the end of the fifteenth century in which the teaching is a synthesis of Hinduism and Islam. The Health, Happy, Holy Organization (3HO) he founded in New Mexico is now represented worldwide. Kundalini yoga is the yoga of energy and aims to awaken kundalini, the serpent, through physical postures and breathing exercises. *Karma* yoga, the chanting of mantras, a vegetarian lifestyle and therapeutic use of yoga and Ayurveda are also part of this.

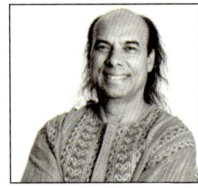

BIKRAM YOGA

Bikram Choudhury (born 1946, India) is happy to call himself 'Yogi to the Stars', having taught yoga to a number of Hollywood actors. He is renowned for teaching physically demanding sequences of twenty-six asanas combined with breathing exercises in a room heated to 40 degrees Celsius (104 degrees Fahrenheit).

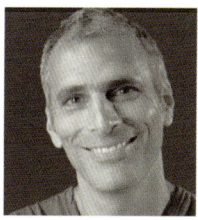

POWER YOGA

Bryan Kest (born 1964, USA), a pupil of Pattabhi Jois, made the name 'power yoga' famous. With less focus on the spiritual, this style of yoga aims for acceptance of oneself and one's own body with highly demanding asana practice. Although pupils are meant to reach their limits during practice, they are taught to listen to their own inner teacher and not cross these, thereby achieving the greatest health benefit for body, spirit and soul.

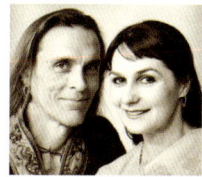

JIVAMUKTI YOGA

Sharon Gannon and David Life (both from the USA) developed jivamukti yoga, which is a spiritual style of yoga. It combines different aspects – studying the basic texts, bhakti yoga, ahimsa, meditation and *nada* yoga (the incorporation of music, chanting and kirtan – singing of mantras as well as the chanting of 'Om' at each lesson).

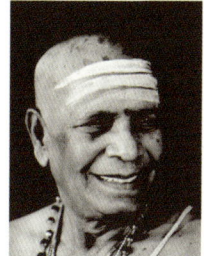

VINYASA YOGA

Vinyasa *Krama* means a step-by-step progression into something. The aim is to fill the unconscious spaces between events that are consciously experienced with attentiveness and awareness. Ahimsa, in particular, plays a central role here, which means that vegetarianism, animal welfare, environmental protection and ethical activism are part of this yoga. Asana practice in the *vinyasa* style is extremely challenging, physically.

The concept of vinyasa krama was adopted for the first time by Krishnamacharya in asana practice. He knew that thoughts could wander between conscious events, for example, anticipating a new asana while practicing a different one. To prevent this and to remain aware, centered and present at all times, Krishnamacharya co-ordinated body movements with breathing techniques.

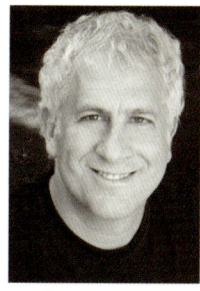

ANUSARA YOGA

Developed by John Friend (born 1959, USA), this style of yoga, along with practicing asanas in the vinyasa style, encourages a life-affirming philosophy focusing on joy and harmony that basically seeks the good in life and in all people.

THE JOURNEY CONTINUES...

New styles of yoga emerge almost daily, with new focuses: hormone yoga, naked yoga, business yoga, acro yoga (yoga with an acrobatic bias), to name but a few. Yoga has also grown to be of economic significance in that there are yoga institutes, studios, seminars, workshops, clothes, accessories, yogi foods and much more. There is no end in sight to the ever-expanding world of yoga. More and more people are recognizing the wide range of benefits associated with it, because everyone can find their own style and path to inner freedom.

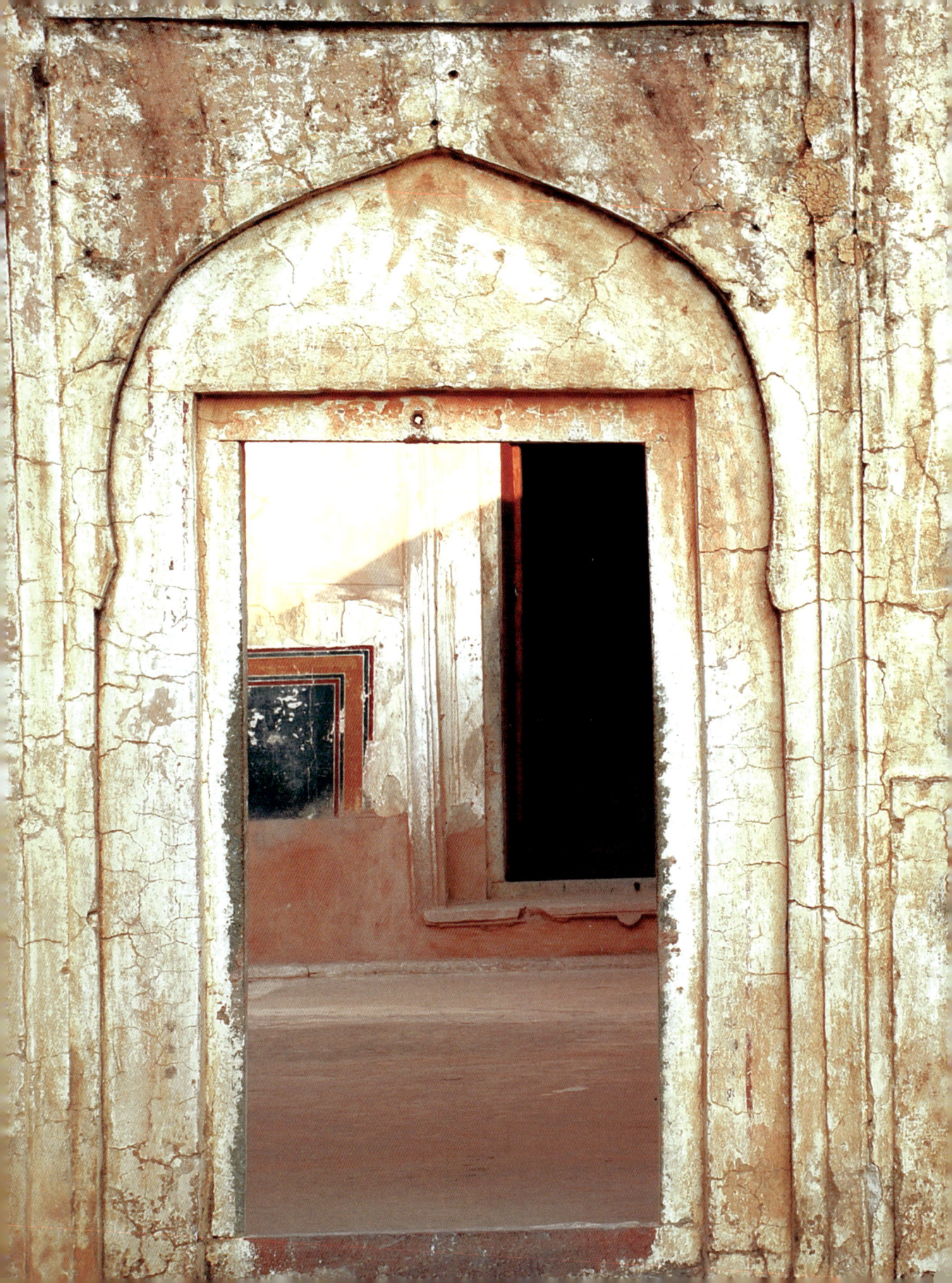

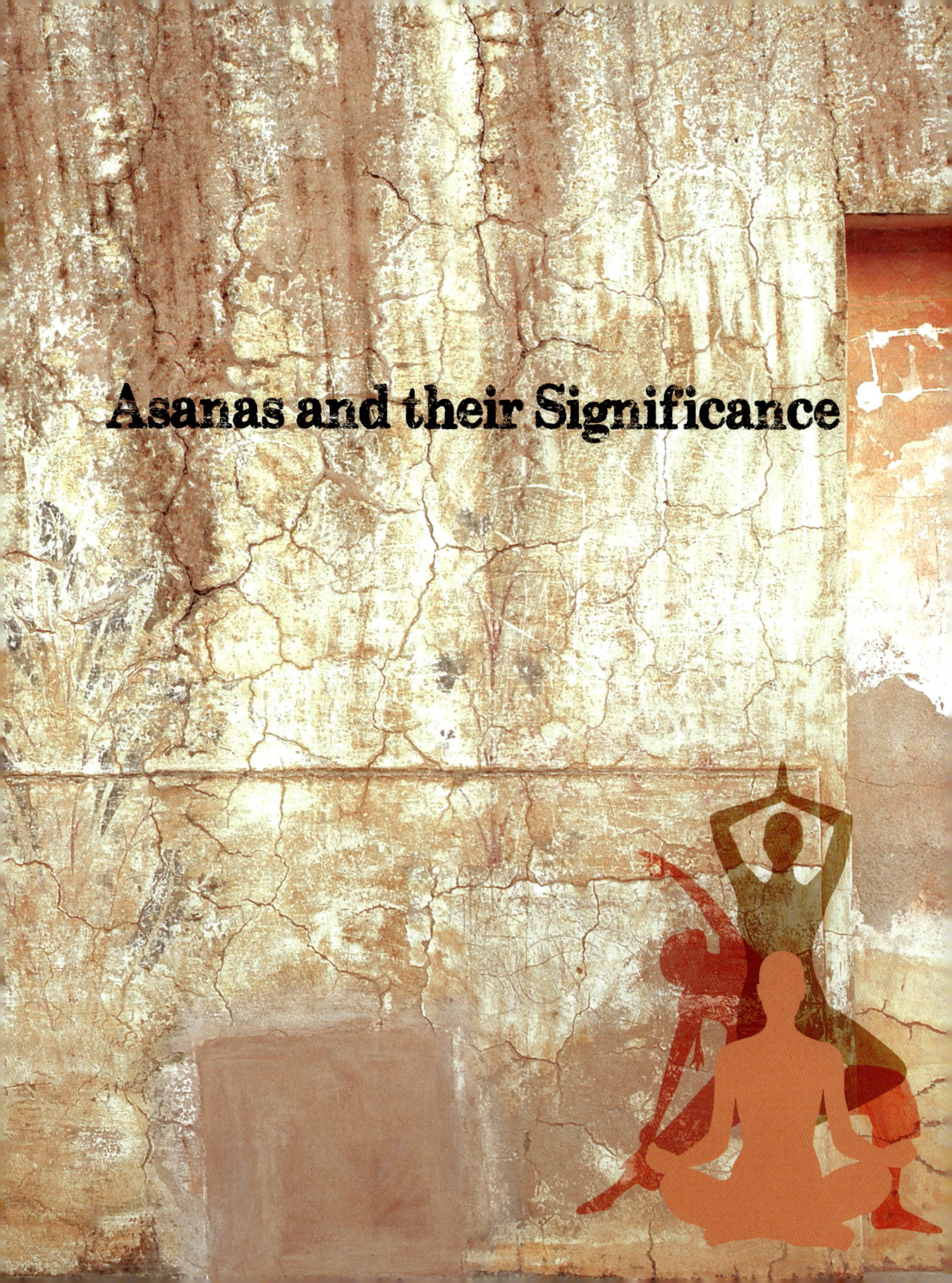

Asanas and their Significance

According to yoga *shastras*, there are 8,40,000 different asanas. Also, there are 8,40,000 species of living organisms in the world, which means that there is one corresponding asana for each of these species. These asanas capture the life experiences and qualities of the corresponding species when they are in a relaxed state. Given the high number of asanas, it would be impossible to learn all of them. Asanas have been adapted by yogis over thousands of years, and currently there are approximately eighty-four important asanas that are practiced and taught.

POSITIVE EFFECTS OF ASANAS

The correct practice of asanas has a positive effect on strength, flexibility and balance. They also improve blood circulation and breathing.

GROUPS OF ASANAS

Depending on the position of their focal point, the asanas are divided into the following categories: sun salutation, standing posture, inverted posture, backbends, sitting, balancing, and supine postures. The details of the various asanas is given in the next chapter.

Principles of Alignment for Asanas

The alignment required for each asana is based on the movement or position of the spinal cord. The requirements for the movement or position of the spine are as follows:

- Twist: turning the spine around its own axis
- Forward bend: bending the spine from the pelvis forward, stretching the back of the body
- Back bend: bending the spine back from the chest, stretching the front part of the body
- Neutral spine: aligning the spine in a neutral curve
- Side bend: stretching the spine to the side

Effortlessness and Stability

The primary goal of the yogi is to find stability and effortlessness in each asana, in equal parts. Yogis aim to establish stability through alignment, which is a fundamental part of the asanas. This helps yogis achieve their other goal, which is the feeling of ease during the asanas. A sense of ease allows yogis to maintain the posture without exerting themselves beyond their capabilities. Yogis can only hold their posture for a short period at first, but with regular practice, they can do it for long intervals. However, posture is not the most crucial thing that the yogis have to master; they must also have complete control over their breathing. The desired feeling of effortlessness is achieved when they breathe calmly and evenly during an asana.

No One is Perfect

Something that is difficult for one person might be easy for another. Everyone has their own personal strengths, weaknesses, preferences and inclinations. Yogis should not feel discouraged if they fail in their first attempts at asanas. They should aim to approach each asana with a new and fresh perspective every time they try it instead of becoming disheartened by the apparent complexity and degree of difficulty. Consistent effort and practice will yield the best results.

Movement and Counter Movement

Each asana involves the extension of the body through movement and counter movement, and different body parts are impacted by this. For example, if a yogi pushes his heels down while standing, it will draw the top of his head up. If he moves his heels forward while sitting, his tailbone will shift back. Therefore, it is critical to turn the body in different directions to create space and comfort even during complex positions.

ASANAS THAT SERVE THE BODY

Here is a brief description of the different kind of asanas:

Bandhas: The Body's Locks

Bandha, a Sanskrit word that means 'lock' or 'seal', relates to the body's lock. Its literal meaning is to close off or to stop. In the practice of a bandha, the energy that travels to a certain part of the body is locked. When this energy is released as a result of increased pressure, it begins to flow more strongly throughout the body. Bandhas are of two types: the first one involves subtle muscle contractions, and the second is based on stronger contractions, which set and hold the muscle contractions of the first type.

Mulabandha

Mulabandha originates from the Sanskrit word *mula* which means 'root' or 'base'; it offers strength and stability to the body.

Starting Position: meditation pose

Concentration: on the muladhara chakra

Breath: deep inhalation followed by holding the breath

Repetition: three to five times

Practice: The yogi must inhale deeply and hold his breath. Then he has to put his hands on his knees, lift his shoulders, and move the upper part of the body slightly forward. The yogi should concentrate on the muladhara chakra, simultaneously contracting his anal muscles.

It is critical to hold the muscular contraction and his breath as long as the yogi can comfortably do so. After exhaling slowly, the yogi should return to the starting position.

Then, the yogi should breathe normally and hold the meditation pose for some time.

Benefits: The mulabandha strengthens the pelvic floor as well as relieves congestion in the pelvic area, and hemorrhoids. It aids with calming down the autonomic nervous system and relaxing the mind. In terms of spirituality, the mulabandha is a way to activate and purify the muladhara chakra. Furthermore, it leads to the awakening of the dormant consciousness and kundalini shakti.

Uddiyanabandha

Uddiyanabandha, from the Sanskrit word *uddiyana* means 'to fly upwards'. This bandha creates stability in the central and upper back portions.

Starting Position: meditation pose or standing
Concentration: on the manipura chakra
Breath: exhale completely and hold the breath
Repetition: three to five times

Practice: In this bandha, the yogi must fully exhale and then hold the breath for some time. Then he must repeat almost the same steps as in mulabandha: putting his hands on his knees, lifting his shoulders, and leaning his body slightly forward. The yogi must keep his back completely straight. For best results, the legs should be slightly parted and the knees should be bent while standing.

The yogi has to keep his concentration on the manipura chakra, and must pull his abdominal muscles in and up and as far as possible into the abdominal cavity. This position should be held for as long as comfortably possible.

After this, the muscular tension should be released, returning to the position where the yogi started, and inhale deeply.

The yogi should breathe normally and remain in the mulabandha position for some time.

Benefits: The uddiyanabandha results in the activation of the manipura chakra and solar plexus. It promotes intestinal activity and stimulates the pancreas, offering relief from constipation and helping diabetics. This bandha strengthens the immune system, balances the mind, alleviates irritability and anger, and drives away depression.

Holding Mulabandha and Uddiyanabandha

For best results towards stability and effortlessness, the two bandhas – mulabandha and uddiyanabandha – are typically performed together. While one is used for inhalation, the other is used for exhalation; either can be used for either purpose. It is challenging to maintain concentration while performing both, but it gets better with practice.

Jalandharabandha

Jalandharabandha, from the Sanskrit word *jalandhara* means 'net' or 'tissue'. It governs the flow of energy between the heart and brain, protecting the heart from pressures. It is performed when the yogi's breath is controlled, his neck vertebrae are extended up, his chin is slightly lowered, and his larynx is drawn in gently.

Starting Position: meditation pose (*siddhasana* or *sukhasana*)
Concentration: on the vishuddha chakra
Breath: inhale deeply and hold the breath
Repetition: three to five times

Practice: Take a deep breath and hold it. Place your hands on the knees, shoulders should be lifted, keeping the body tilted forward. Back should be straight. Now press your chin tightly against the chest, holding the breath till you can. Come to the starting position by exhaling deeply and raising the head. Breathe normally and remain in this position for some time.

Benefits: The practice regulates thyroid function and cures throat diseases. It awakens the visuddha chakra.

Outer Props

If you are unable to reach the floor, you will not achieve good stability; you will not be mobile enough for the alignment required. This is where outer props such as a belt, cushion, wooden or foam block, or blanket come in handy. You can learn to use different props for each asana.

Namaste and Drishti: Improving Concentration

In Sanskrit, 'namaste' suggests 'the divinity in me bows to the divinity in you'. It is a gesture that is often used as a greeting, while taking leave, or for thanking someone. It also has the additional benefit of improving concentration during asanas.

'Drishti' is defined as 'gaze' in Sanskrit, signifying the point of focus of the gaze. Drishti is not an actual object. Instead, it provides support for movement in the direction of the gaze and keeps the consciousness from getting distracted. Thus, the consciousness and gaze follow the movement.

Preparatory Exercise

Before you begin your asana practice, you must mobilize your body. Give special attention to your joints and spine. Combine the following preparatory exercises to suit your personal needs:

- Sit in a comfortable position that allows you to effectively align your spine.
- Move your head gently to the right.
- Then move your head gently to the left.
- Allow your head to fall back without bending your neck vertebrae.
- Stretch your neck and then allow it to drop towards your chest.
- Bring your fingers together, stretch your arms out in front of you (your elbows will turn in slightly).
- Gently rotate your wrist joints in both directions.
- Gently rotate one foot at a time, move both hands to your knee, and turn the knee joint. Repeat on the other side.
- Draw circles in the air with your raised feet. Do it again, changing direction this time.
- Raise your shoulders.
- Lower your shoulders.
- Move your shoulders back, without causing your back to hollow.
- Move your shoulders forward, without rounding your back.
- Sit comfortably upright with your legs crossed, straightening your spine. Then inhale and raise your arms.
- Exhale and turn to the right.
- Put your right hand close to your tailbone and your left hand lightly on your right thigh.
- Don't use force to turn.
- Switch sides and repeat the exercise.

In India, every day of the week is committed to a specific God or planet. There are special *vratas* and *upvaas* or fasts, for each day. Similarly, there are specific asanas and yoga practices corresponding to each day, featuring different bends, depending on the anatomical focus of the poses.

You can build up your routine over time by adding different postures, starting with the simple ones and then going on to the advanced postures.

If in doubt, always refer to a yoga teacher who will guide you on the correct posture and work with you on your alignment.

Practicing a little everyday is better than practicing once or twice a week.

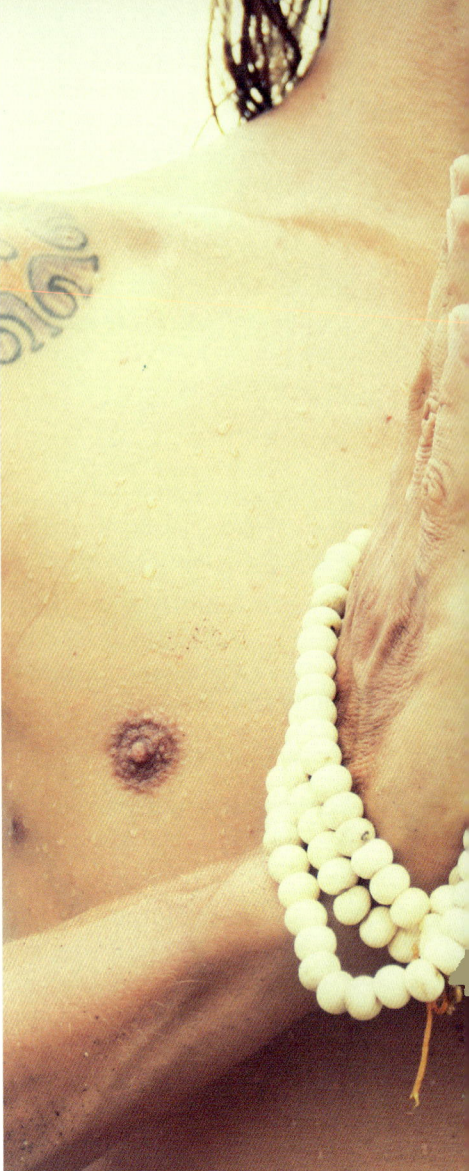

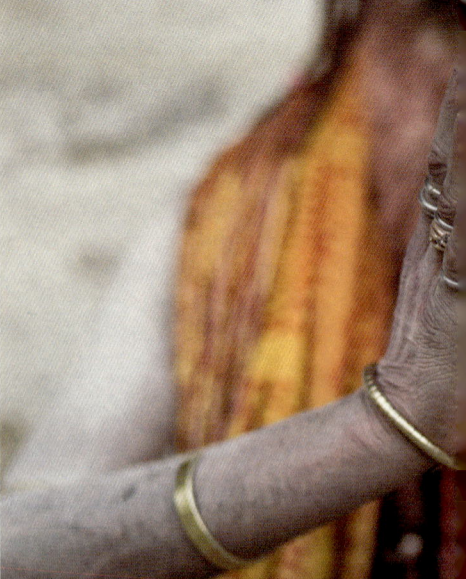

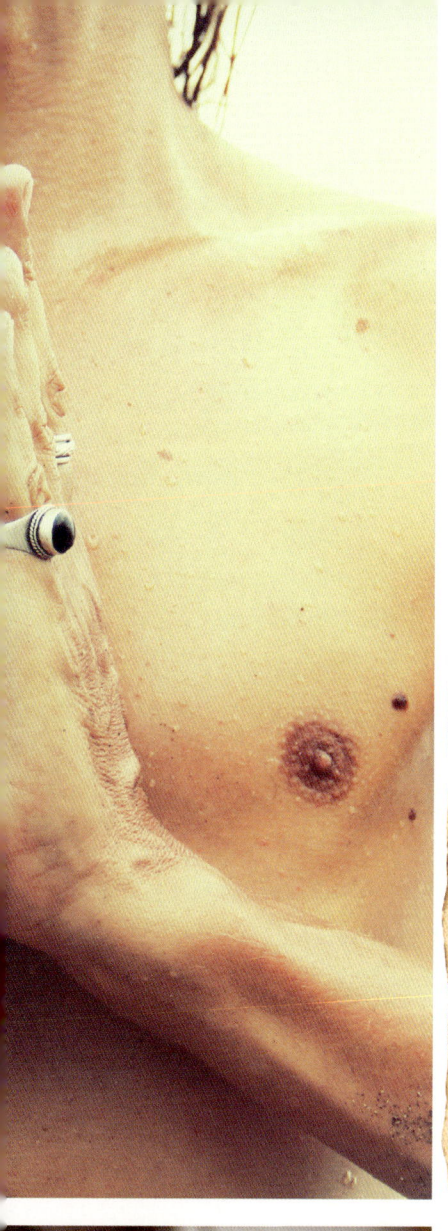

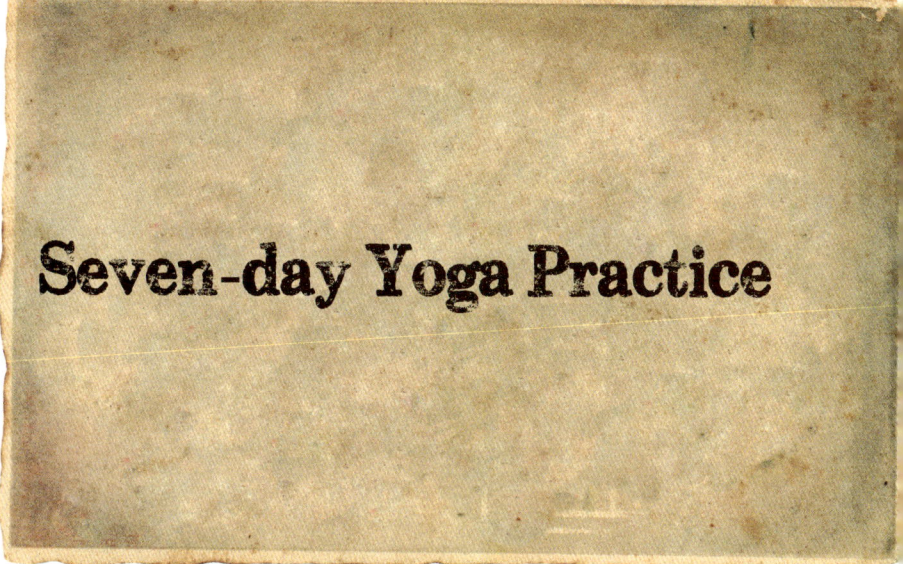

Seven-day Yoga Practice

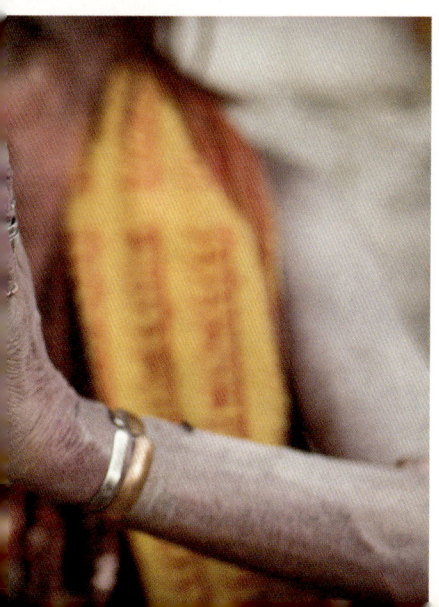

WEEKLY ROUTINE

Monday: Standing Poses

Samasthiti – Mountain pose
Virabhadrasana 1 – Warrior pose 1
Virabhadrasana 2 – Warrior pose 2
Uttanasana – Forward bend pose
Gurudrasana – Eagle pose
Natrajasana – Dancer's pose
Balasana – Child's pose

Tuesday: Seated Poses

Paschimottasana – Back stretch forward bend pose
Ardha Matseyendrasana – Half spine twist pose
Gomukhasana – Cow face pose
Paripurana Navasana – Boat pose
Sukhasana and *Saiddhasana* – Pleasant pose
Padmasana – Lotus pose

Wednesday: Back Bending Poses

Chakrasana – Wheel pose
Ustrasana – Camel pose
Dhanurasana – Bow pose
Salabhasana – Locust pose or grasshopper pose
Bhujangasana – Cobra pose

Thursday: Balancing Poses

Kakasana – Crow pose
Mayurasana – Peacock pose
Vasisthasana – Side plank pose
Chaturanga Dandasana – Four-limbed staff pose

Friday: Inverted Poses

Sirsasana – Head stand pose
Sarvangasana – Headstand pose
Halasana – Plow pose

Saturday: Supine Poses

Matsayasana – Fish pose
Advanced variation – Bound fish pose
Supta Virasana – Reclining pose
Yoga Nidrasana – Sleeping yogi pose
Shavasana – Corpse pose

Sunday: Surya Namaskar (Sun Salutation)

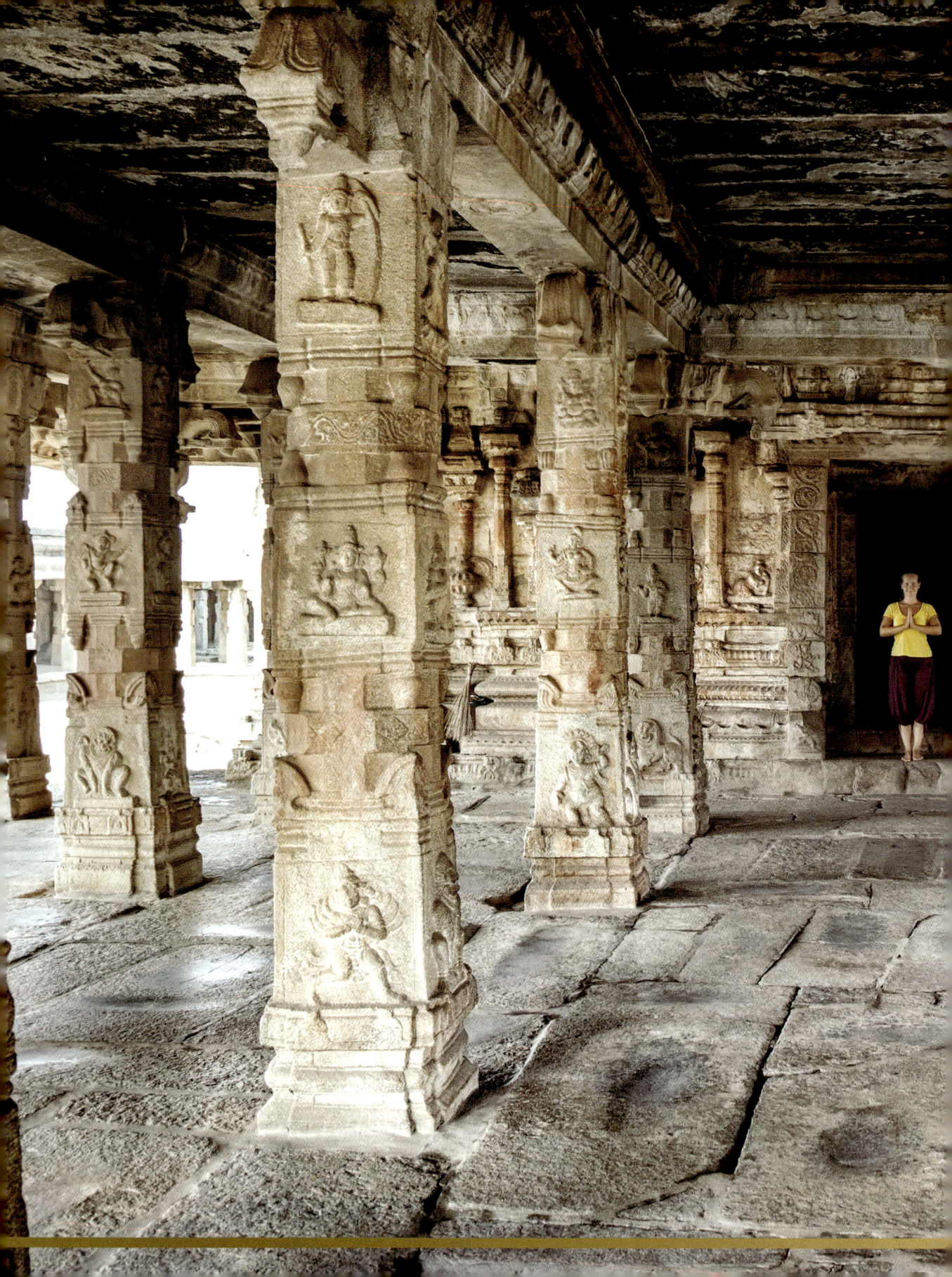

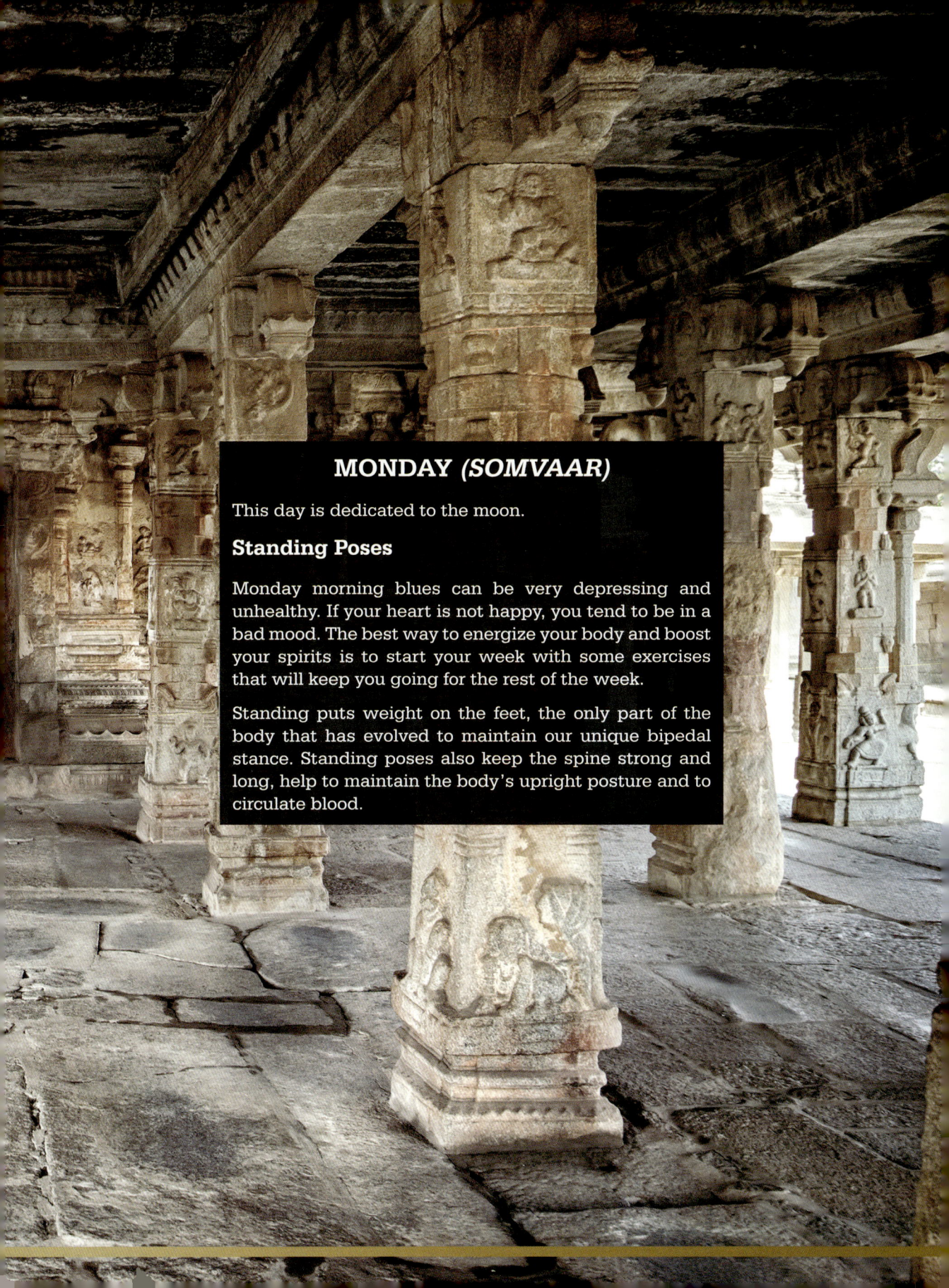

MONDAY (SOMVAAR)

This day is dedicated to the moon.

Standing Poses

Monday morning blues can be very depressing and unhealthy. If your heart is not happy, you tend to be in a bad mood. The best way to energize your body and boost your spirits is to start your week with some exercises that will keep you going for the rest of the week.

Standing puts weight on the feet, the only part of the body that has evolved to maintain our unique bipedal stance. Standing poses also keep the spine strong and long, help to maintain the body's upright posture and to circulate blood.

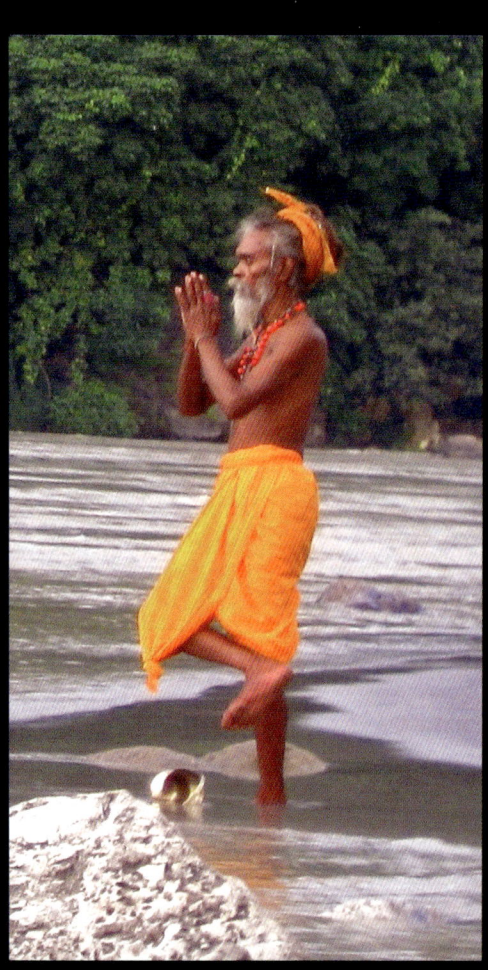

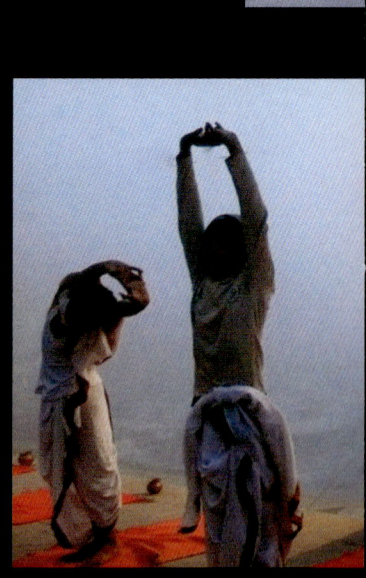

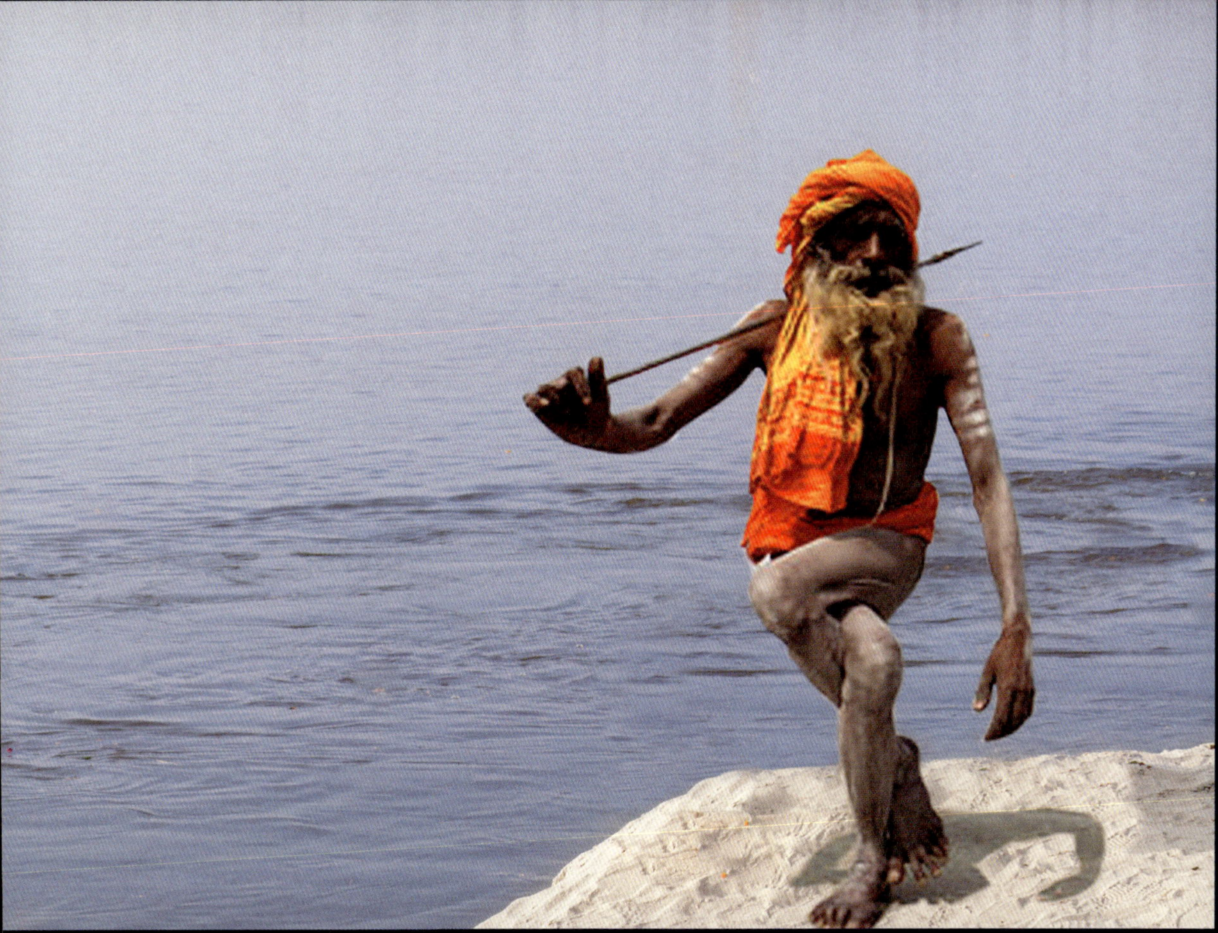

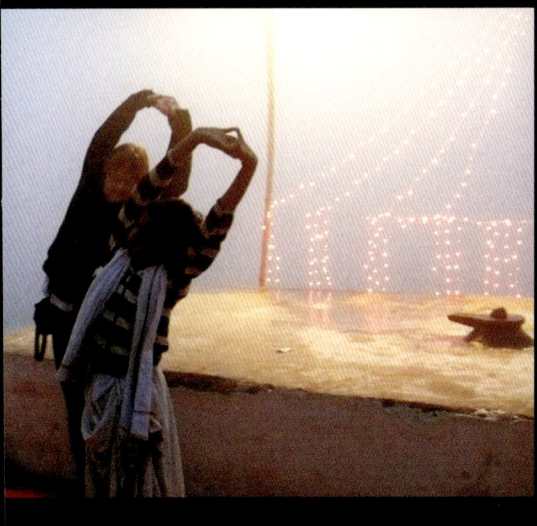

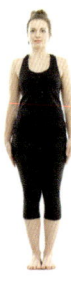

SAMASTHITI OR MOUNTAIN POSE

This is also known as *tadasana*. The Sanskrit word 'tadasana' or 'samasthiti' refer to the same thing – mountain posture. This is the basic standing pose and starting position for the standing poses, as well as for the sun salutation sequence. The aim of this pose is alignment: to stand as firm and erect as a mountain.

1. Stand with feet together, big toes touching with heels apart. Lift toes and balls of feet, while spreading your feet at the same time. Then gently lower them to the floor. Swaying back and forth and side to side at first, slowly come to a standstill pose until you are able to balance your weight evenly.

2. Stand straight, with chest lifted and abdomen in, spine and neck too should be in a straight line. Let arms hang straight down next to torso, palms beside thighs, shoulders relaxed and pulled away from ears. Hold for thirty to sixty seconds.

Benefits

1. Helps you learn to maintain balance through a higher degree of control on your own body.

2. Helps you tone, strengthen and stretch your knees, back, arms and thighs. It also works on your core stomach muscles.

3. Improves posture.

4. Strengthens the knees, thighs and ankles.

5. Firms the abdomen and buttocks.

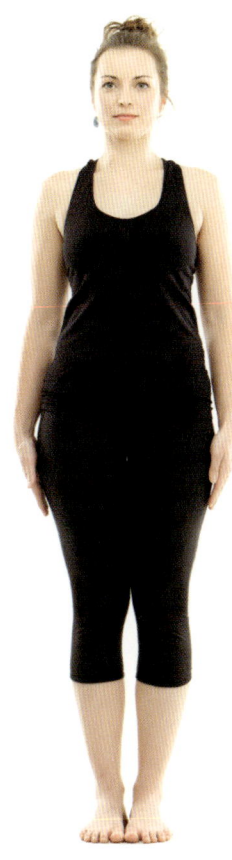

Anatomical Focus

- The abdominal and back muscles support and balance the torso.

- The rhomboids work with the middle part of the trapezius muscle, drawing the shoulder blades in and opening the chest.

- The psoas and glutei muscles lengthen in order to keep the pelvis upright and balanced.

- The knees are kept straight by the shortening of the quadriceps muscles on the front of the thighs.

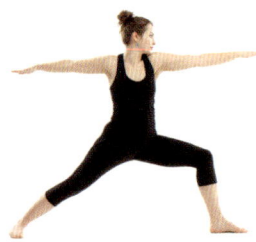

VIRABHADRASANA 1 OR
WARRIOR POSE 1

Virabhadra is the name of a mythical warrior, and the pose Virabhadrasana is dedicated to him. This iconic lunging pose extends the torso and opens the chest upwards.

1. From tadasana, place your feet wide apart and take the arms out to your side.

2. Turn the left foot to the left and turn the right foot by forty-five degrees.

3. Bend the left knee and draw the left hip back and the right hip forward, so that the pelvis is square.

4. Raise the arms and bring the palms together, drawing the shoulders down.

5. Keep the head in a neutral position, or tilt it back and look up. Hold for thirty to sixty seconds.

6. Exhale and let the arms down, straighten the right knee and turn the feet forward.

7. Take a few breaths, then repeat the pose on the left side.

Benefits

1. The chest is fully expanded to enable deep breathing.

2. Strengthens the arms, shoulders and back as well as stretches the thighs, calves and ankles.

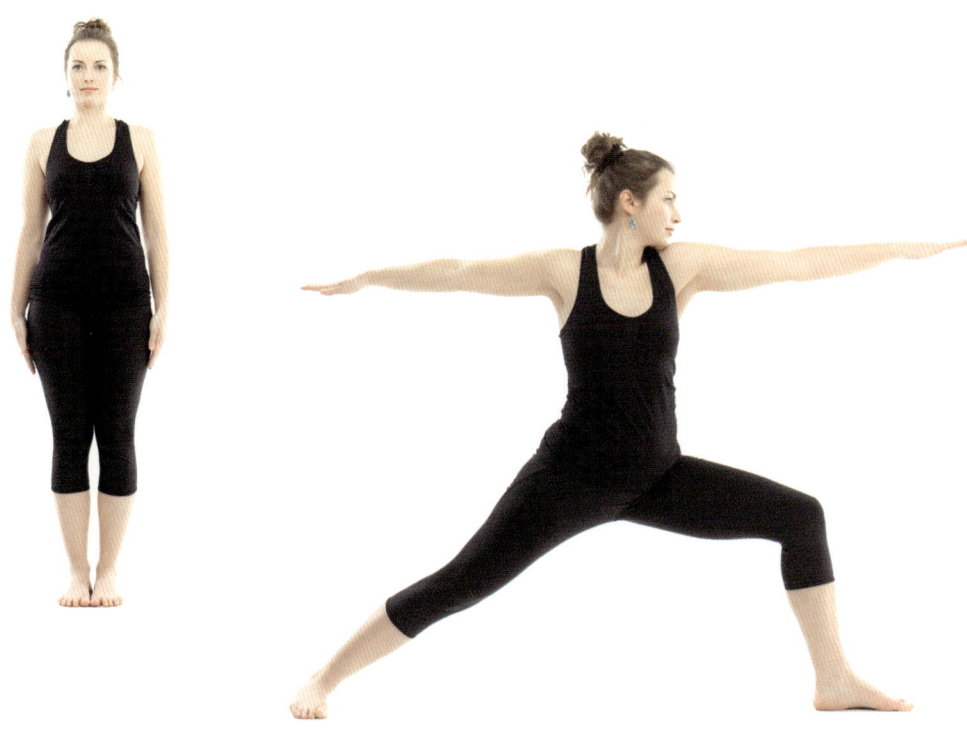

Anatomical Focus

- Spinal rotation; scapular abduction and upwards rotation as the triceps assist in rotating the shoulder blade.

- Front leg: hip flexion; the quadriceps contract to support the body weight; also knee flexion and ankle dorsiflexion.

- Back leg: hip extension; the quadriceps straighten the knee; also ankle dorsiflexion and stretching of the calf muscles.

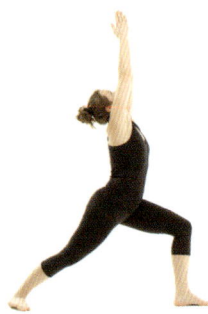

VIRABHADRASANA 2 OR
WARRIOR POSE 2

This pose develops strong muscles in the legs. The warrior series is good preparation for the advanced standing poses and forward bending.

1. From tadasana, place your feet wide apart and take the arms out to your side.
2. Turn the left foot to the left and turn the right foot by forty-five degrees.
3. With the left knee bent, position thigh in a parallel line to the floor. Pull the right hip back, keeping the right leg straight.
4. Look over the left hand. Keep the shoulders level. The legs, dorsal region and hips should be in a straight line.
5. Hold for thirty to sixty seconds.
6. Exhale and let your arms down, straighten the right knee and turn the feet forward.
7. Take a few breaths, then repeat the pose on the left side.

Benefits

1. Strengthens and tones the calf and thigh muscles and relieves cramps in these muscles.
2. Tones the back muscles and the abdominal organs.

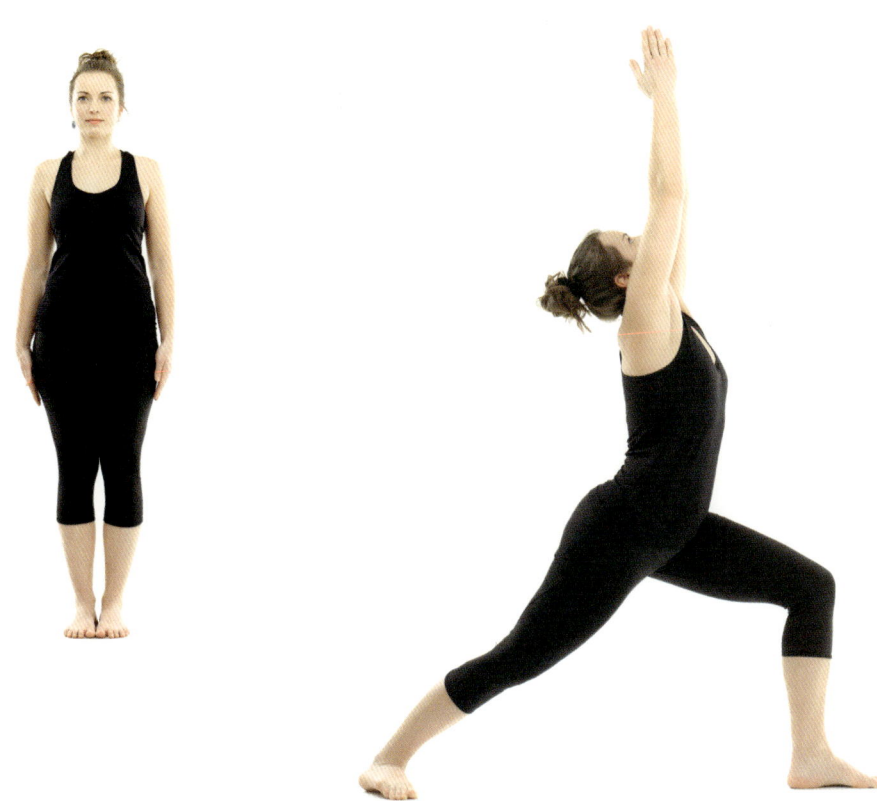

Anatomical Focus

- Lift the back and arch it slightly, and the abdominal muscles contract to protect the lower back.

- The triceps straighten the elbows; the deltoids and rotator cuff muscles raise the arms and open the chest.

- Front leg: hip flexion; the quadriceps contract to support the body weight; also knee flexion and ankle dorsiflexion.

- Leg: the buttock muscle of the back leg extends to enable hip extension.

- The quadriceps straighten the knee and the muscles, as well as shorten the front shin to enable ankle dorsiflexion and to stretch the calf muscles on the back of the leg.

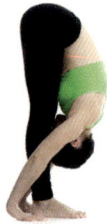

UTTANASANA OR FORWARD BEND POSE

This comes from Sanskrit word 'Uttana' meaning intense stretch and asana which means posture or seat.

This pose helps identify any imbalances or asymmetry in the body, but the main purpose is to give the spine an intense stretch. Uttanasana can be practiced either as a pose by itself or as a resting position in-between the standing poses.

1. Stand in tadasana position while exhaling and pulling in the abdomen.

2. Fold forward from the hips and reach for the floor. While inhaling, lift the hips forward, lengthen the front torso and try to straighten the legs.

3. While exhaling bring the belly onto the thighs. Let the head hang and allow the neck to lengthen. The forehead should eventually rest against the knees or shins. Keep drawing the kneecaps up as you lengthen over the legs.

Benefits

1. Stretches the calves, hamstrings and hips.

2. Stimulates the kidneys and liver.

3. Strengthens the knees and thighs.

4. Aids digestion.

5. Reduces stress, fatigue and anxiety.

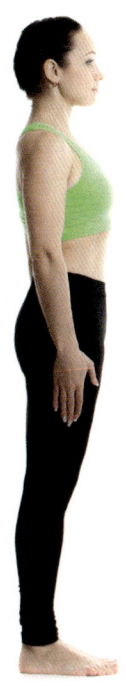 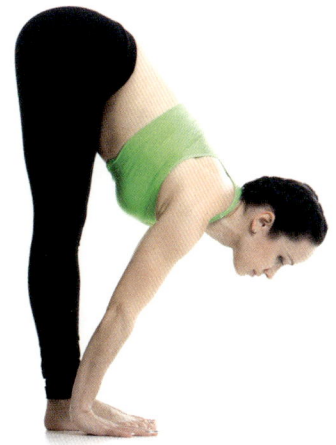 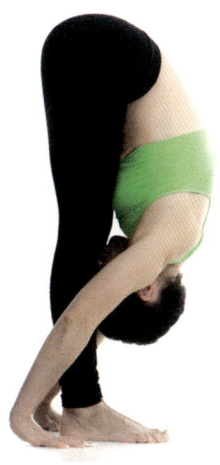

Anatomical Focus

- When we do a forward bend from the hips, the gluteus maximus stretches.

- This produces a pull on the femurs that can externally rotate them and turn the kneecaps slightly outwards.

- Ideally we would like the kneecaps to face directly forward. An added benefit of engaging gluteus medius is that it internally rotates the thighs.

- The gluteus minimus contributes to this action when the hips are flexing.

- This counteracts the pull of the stretching gluteus maximus and brings the kneecaps to face forward – the optimal form of the pose.

- Access this fringe benefit by fixing the feet on the mat and gently attempting to drag them apart, as we did for sacral nutation. Feel how this internally rotates the thighs.

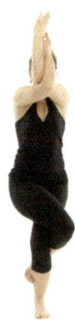

GARUDASANA OR EAGLE POSE

In Sanskrit, 'garuda' means an eagle. This pose is particularly effective for improving balance and coordination, as the balance over one leg and folding and twisting of the arms challenge the way the brain sees the body.

1. Stand in tadasana. With knees bent, balance on the left foot while lifting the right foot. Cross the right thigh over the left.

2. With the right toes pointed to the floor, and the foot pressed back, the top of the foot should be hooked over the lower left calf. Balance on the left foot.

3. Lift arms straight in front of you. Place the left arm on top of the right arm, and bend your elbows.

4. Bring the back of each hand facing the other. Press the backs of your hands together. Bring palms together as much as you can by crossing at the wrists, then cross and raise elbows and let fingers extend upwards towards the ceiling.

5. Hold the pose for fifteen to thirty seconds.

6. Release slowly and repeat steps with the legs and the arms reversed.

Benefits

1. Stretches and strengthens the calves and ankles.

2. Stretches the hips, upper back, and shoulders.

3. Improves the sense of balance.

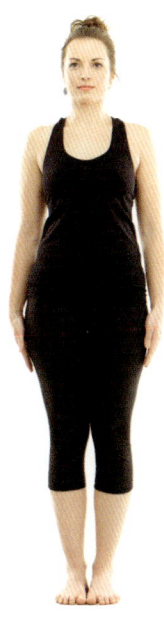 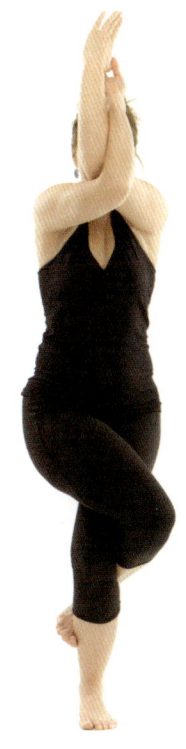 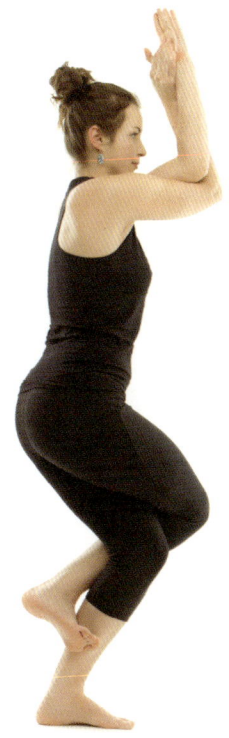

Anatomical Focus

- Eccentric contradiction of the deltoid in the upper arm deepens the stretch of the rotator cuff.

- The pose is stabilized by the gastrocnemius/soleus of the calf, which flexes the standing ankle to press the foot down.

- Adductor muscles squeeze the thighs together and the tenser fascia lata and gluteus medius rotate the fermus internally.

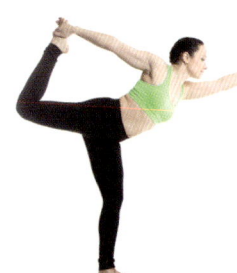

NATRAJASANA OR DANCER'S POSE

In Sanskrit, 'nat' means dancer, 'raja' means king – the dancing posture of the king. This is an asymmetrical standing backward bend pose, requiring good balance and concentration. If you practice this pose at home, try holding on to a door handle as you pull the raised leg up as high as you can.

The natarajasana pose needs to be done gracefully and slowly, almost like a dance, in order to derive maximum benefit from it.

1. Stand in the tree pose. As you inhale, shift your weight to the left foot and lift your right heel towards your buttock.

2. Put additional pressure on the straight left leg, thigh, hip and knee to ensure your legs are properly balanced.

3. Now reach your right hand behind the raised leg and grasp the right ankle. Lift your hip and pubic area accordingly to avoid additional strain.

4. Try to straighten the knee and stretch the left arm forward, in front of the torso and parallel to the floor.

5. Hold the pose for twenty to thirty seconds.

6. Then let go of the foot, place it back on the floor.

7. Repeat for the same length of time on the other side.

Benefits

1. Stretches the shoulders, chest, abdomen, thighs and groin.

2. Strengthens the legs and ankles.

3. Helps to center mind and body.

4. Improves concentration.

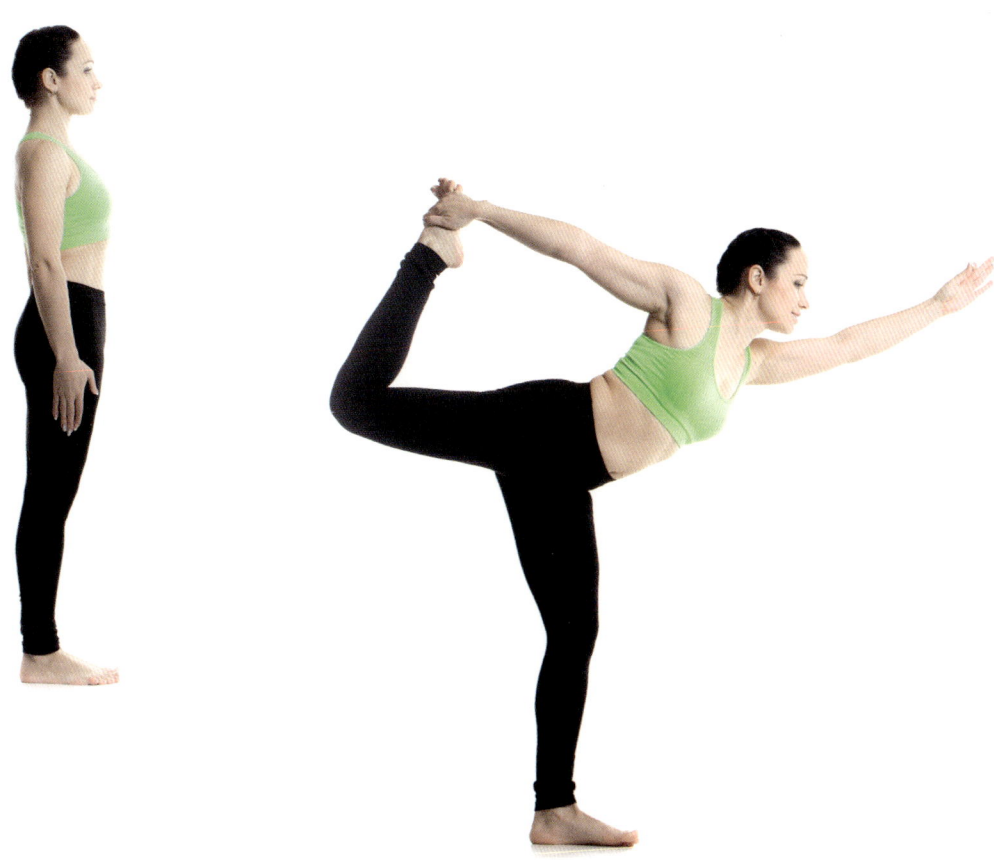

Anatomical Focus

- The forearms supinate.

- On the standing leg, the action of the psoas muscle creates hip flexion and the quadriceps create knee extension.

- On the raised leg there is hip extension and knee flexion due to the quadriceps extension, and hamstring contraction and ankle plantar flexion as a result of the action of the gastrocnemius muscles.

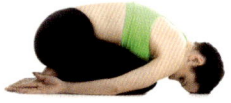

BALASANA OR CHILD'S POSE

The Sanskrit word 'bala' means child. This restorative pose can be practiced at any time, especially during a dynamic practice of standing poses. Here, the body faces the floor in a fetal position.

1. Start with table pose – kneel down and put your hands on the floor.

2. Maintaining the position of the hands, exhale while you sit back on your heels and rest your upper body on the thighs.

3. Let your forehead rest on the floor.

4. Place your arms next to you with hands adjacent to feet and palms facing up.

5. Exhale when you release the hips to the heels and feel your spine lengthening.

6. Balasana is a resting pose. Stay in this position for thirty seconds up to a few minutes.

7. To release the pose, press your hands down on the floor while inhaling and lift yourself to a seated position.

Benefits

1. Stretches and relaxes spine and lower back.

2. Stretches the ankles, thighs and hips.

3. Alleviates fatigue and stress.

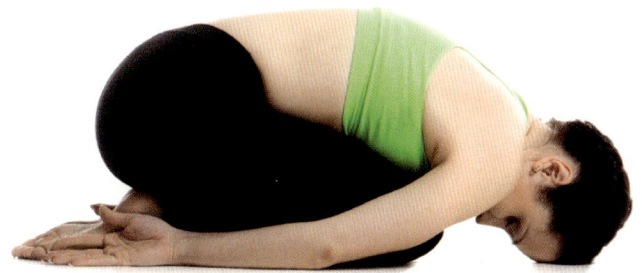

Anatomical Focus

- Knee flexion.

- Spinal flexion. The muscles of the back are passively stretched.

- Hip flexion due to the psoas muscle and abduction.

- Ankle plantar flexion.

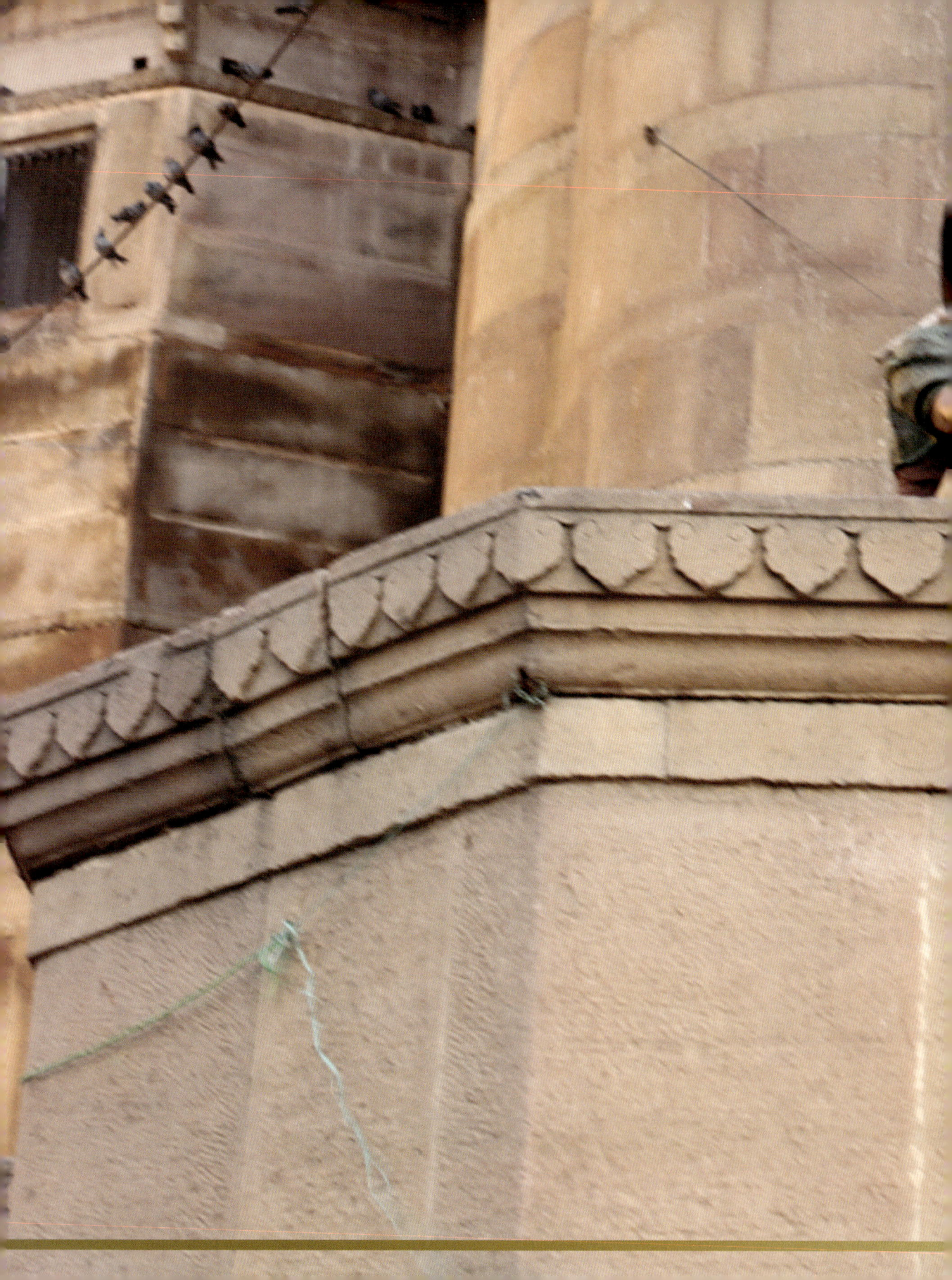

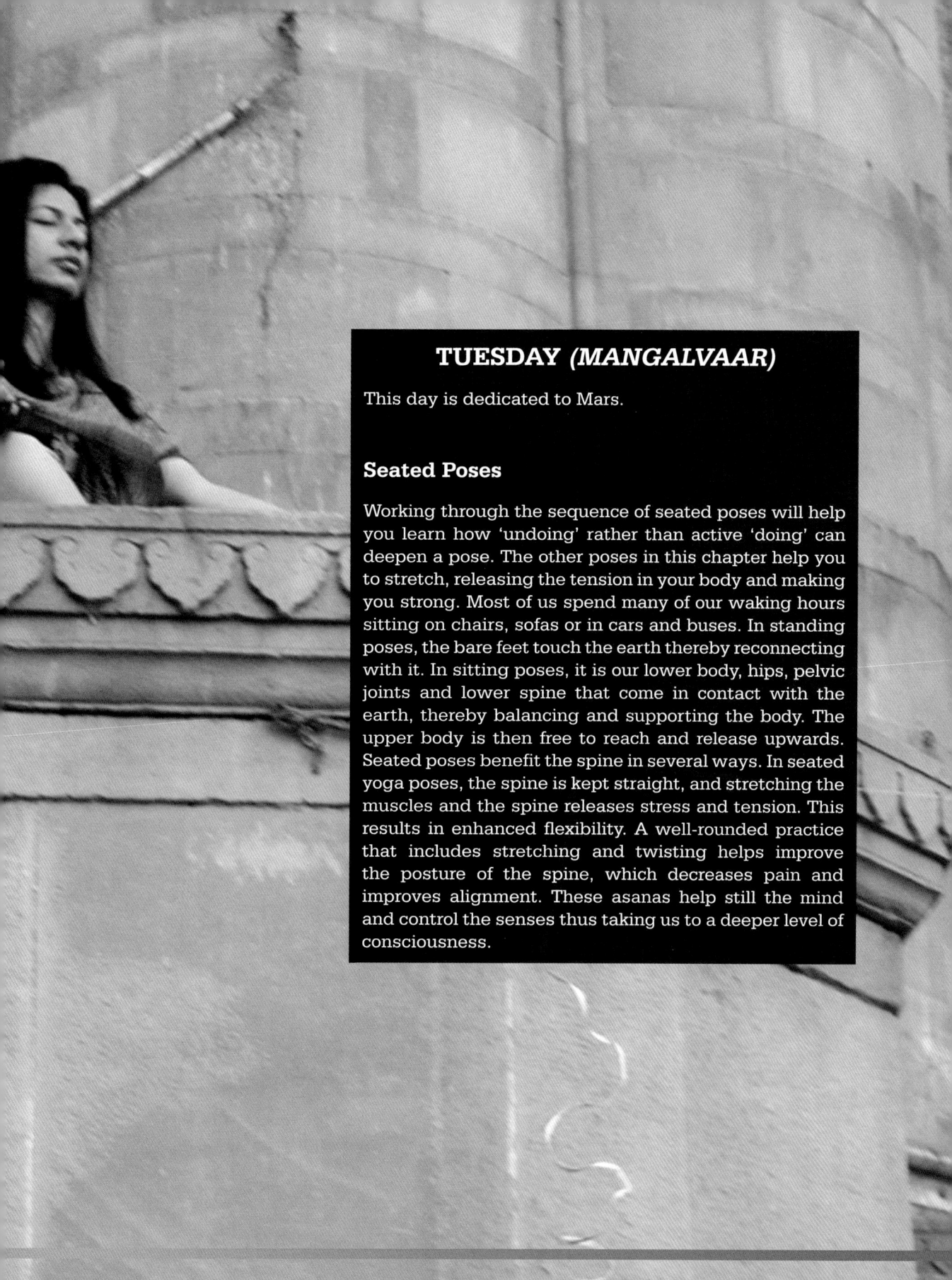

TUESDAY (MANGALVAAR)

This day is dedicated to Mars.

Seated Poses

Working through the sequence of seated poses will help you learn how 'undoing' rather than active 'doing' can deepen a pose. The other poses in this chapter help you to stretch, releasing the tension in your body and making you strong. Most of us spend many of our waking hours sitting on chairs, sofas or in cars and buses. In standing poses, the bare feet touch the earth thereby reconnecting with it. In sitting poses, it is our lower body, hips, pelvic joints and lower spine that come in contact with the earth, thereby balancing and supporting the body. The upper body is then free to reach and release upwards. Seated poses benefit the spine in several ways. In seated yoga poses, the spine is kept straight, and stretching the muscles and the spine releases stress and tension. This results in enhanced flexibility. A well-rounded practice that includes stretching and twisting helps improve the posture of the spine, which decreases pain and improves alignment. These asanas help still the mind and control the senses thus taking us to a deeper level of consciousness.

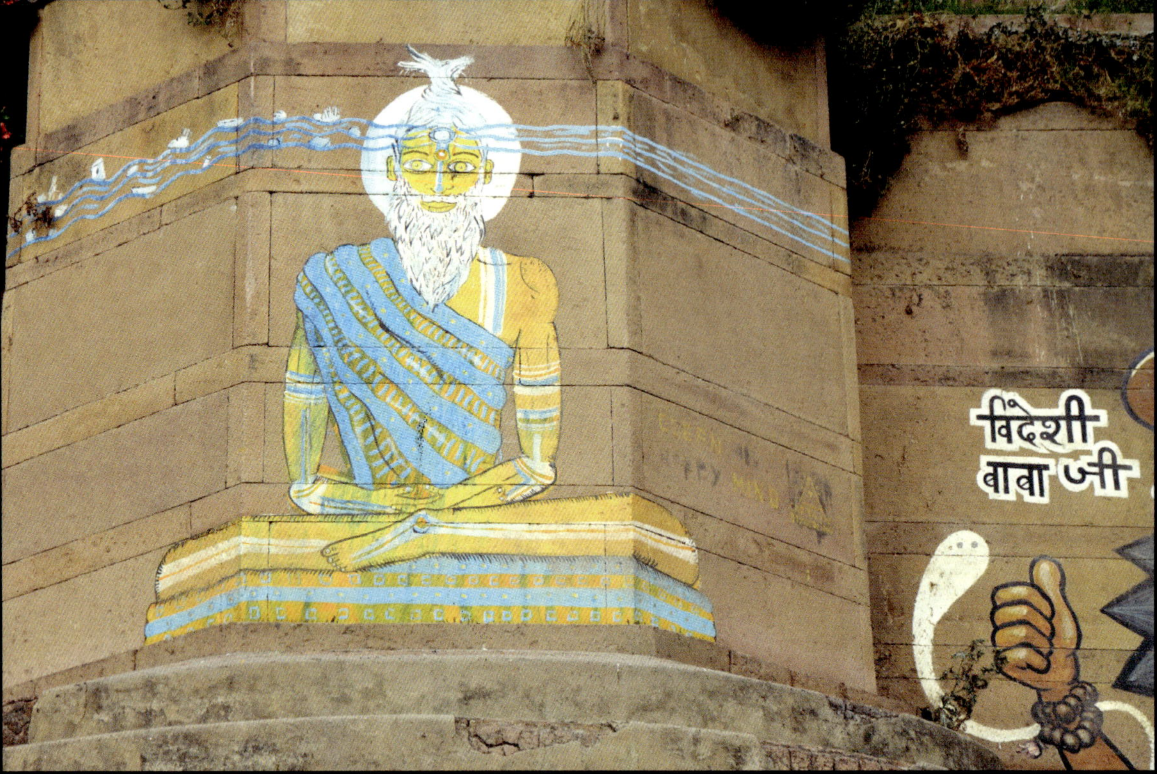

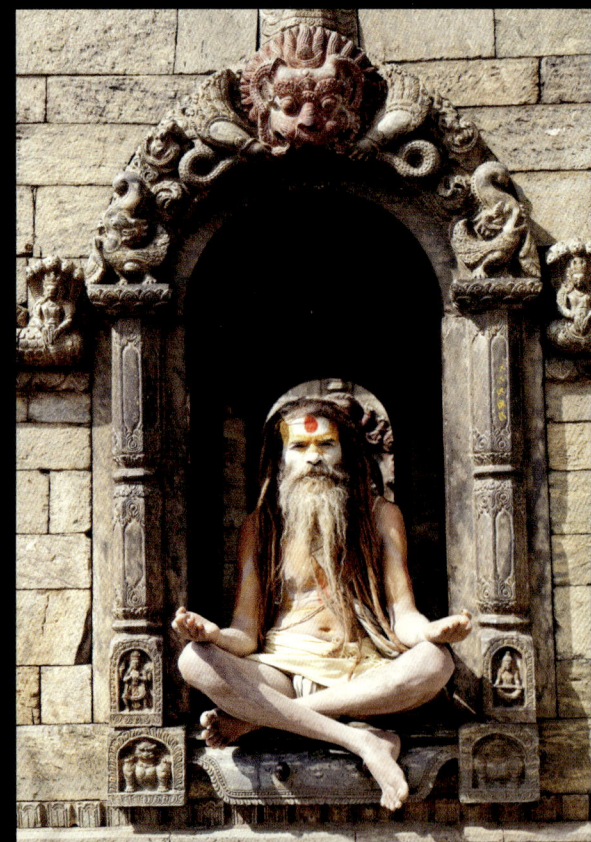

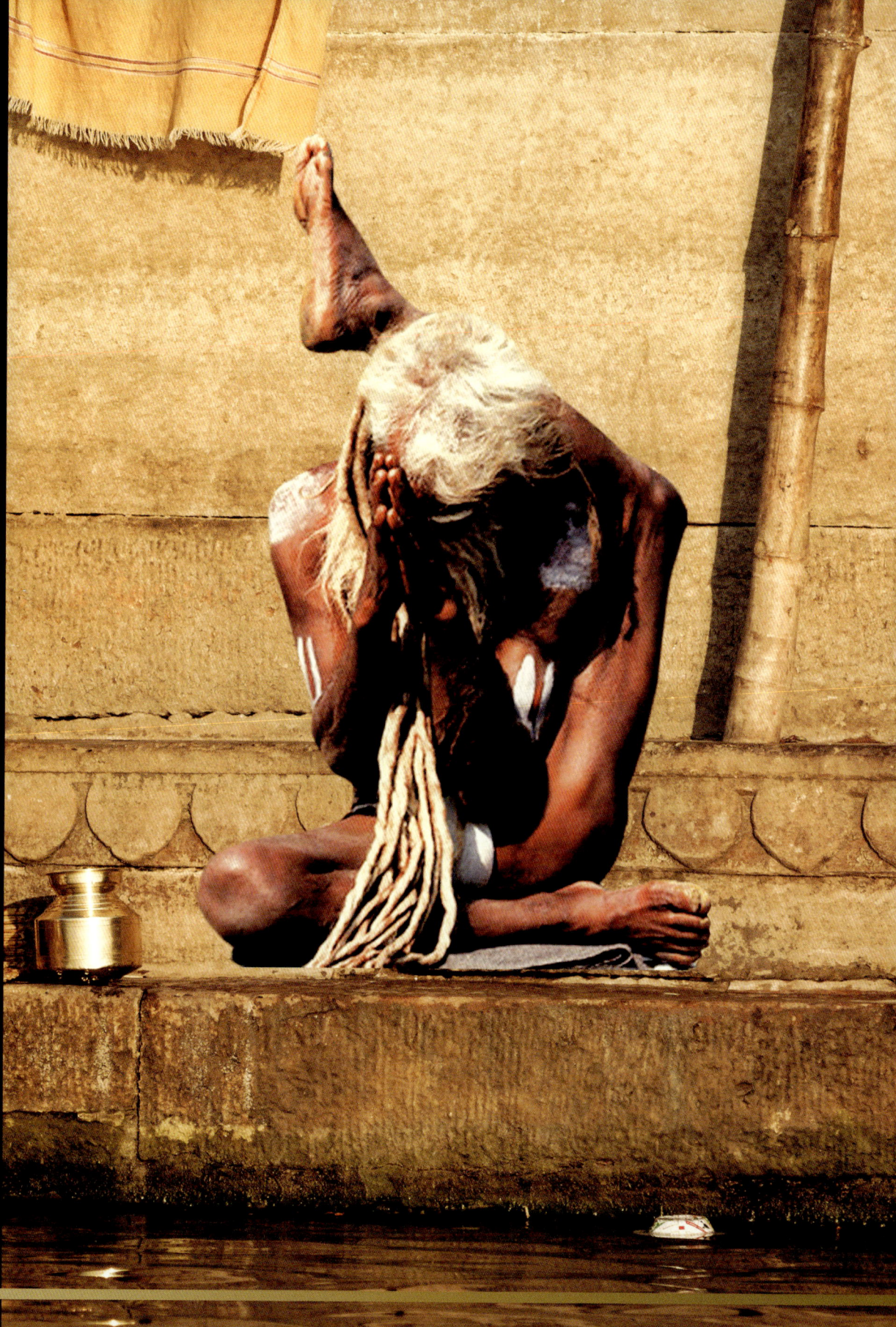

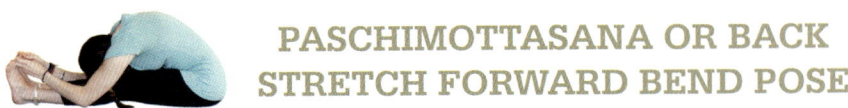

PASCHIMOTTASANA OR BACK STRETCH FORWARD BEND POSE

The word 'paschima' means west, back or back body, and 'uttana' means intense stretch or extended. The spine should lengthen and not be rounded when performing this back stretching pose.

1. Sit with the back straight and keeping legs together, stretch them out in front of you, with feet pointing upwards and towards the ceiling. Keeping the spine straight is the key to this pose.

2. While breathing in, raise and stretch arms overhead, and lengthen the spine upwards in the same direction.

3. From the hips, bend forward, while exhaling. Elongate the spine and as you come down, reach for the feet with your hands.

4. If possible, hold your big toes in a way that the index fingers wrap around them and the thumbs rest on top. If not, then your hands can rest alongside your legs on the floor or on top of the shins or thighs. As much as possible, keep the back straight while bending from hip area with feet pointing up.

5. Once position is established, gently pulling on legs and feet with the arms, giving the back and spine extra stretch as the head moves further towards the feet and legs.

6. While holding the posture, relax your shoulders and hips. While exhaling, bring your abdomen close to the thighs, lower the chest closer to the knees and ensure that your head is nearer to the feet.

7. Hold the asana for thirty seconds to begin with and then work up to five minutes or more, if possible.

Benefits

1. Helps alleviate stress and depression.

2. Stretches the hamstrings, shoulders and spine.

3. Stimulates the ovaries, uterus, liver and kidneys.

4. Improves digestion.

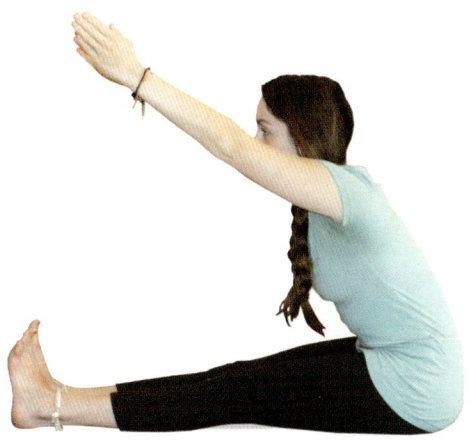

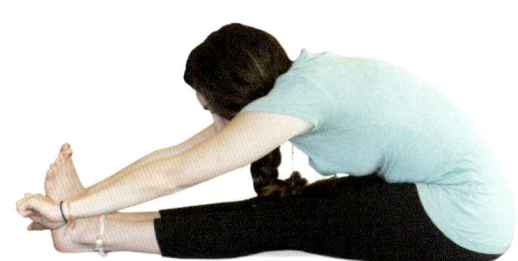

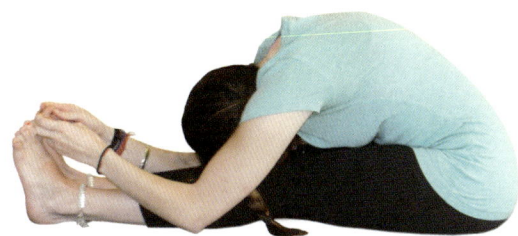

Anatomical Focus

- The rectus abdominis muscle bends the trunk forward.

- The biceps bend the elbows to deepen the stretch by bringing the torso over the thighs.

- The psoas, pectineus, rectus femoris and sartorius muscles flex the hips.

- The abductor muscles draw the thighs together.

- The knees are straightened by the action of the quadriceps, and the hamstrings are stretched.

- Flexing the ankles stretches the calf muscles.

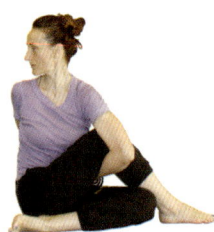

ARDHA MATSYENDRASANA OR HALF SPINE TWIST POSE

In Sankrit, 'ardha' means half, 'matsya' means fish, 'endra' means king, and 'asana' means posture. As per ancient texts, ardha matseyndrasana enhances appetite, destroys most deadly diseases and stimulates kundalini. It effectively stretches, strengthens and enhances flexibility of the entire spinal cord.

1. Sit in vajrasana pose with legs stretched in front of you.

2. Bend your right leg at the knee and place the foot over the left leg.

3. Fold your left leg at the knee so that it is touching your right buttock.

4. Keeping spine straight gently turn the upper body to the right, and exhale; with left hand hold right foot while the right hand is placed on the ground behind you.

6. Hold the posture for twenty to thirty seconds while breathing normally. With practice, you will be able to hold the posture longer, for three to five minutes.

7. Gently release posture and repeat steps with other side.

Benefits

1. Stimulates the liver and kidneys.

2. Stretches the shoulders, hips and neck.

3. Stimulates the digestive juices in the belly.

4. Relieves menstrual discomfort, fatigue, sciatica and backache.

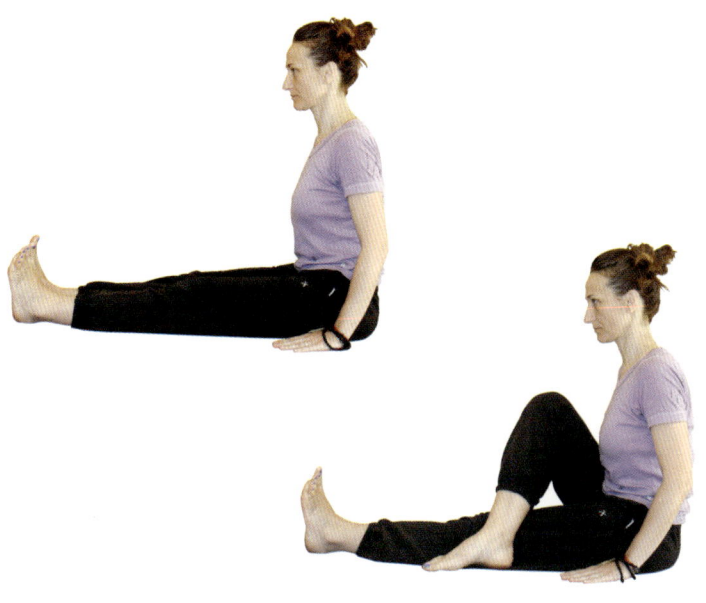

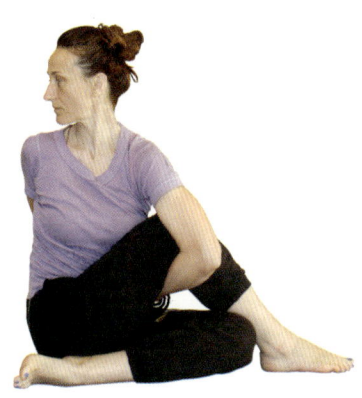

Anatomical Focus

- There is a spinal rotation due to the erector spinae muscles.

- Front arm: rhomboids are active to hold the scapulae over the ribcage. The arm externally rotates the arm while the deltoids laterally abduct the arm against the raised leg. Biceps flex the elbow.

- Back arm: the shoulder extends and the arm externally rotates. The elbow is flexed in the bind due to the biceps.

- Deep hip flexion with the top leg, which internally rotates, knee flexion.

- Hip flexion with the bottom leg, which also abducts.

- Knee flexion is due to the action of the hamstrings.

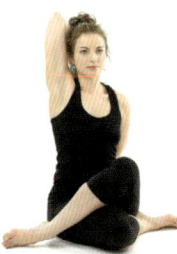

GOMUKHASANA OR COW FACE POSE

In Sanskrit, 'go' means cow and 'mukha' means face. This pose resembles the face of a cow. The pose stretches the leg muscles, opens the chest and shoulders and straightens the spine.

1. Cross your knees and sit with legs straight. Cross the right leg over the left, stacking the knees, and bring the heels beside the thighs.

2. Inhale and reach the left arm behind your back. Bend the elbow and turn the palm to face away, with the fingers pointing upwards. If required, reach the right arm behind the back to grab the left elbow and gently pull it in towards the middle of the back.

3. As you inhale, raise the right arm and reach back to clasp the fingers on the left hand. Position the right elbow behind the head.

4. Hold the posture for about a minute, then lower the arms, uncross the legs and switch sides.

Benefits

1. Stretches the armpits, shoulders, hips, thighs, ankles, triceps and chest.

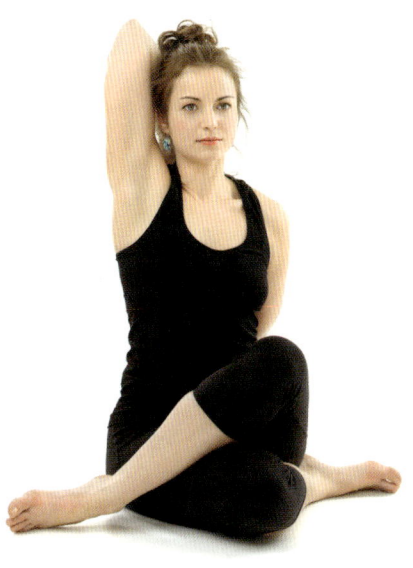

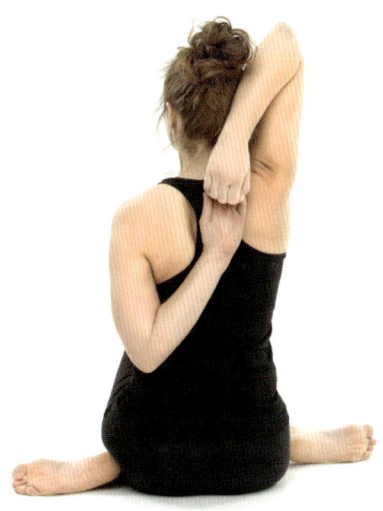

Anatomical Focus

- Extends latissimus dorsi.

- The serratus anterior and rhomboids rotate the shoulder blade upwards; lateral rotation and flexion of the shoulder is due to the infraspinatus and teres minor. Biceps create elbow flexion.

- Downward rotation and abduction of the shoulder blade, due to the lower trapezius and rhumboids. Internal rotation abduction of the shoulder are the action of the suscapularies.

- Hip and knee flexion.

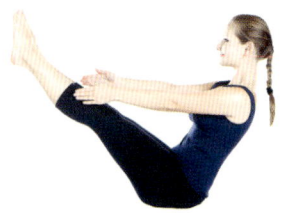

PARIPURANA NAVASANA
OR BOAT POSE

The posture resembles the shape of a boat. Keep arms stretched alongside the legs with hands placed on the floor next to hips or alternatively holding the back of thighs.

1. Sit on the floor with legs stretched out straight in front of you. With fingers pointed to the feet, place hands a little behind the hips and press down on the floor, strengthening the arms. Lean back a little while raising the top of the sternum. Keep your back straight and not rounded while lengthening the torso all the way between sternum and pubis. Let the tailbone and your sitting bones be a 'tripod' for your sitting position.

2. Bend knees while exhaling; raise feet from the floor to achieve a forty-five to fifty degree angle of the thighs to the floor. Stretch your tailbone towards floor and raise pubis towards navel. If you can, straighten knees slowly so that the toes are a little above eye level.

3. Keep your arms stretched and parallel to each other next to the legs and reach out with your fingers as strongly as you can, while spreading the shoulder blades. Alternatively, place hands on the floor next to your hips or you can hold the back of your thighs.

4. Keep lower belly firm and flat but not thick and hard. To anchor yourself in the pose, breathe easily while pressing down the top of the thigh bones towards the floor and raising top sternum. Lift base of skull away from back neck so that chin tips towards the sternum.

5. When first learning the pose, hold for ten to twenty seconds, and then as you become more confident increase length of time to upto a minute.

6. Release legs while exhaling and sit upright when inhaling.

Benefits

1. Strengthens the spine, abdomen and hip flexors.

2. Stimulates the thyroids, kidneys, intestines and prostrate glands.

3. Improves digestion.

4. Tones and strengthens the abdominal organs.

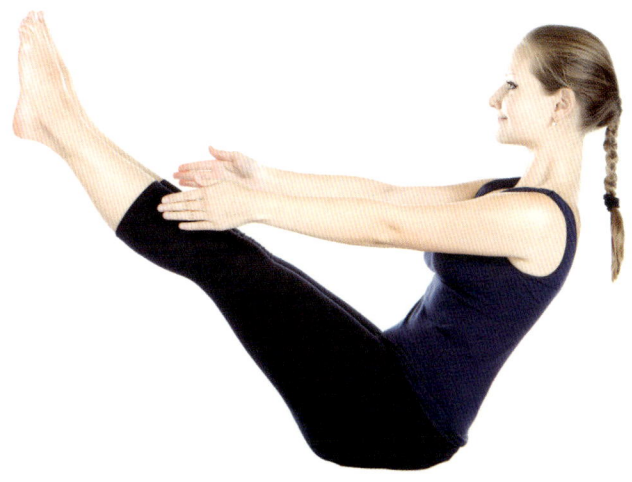

Anatomical Focus

- Shoulder flexion through activation of the anterior deltoids; rhomboid and trapezius muscles draw the shoulders down.

- Tricep muscles extend the elbows.

- Hip flexion due to the psoas major and rectus femoris.

- Rectus abdominis bends the trunk. Abduction of the legs; knee extension due to the quadriceps.

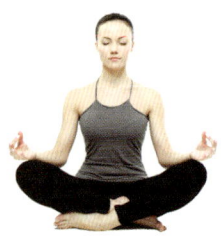

SUKKHASANA AND SIDDHASANA OR PLEASANT POSE

In Sanskrit, 'sukha' means pleasure. Ideal alternatives to padmanasana, these poses are recommended for pranayama practice and meditation. The crossed legs and erect spine keep the mind alert while the body is rested.

1. Take a sitting position on the floor with your legs stretched out straight. Cross legs in a way that each foot is placed under the opposite knee and the sides of the feet are resting on the floor with a gap between pelvis and feet.

2. With hands placed on top of the knees and the palms facing upwards or assuming a mudra, straighten the spine while drawing the tailbone towards the floor.

3. This seated position can be practiced for any length of time, but alternate leg position in a way that each leg gets a chance to be on top.

Benefits

1. Stimulates the abdomen, pelvis, spine and bladder.
2. Stretches the knees and ankles.

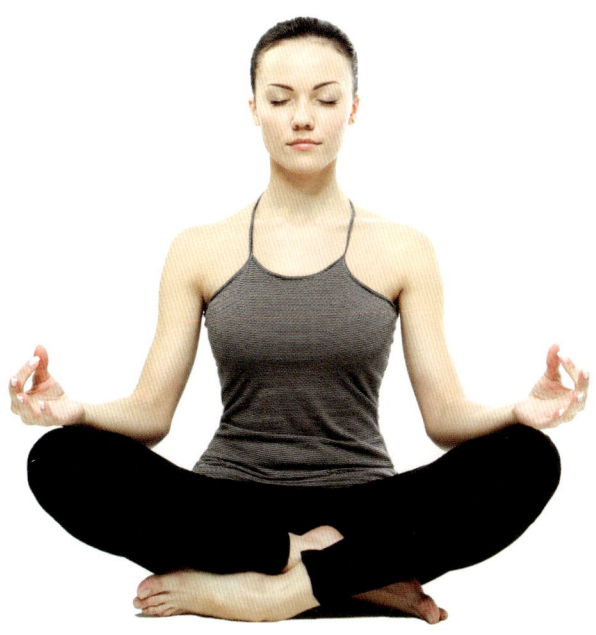

Anatomical Focus

- Axial spine extension: the erector spinae muscle keeps the spine straight.

- Knee flexion: the hamstrings flex the knees.

- Hip flexion due to the action of the psoas muscle.

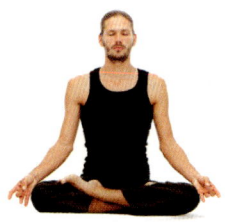

PADMASANA OR LOTUS POSE

Padmasana means a lotus throne. It is the ultimate position for meditation and pranayama practice. The pose brings flexibility to the knees and ankles, but is more difficult to master than it appears, as it requires hip flexibility. Many find it difficult to hold for long periods.

1. Sit on the ground with legs spread forward.
2. Place each foot on opposite thigh, right foot on left and the left foot on the right thigh.
3. Place the hands on the knees.
4. Keep the body, back and head straight and erect.
5. Keep eyes closed.
6. This pose is mainly for pranayama or meditation.

Benefits

1. Stimulates the pelvis, spine, abdomen and bladder.
2. Stretches the ankles and knees.

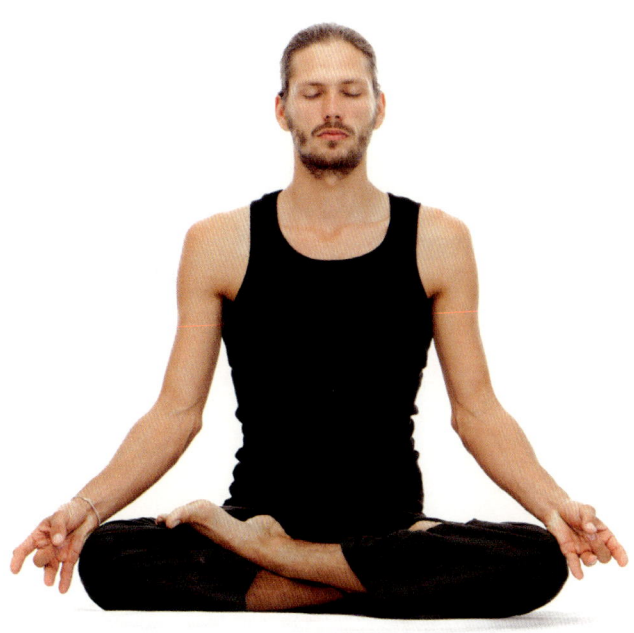

Anatomical Focus

- Axial extension of the spine: the erector spinae muscle keeps the spine straight.

- Knee flexion: the hamstrings flex the knees.

- Hip flexion due to the action of the psoas muscle.

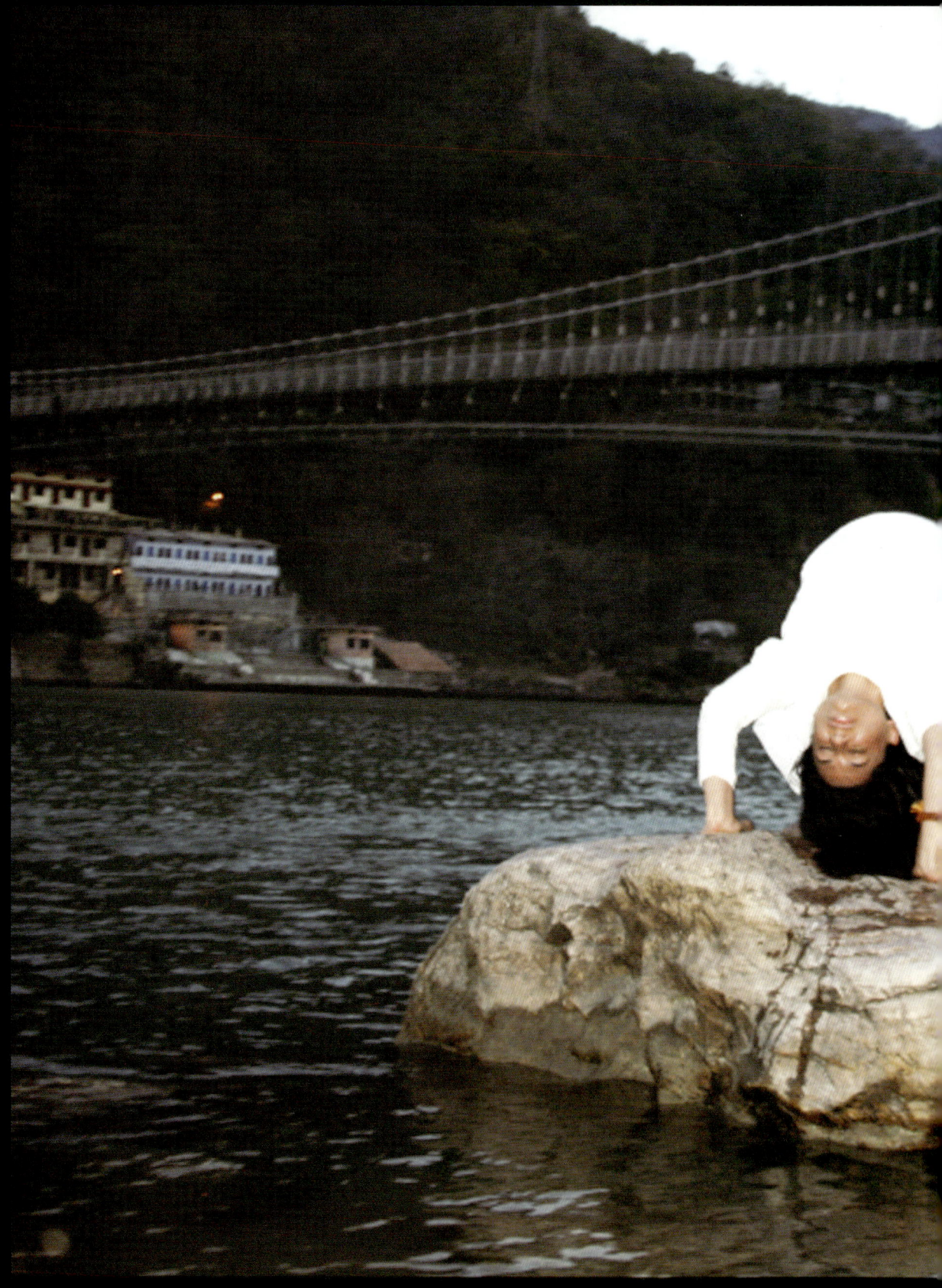

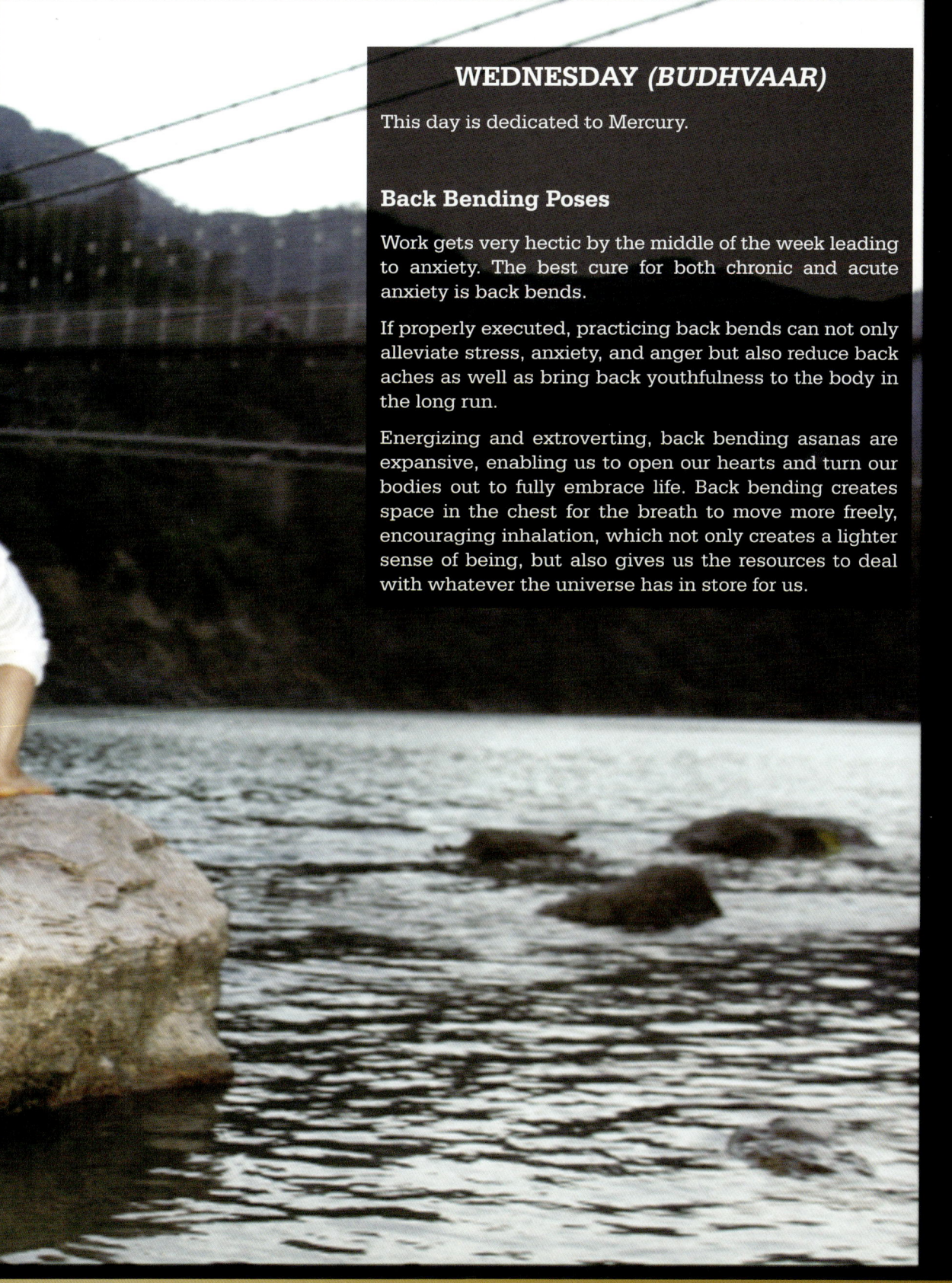

WEDNESDAY *(BUDHVAAR)*

This day is dedicated to Mercury.

Back Bending Poses

Work gets very hectic by the middle of the week leading to anxiety. The best cure for both chronic and acute anxiety is back bends.

If properly executed, practicing back bends can not only alleviate stress, anxiety, and anger but also reduce back aches as well as bring back youthfulness to the body in the long run.

Energizing and extroverting, back bending asanas are expansive, enabling us to open our hearts and turn our bodies out to fully embrace life. Back bending creates space in the chest for the breath to move more freely, encouraging inhalation, which not only creates a lighter sense of being, but also gives us the resources to deal with whatever the universe has in store for us.

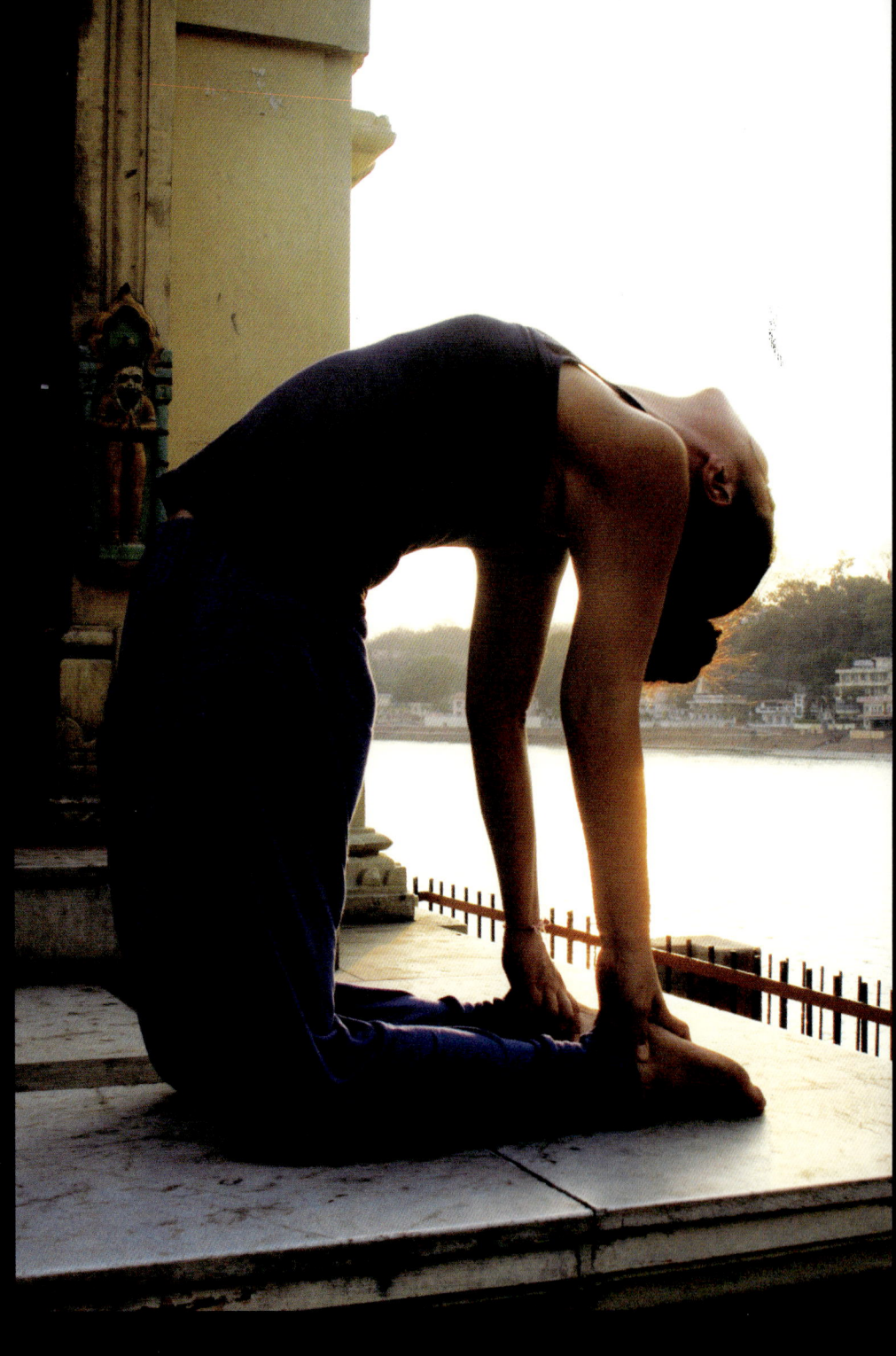

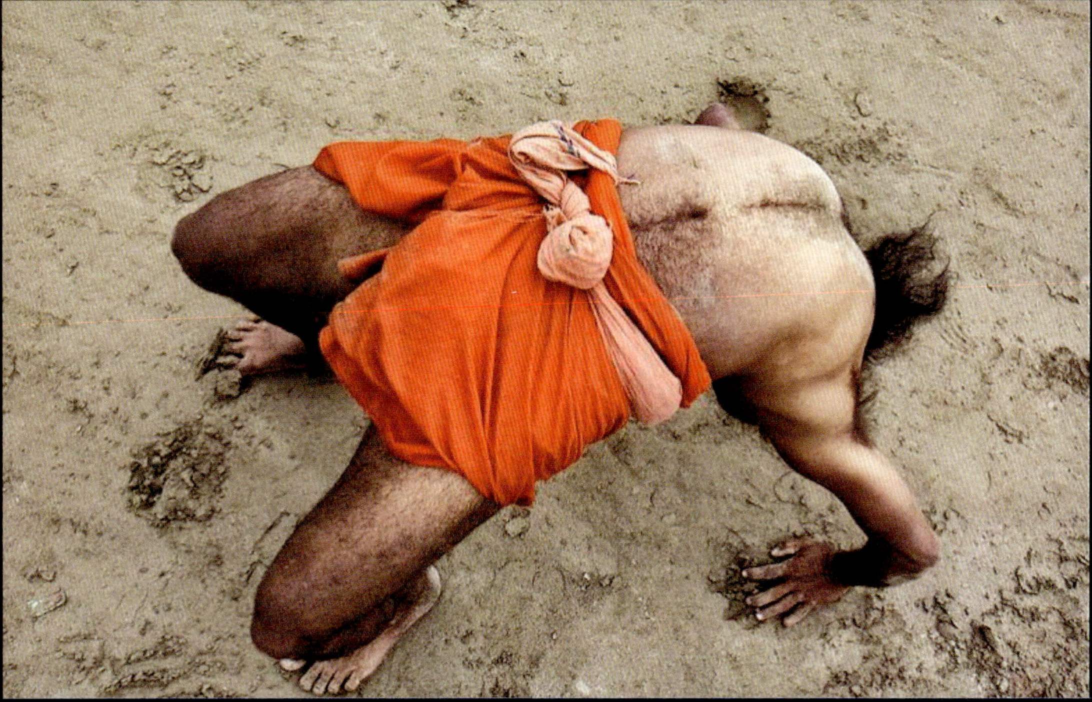

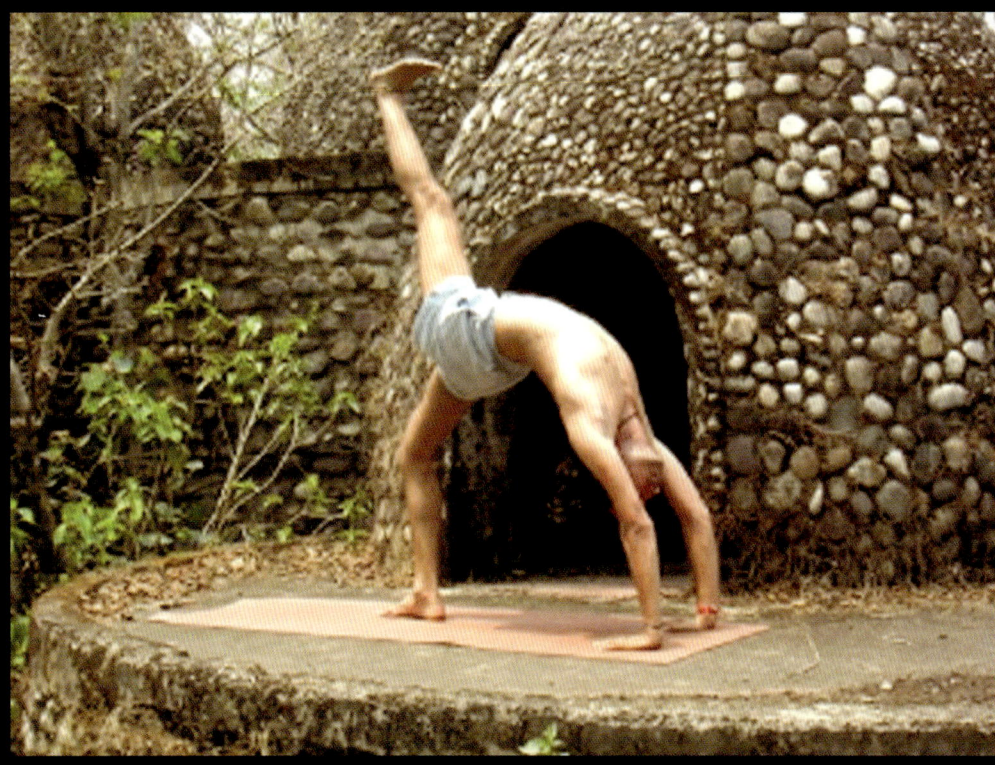

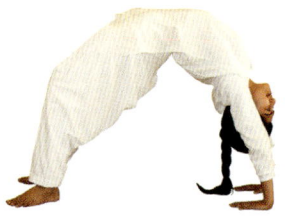

CHAKRASANA
OR WHEEL POSE

'Chakra' means wheel. This particular asana opens the chest and heart center – the anahata chakra – leading to vitality. Bending backwards turns the body out to face the world and helps you to see things from a different perspective, an action associated with embracing life.

1. Lie on the floor facing upwards. With knees bent, place feet on the floor with heels next to sitting bones. Bend elbows and place palms alongside the head on the floor. Forearms should be perpendicular and fingers pointed to shoulders.

2. While exhaling, press inner feet into the floor, raise tailbone up towards pubis, and lift buttocks off the floor, keeping them firm. Thighs and inner feet should be parallel. After two or three breaths, lift crown of head, with inner hands pressed into floor, and shoulder blades pressed against the back.

3. With hands and feet pressed into the floor, exhale. Press shoulder blades and tailbone against the back. Raise head off the floor and straighten arms as you do so. Firm outer thighs and turn inner thighs inwards slightly. Hip points should be narrowed and tailbone lengthened towards the back of knees, while pubis is raised towards navel.

4. Turn upper arms outward with weight on the hands. Spread shoulder blades and either lift head to look down on the floor or let it hang.

Benefits

1. Stretches the lungs and chest.

2. Strengthens the legs, buttocks, abdomen, spine, arms and wrists.

3. Stimulates the pituitary glands and thyroid.

4. Counteracts depression.

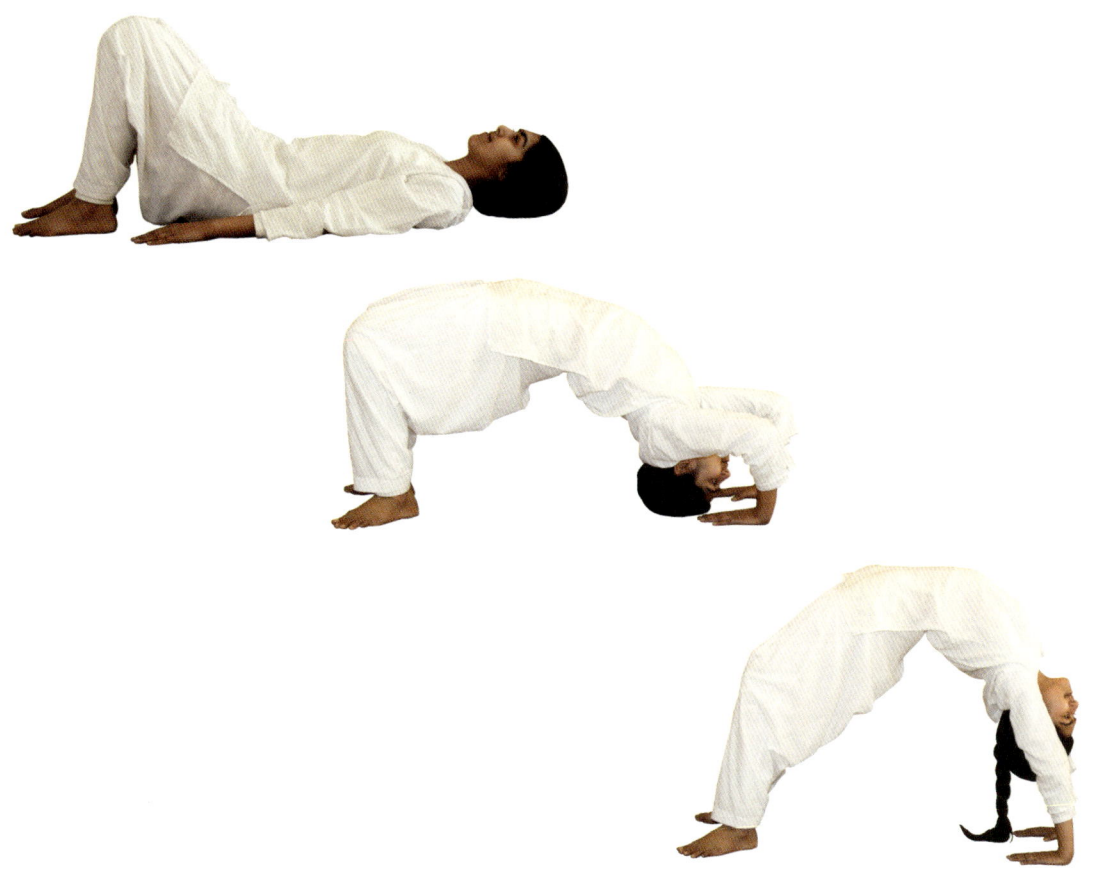

Anatomical Focus

- The erector spinae arches the back. The quadratus lumborum works with the psoas muscle and the rectus abdominis to stabilize the lower back.

- Upward rotation and elevation of the shoulder blade takes place due to the action of the serratus anterior.

- Shoulder flexion occurs due to the anterior deltoids and biceps. The rotator cuff and deltoids stabilize the shoulder joint.

- Elbow extension involves the triceps.

- The action of the pronator quadratus and teres causes forearm pronation.

- Wrist dorsiflexion is caused by the wrist extensors.

- Hip extension and abduction involve the hamstrings and gluteus maximus.

- Knee flexion involves the quadriceps.

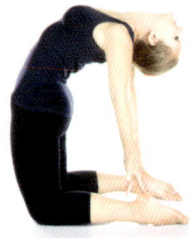

USTRANASANA OR CAMEL POSE

The Sanskrit word 'ustra' means camel. This is a deep back bending pose that can be challenging at first. The hands and feet connect the upper and lower appendicular skeleton.

1. Kneel down on the floor with knees, hips and thighs perpendicular to the floor.

2. Now try to move your thighs inwards.

3. Place your hands on your hips with palms placed on buttocks and fingers pointing towards the floor.

4. Try to bend your body backwards by raising your chest in the upward direction and lower your arms a little.

5. Keep your chest raised, and your chin tucked as you drop your hands toward your heels.

6. Balance your body on your palms and feet.

7. Stay in this pose for 30 seconds to one minute.

Benefits

1. Stretches the ankles, thighs and groin and entire front of the body.

2. Stretches the deep hip flexors.

3. Strengthens the back muscles.

4. Stimulates the abdominal organs.

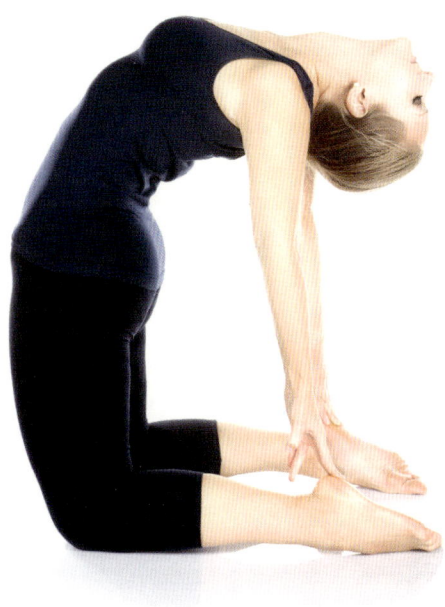

Anatomical Focus

- Scapular abduction and download rotation occurs through the action of the rhomboids and trapezius muscles.

- Shoulder extension occurs due to the action of the posterior deltoids at the back of the shoulders and abduction.

- Elbow extension involves the triceps.

- The spine is protected from over-mobilization by the psoas and abdominal muscles.

- Hip extension and abduction occurs due to the gluteus maximums hamstrings.

- Knee flexion and ankle plantar flexion takes place due to the gastrocnemius and soleus muscles.

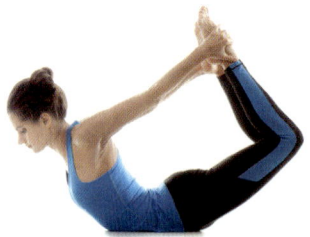

DHANURASANA
OR BOW POSE

Dhanurasana comes from the Sanskrit word 'dhanu' which means bow. This pose resembles an archer's bow with the arms representing the strings while the torso and legs represent the body of the bow.

1. Lie on your belly, with hands resting alongside the body and palms facing upwards. While exhaling, bend knees and bring heels close to buttocks. Reach back with your hands to hold ankles. The distance between the knees should not be more than the width of your hips. Maintain this distance throughout the pose.

2. While inhaling, push strongly to move heels away from buttocks and thighs up from the floor. This will stretch and pull the head and upper torso away from the body. Keep pushing the tailbone down into the floor, and try to avoid hardening the back muscles, keep them relaxed. Press shoulder blades into your back as you lift heels and thighs higher. Pull back your shoulders and look forward.

3. Keep breathing. This may be difficult to do so with belly pressed onto the floor, so try to breathe into the back of your torso.

4. Maintain pose for thirty seconds to a minute.

5. Exhale while releasing pose and rest by lying quietly and breathing gently. Repeat pose once or twice more.

Benefits

1. Stretches the ankles, thighs and groin, entire front of the body, abdomen and chest, throat and deep hip flexors.

2. Strengthens the back muscles.

3. Improves posture.

4. Stimulates the organs of the neck and abdomen.

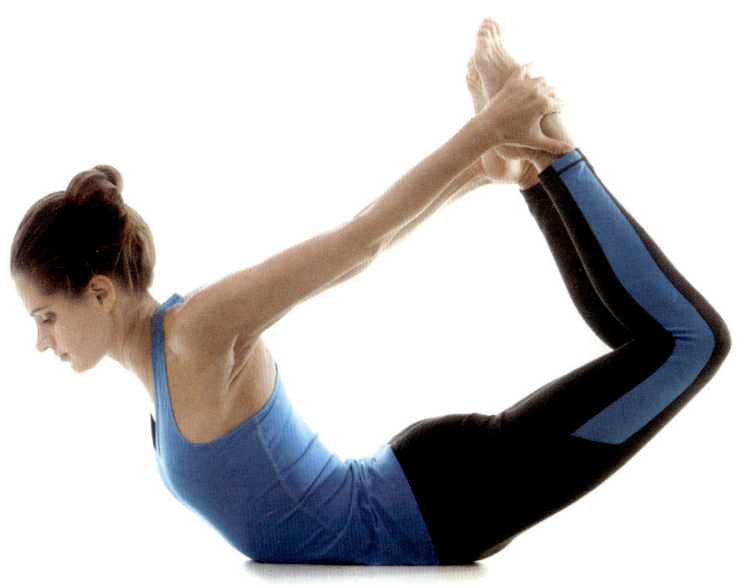

Anatomical Focus

- Spinal extension occurs due to the erector spinae and quadratus lumborum muscles.

- Scapular abduction, shoulder extension and internal rotation occur due to lower trapezius and rhomboids. Elbow extension occurs due to posterior deltoids and triceps.

- Elbow extension occurs due to posterior deltoids and triceps.

- Hip extension and abduction occurs as the hip flexors and rectus abdominis are stretched.

- Knee flexion takes place due to the action of the hamstrings.

- Ankle plantar flexion occurs due to the soleus muscle.

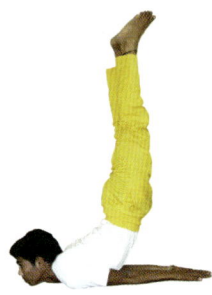

SALABHASANA OR LOCUST/GRASSHOPPER POSE

'Salabh' means grasshopper in Sanskrit. An advanced prone back bending pose, this asana strengthens the muscles in the back.

1. Lie down, resting on the abdomen and place the chin on the floor or, if it is more comfortable, turn the head to the side and lay one cheek on the floor.

2. Place arms underneath the abdomen. The hands should be under the thighs with palms facing down.

3. Press the palms against the floor while inhaling. Keep the legs straight and raise them as high as possible.

4. Hold your breath and remain in this position for as long as it feels comfortable. Exhale and return to the first position.

Benefits

1. Strengthens the muscles of the spine, buttocks and backs of the arms and legs.

2. Stretches the shoulders, chest, belly and thighs.

3. Improves posture.

4. Stimulates the abdominal organs.

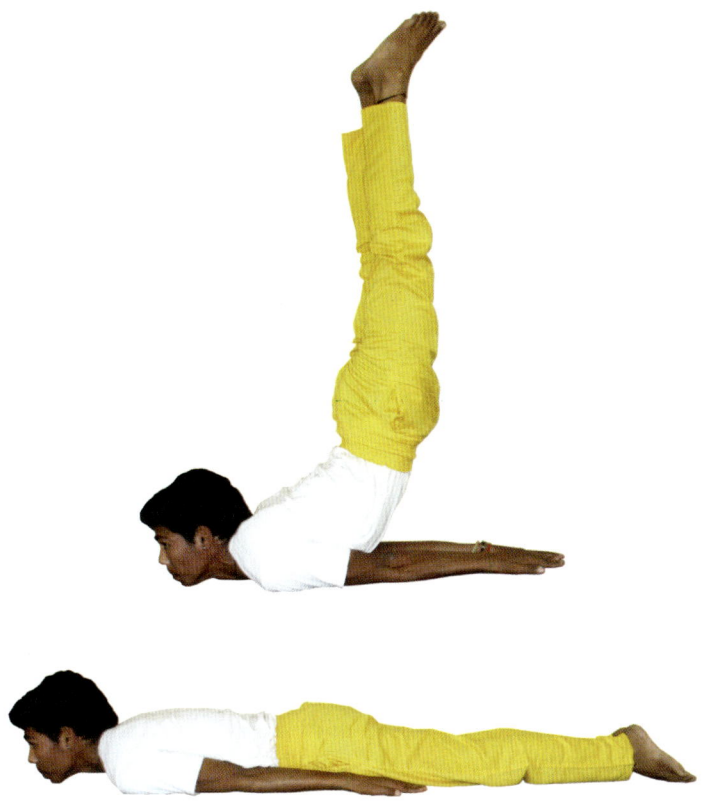

Anatomical Focus

- Spinal extension occurs due to the erector spinae, which arch the back.

- Scapular downward rotation and abduction takes place due to the lower trapezius and rhomboids. Elbow extension occurs due to the triceps. Pectoralis muscles open the chest.

- Hip extension occurs due to the gluteus maximums and abduction takes place due to the abductor muscles.

- Knee extension occurs due to the quadriceps; abduction takes place due to the hamstrings and abductors.

- Ankle plantar flexion arises due to the soleus muscle.

BHUJANGASANA OR COBRA POSE

In Sanskrit 'Bhujanga' means serpent. This asana resembles a serpent with its hood raised. Cobra pose or bhujangasana is part of the sequence of surya namaskar, the sun salutation.

1. Lie on your stomach with your toes flat on the floor and forehead resting on the ground.

2. Keep your legs close together, with your feet and heels lightly touching each other.

3. Place your hands with palms facing downwards under your shoulders, keeping your elbows parallel and close to your torso.

4. Taking a deep breath in, slowly lift your head, chest and abdomen while keeping your navel on the floor.

5. Pull your torso back and off the floor with the support of your hands.

6. Distribute the back bend evenly through the spine. Hold the pose for fifteen to thirty seconds, breathing easily. Release back to the floor with an exhalation.

7. Repeat a few times.

Benefits

1. Strengthens the spine.

2. Stretches the chest, lungs, shoulders and abdomen.

3. Firms the buttocks.

4. Stimulates the abdominal organs.

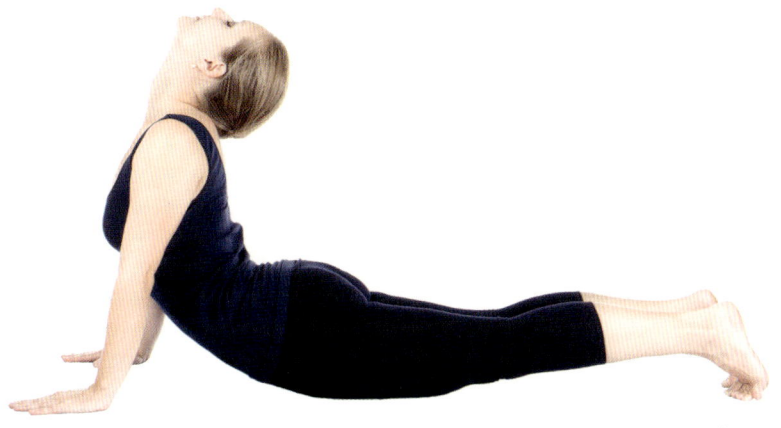

Anatomical Focus

- The spine extends due to the erector spinae muscles. The lower trapezius draws the shoulders back and down and the pectoralis major opens the chest.

- Elbow extension occurs by the action of the triceps, and forearm pronation due to the pronator quadratus.

- Hip extension and abduction are activated by the gluteus maximus; the deep hip flexors stretch the psoas, pectineus and abductor longus muscles.

- Knee extension occurs due to the quadriceps and ankle plantar flexion due to the soleus muscle.

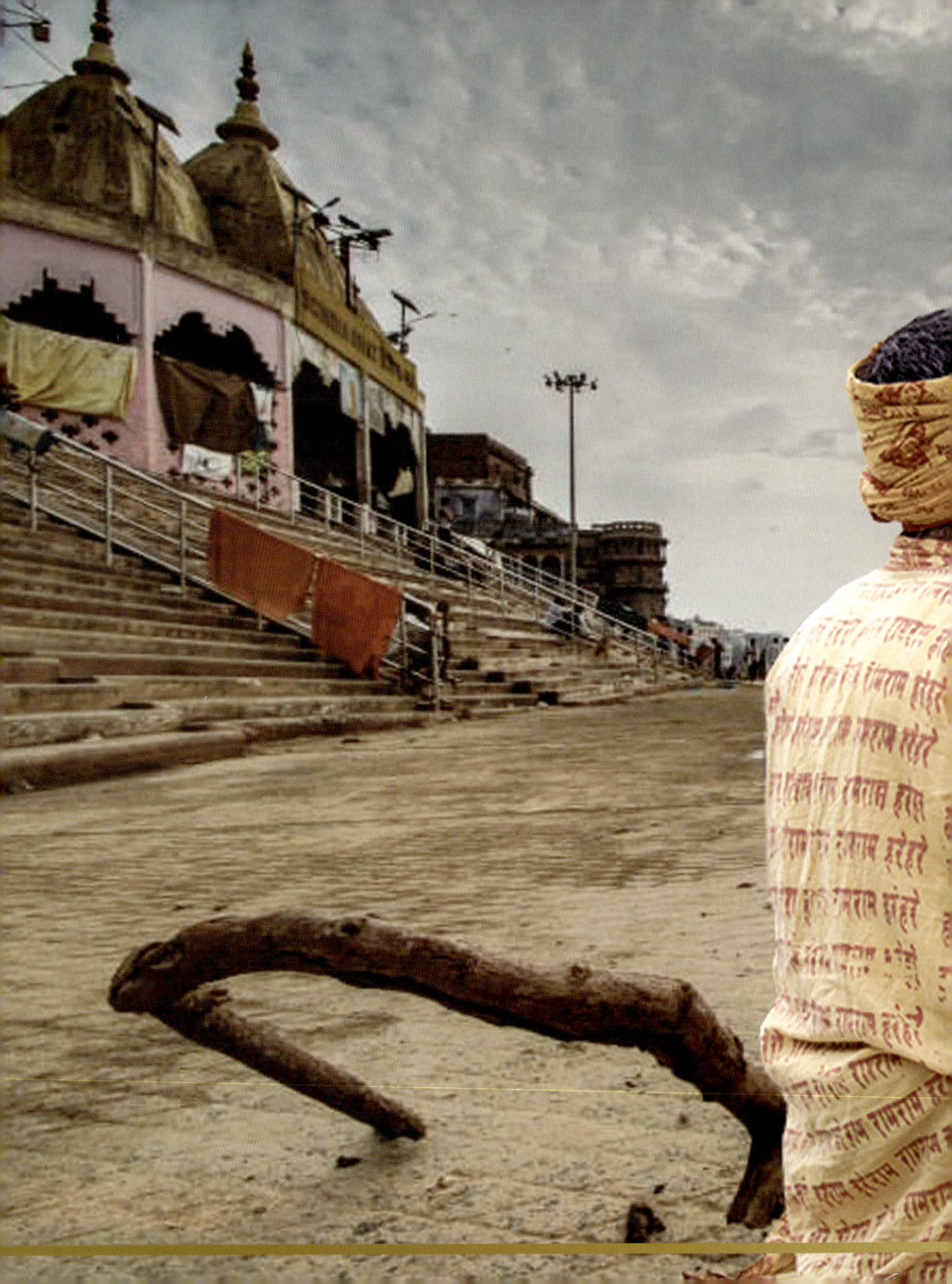

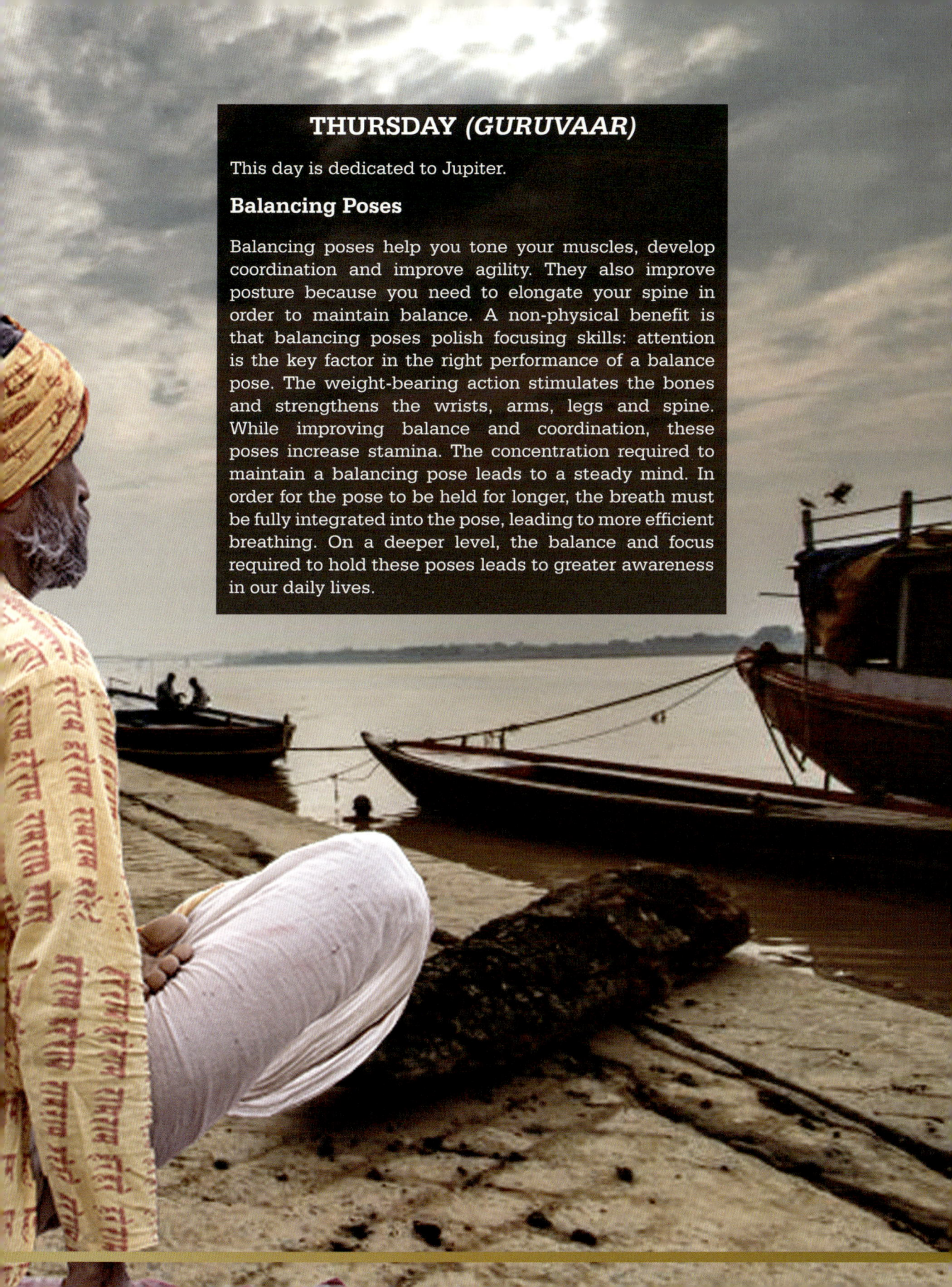

THURSDAY *(GURUVAAR)*

This day is dedicated to Jupiter.

Balancing Poses

Balancing poses help you tone your muscles, develop coordination and improve agility. They also improve posture because you need to elongate your spine in order to maintain balance. A non-physical benefit is that balancing poses polish focusing skills: attention is the key factor in the right performance of a balance pose. The weight-bearing action stimulates the bones and strengthens the wrists, arms, legs and spine. While improving balance and coordination, these poses increase stamina. The concentration required to maintain a balancing pose leads to a steady mind. In order for the pose to be held for longer, the breath must be fully integrated into the pose, leading to more efficient breathing. On a deeper level, the balance and focus required to hold these poses leads to greater awareness in our daily lives.

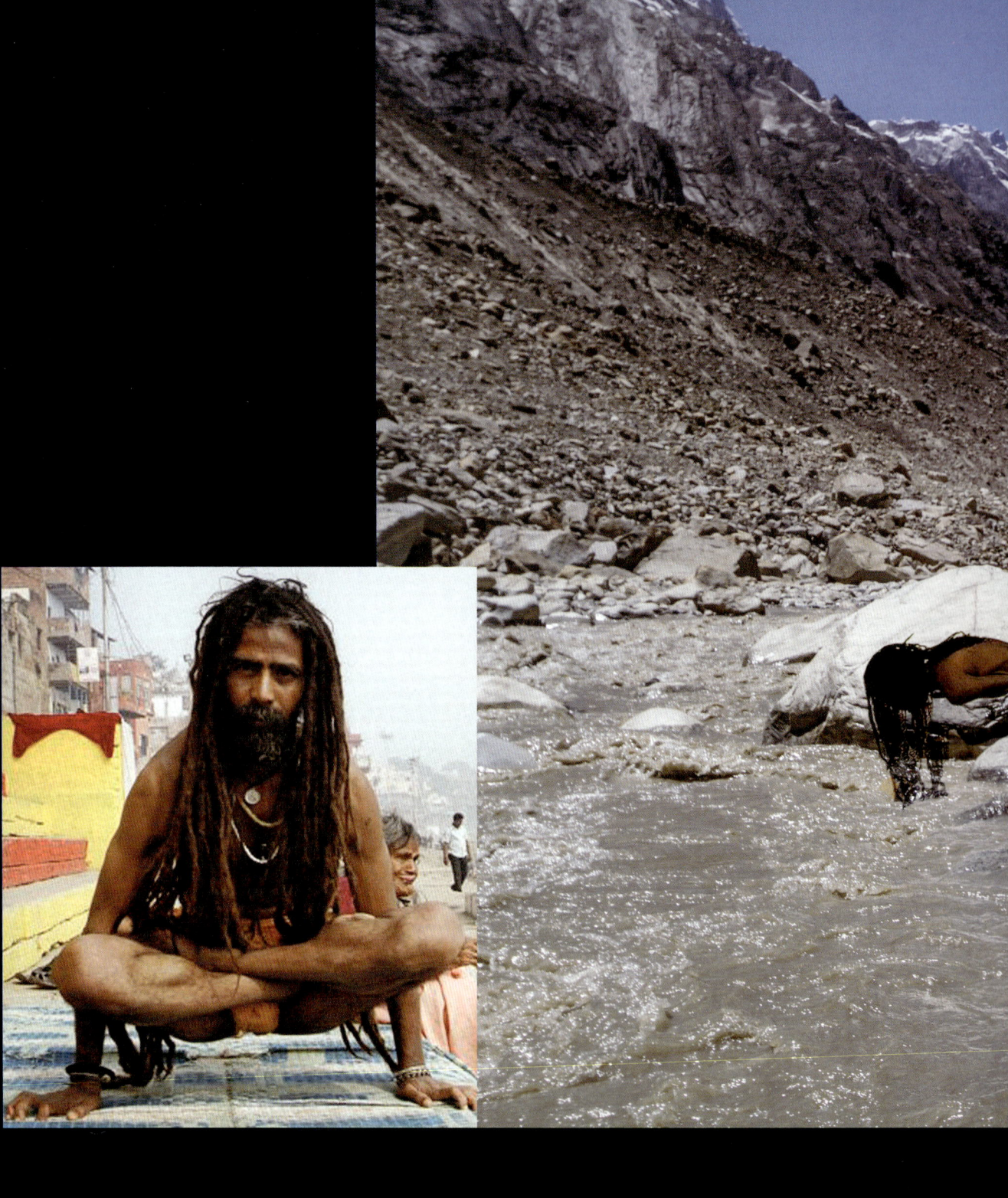

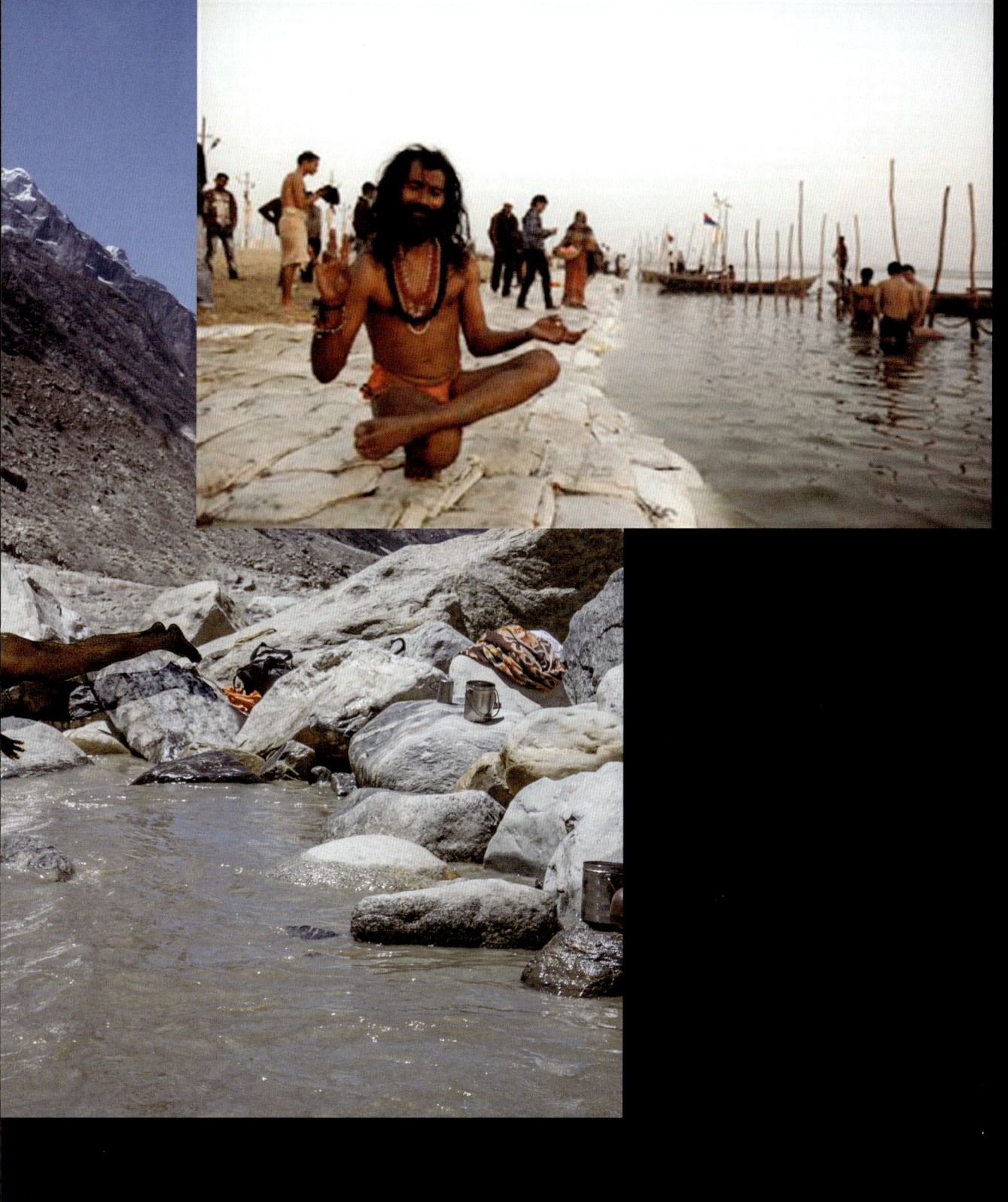

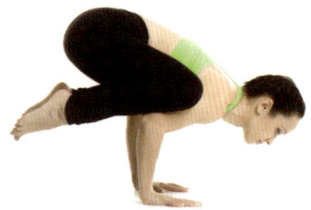

KAKASANA OR CROW POSE

Kakasana is a Sanskrit word where 'kak' means crow, and 'asana' means posture. The crow pose looks harder than it is. It requires more coordination, concentration and awareness than muscular strength in the upper arms. As you hold the pose, the chest is immobilized so you can only breathe abdominally.

1. Come into a squatting position with feet apart and heels on the floor. Separate your knees and lean the torso forward, bringing the upper arms between the knees.

2. Place your palms to the floor with fingers spread out and elbows bent. Lean shins against the back of the upper arms, so that a shelf is created for the shins to rest on.

3. While inhaling, look forward, lift the heels and seat, and bend the elbows, to bring weight onto the back of the arms.

4. Exhale and lift your weight forward, so that the elbows are in alignment over the wrists and the feet begin to rise from the floor, either one at a time or else both together. Once you feel steady, bring the heels closer to the buttocks and point the toes.

5. Keep breathing and hold the pose for twenty to thirty seconds. While releasing, exhale and slowly and gently bring the feet to the floor, and into a squat.

Benefits

1. Strengthens wrists and arms.

2. Stretches the upper back.

3. Strengthens the abdominal muscles.

4. Opens the groin.

5. Tones the abdominal organs.

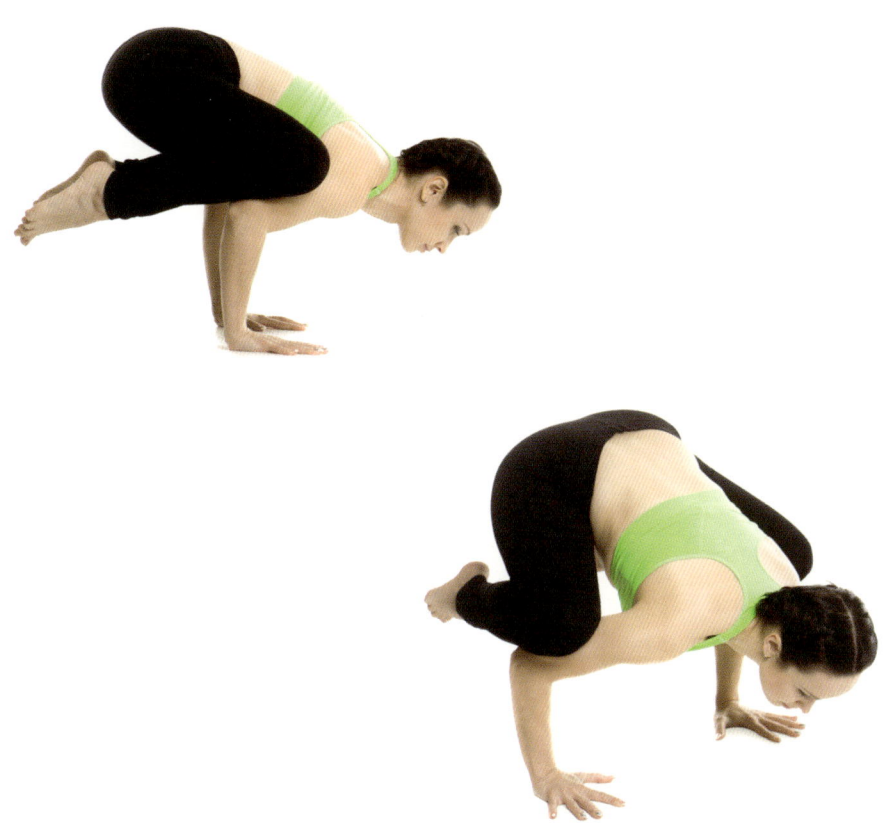

Anatomical Focus

- The serratus anterior muscle draws the shoulder blades forward while the pectoralis and deltoid muscles stabilize the shoulders.

- The lower trapezius, which spans the back, presses down on the shoulder blades.

- The tricep muscles straighten the elbows.

- The hamstring muscles bend the knees.

- The abductor muscles squeeze the knees into the upper arms to link the upper and lower extremities.

- The psoas and rectus abdominis muscles combine to flex the trunk and hips.

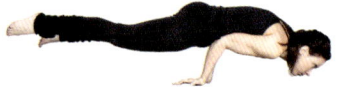

MAYURASANA OR PEACOCK POSE

In Sanskrit, 'mayura' means peacock. In Hindu lore, the peacock is a symbol of immortality and love. This asana tones the abdominal region. The pressure from the elbows stimulates blood circulation in the abdominal organs thus improving digestion and stomach ailments and removing toxins in the body.

1. Place your hands between your knees on the floor, palms facing down, fingers pointing backwards, towards the feet.

2. Keeping elbows together, place them on the abdomen.

3. Rest your forehead on the mat in front of you.

4. Straighten and stretch out legs behind you so that the body is resting on the hands, feet and head.

5. With head up, slowly move the weight of your body forward while lifting feet at the same time so that body is parallel to the floor. As a beginner, you will find it easy to lift one foot at a time, until your arms are stronger and you are able to move body weight forward.

6. Maintain posture for about ten seconds when initially learning and then hold for upto thirty seconds or more.

Benefits

1. Strengthens wrists and forearms.

2. Tones abdominal muscles.

3. Strengthens the back torso and legs.

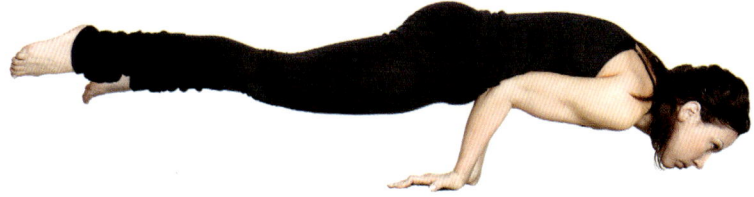

Anatomical Focus

- There is cervical extension in the spine; thoracic flexion and lumbar extension, the erector spinae, quadratus lumborum and rectus abdominis muscles hold the trunk solid.

- Scapular abduction occurs due to the action of the serratus anterior and pectoralis major and minor. Rotator cuff and deltoids protect the shoulder joint.

- There is elbow flexion as the biceps and triceps keep the elbows at right angles.

- The supinator causes forearm pronation.

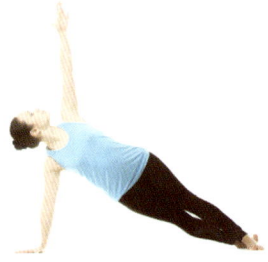

VASISTHASANA
OR SIDE PLANK POSE

Vasisthasana is a Sanskrit word in which 'vasisth' refers to 'excellence, the best and the most rich'. Many well-known sages in the yoga tradition are named Vasisth. As the level of excellence is an attribute of many sages, the side plank pose is also referred to as the sage pose.

1. Bring the right knee and hand to the floor with left leg straight and left hand on the side of the left thigh and straighten the left leg. Place the left hand on the side of the left thigh.

2. Press down into the floor with the right hand while raising the right knee off the floor. Place the left foot on top of the right foot. Align the entire body into a diagonal line from head to toe.

3. Keep breathing and hold the pose for thirty seconds to one minute.

Benefits

1. Strengthens the belly, arms and legs.

2. Strengthens and stretches the wrists.

3. Stretches the back of the legs.

4. Improves the sense of balance.

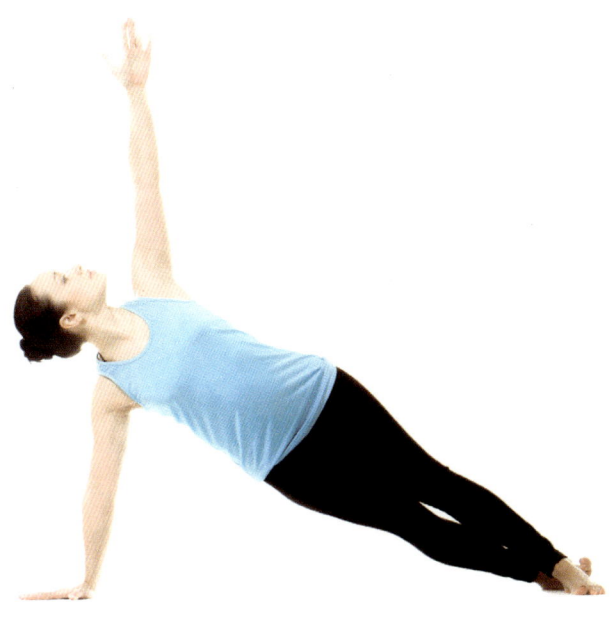

Anatomical Focus

- The erector spinae and rectus abdominis muscles stabilize the spine.

- Shoulder abduction involves the deltoid muscle of the top arm.

- Elbow extension involves the triceps of the lower arm.

- The hip remains in neutral extension and abduction.

- Knee extension occurs due to quadriceps action.

- Ankle dorsiflexion involves the tibialis anterior.

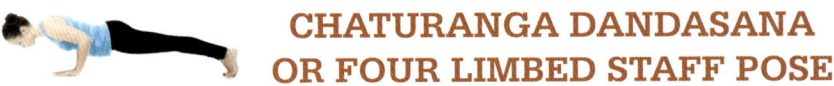

CHATURANGA DANDASANA OR FOUR LIMBED STAFF POSE

Chaturanga Dandasana is a Sanskrit word where 'chatur' means four, 'anga' means limb, 'danda' means the spine, and 'asana' means posture. This pose is commonly used as a transition pose during dynamic vinyasa practice.

1. Start in the plank pose. Keeping shoulders aligned and slightly ahead of the wrists, rest on the balls of your feet and press back the soles of your feet, as if there is a wall behind the feet.

2. At the same time, while on the heels, push back so that the quadriceps and lower body get engaged. Stretch the sternum forward to create a line of energy straight to your feet from the top of the head.

3. Inhale and pull the shoulders and the top of the thighs away from the floor. Lower body should be pulled in and pelvis should go towards the floor.

4. Bend elbows while exhaling. Keep them over your wrists and against the body. Gently lower your body towards the floor, staying as straight as possible.

5. Lower gaze to the floor, approximately six inches in front of you. Lower your shoulders till they are same height as elbows. Continue to stretch heels, sternum and top of head while you breathe.

6. To release pose, exhale and either push back to plank pose or lower down to belly.

Benefits

1. Strengthens arms, wrists and abdominal muscles.

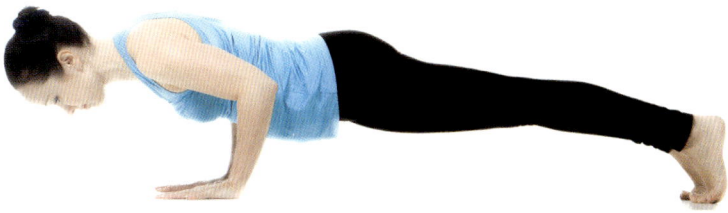

Anatomical Focus

- The erector spinae, quadratus lumborum and rectus abdominis muscles hold the trunk solid.

- Scapular abduction occurs due to the rotator cuff and deltoids.

- The biceps and triceps keep the elbows at right angles.

- Hips are in neutral extension. Abduction is caused by the hamstrings and abductor magnus.

- Knee extension is due to the quadriceps.

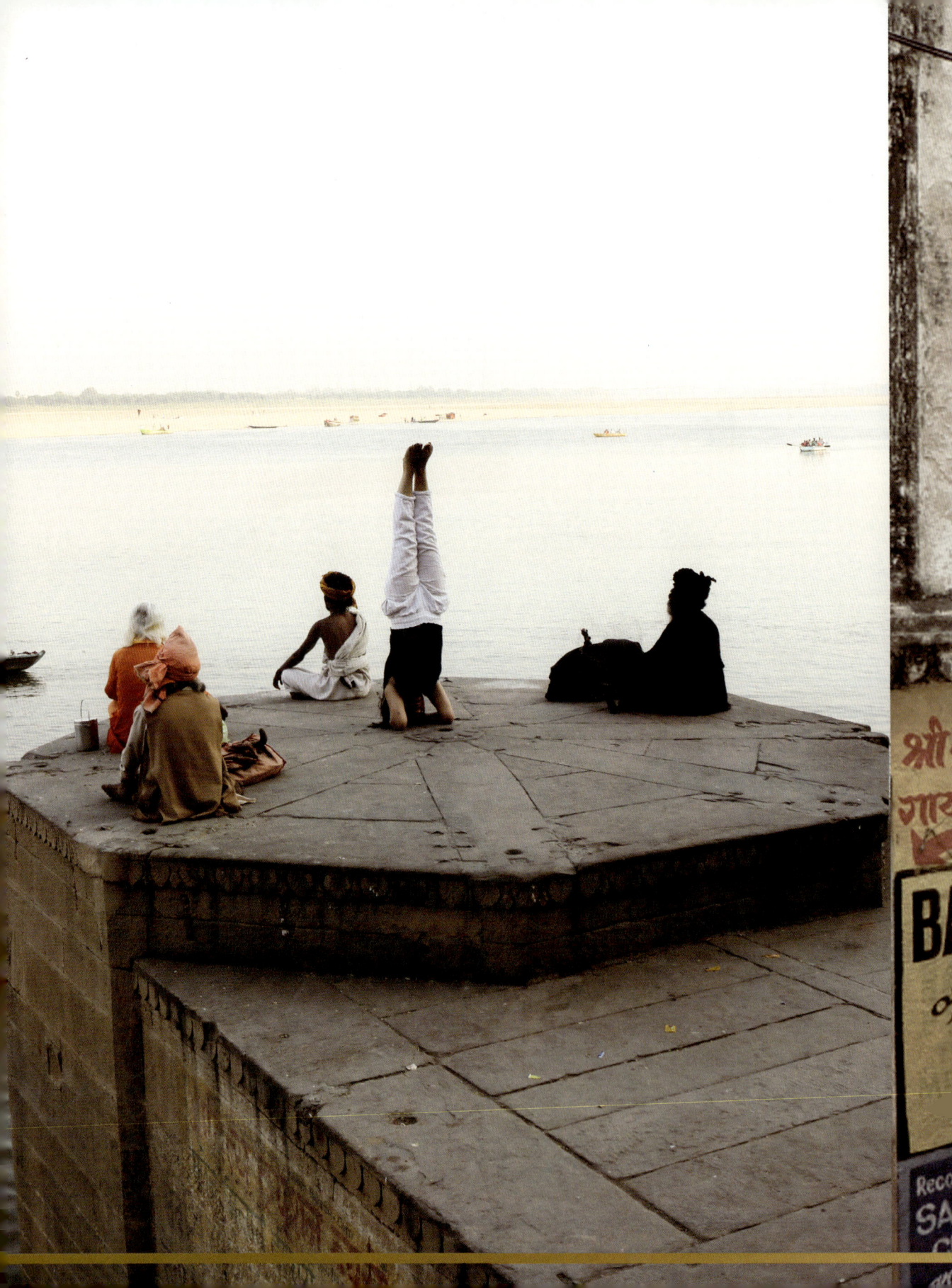

FRIDAY *(SHUKRVAAR)*

This day is dedicated to Venus.

Inverted Poses

Turning our world upside down on a Friday enables us to remain grounded and present. The inverted poses energize and stabilize the body.

There are many benefits of turning ourselves upside down, even though upending oneself as such is against our physical nature. Yoga inspires us to move away from habits which have unconsciously become a part of our daily lives, and upending is just one of the ways in which yoga invites us to move away from the usual and shake things up a bit. Since bipedalism is the one most obvious trait of humankind, so inverting our body and balancing on our hands is bound to have a positive effect on our well-being.

On a physical level, inversions are a boon to our circulatory and endocrine systems. By reversing our relationship with gravity, we allow fresh, oxygenated blood to circulate and replace stagnant blood in the veins and arteries. Psychologically, inversions are a great way to clear the mind and bring a renewed sense of balance and focus.

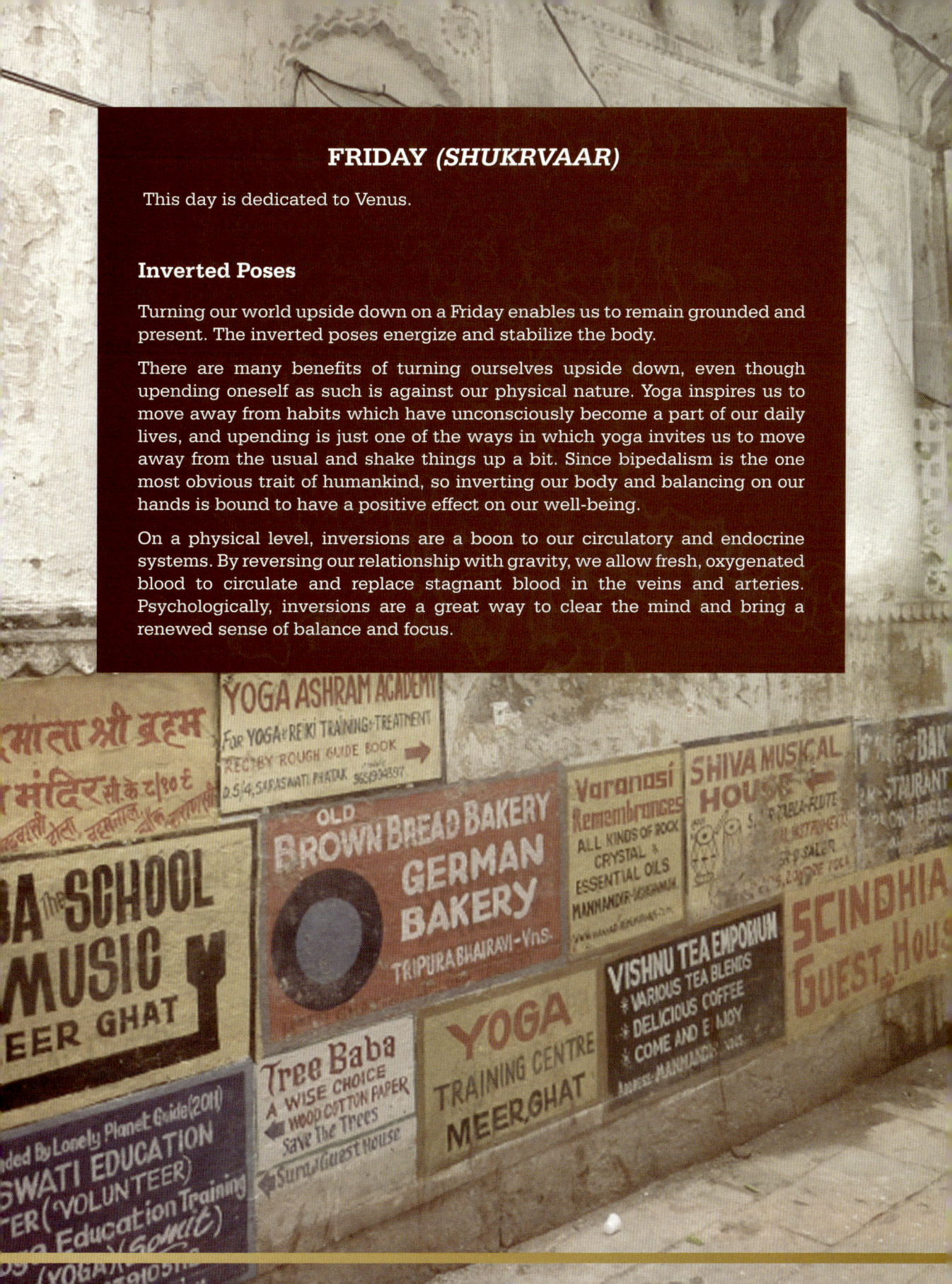

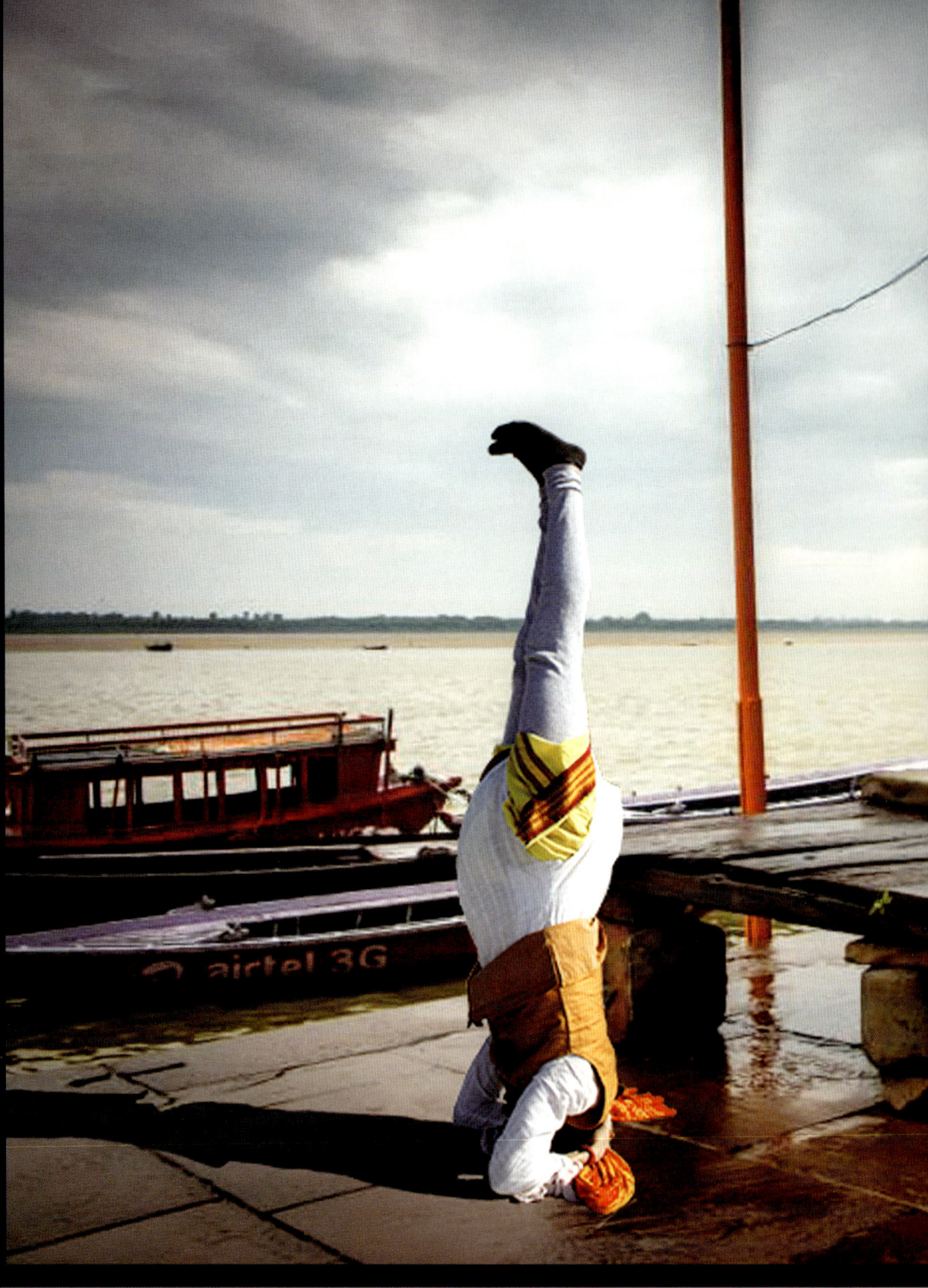

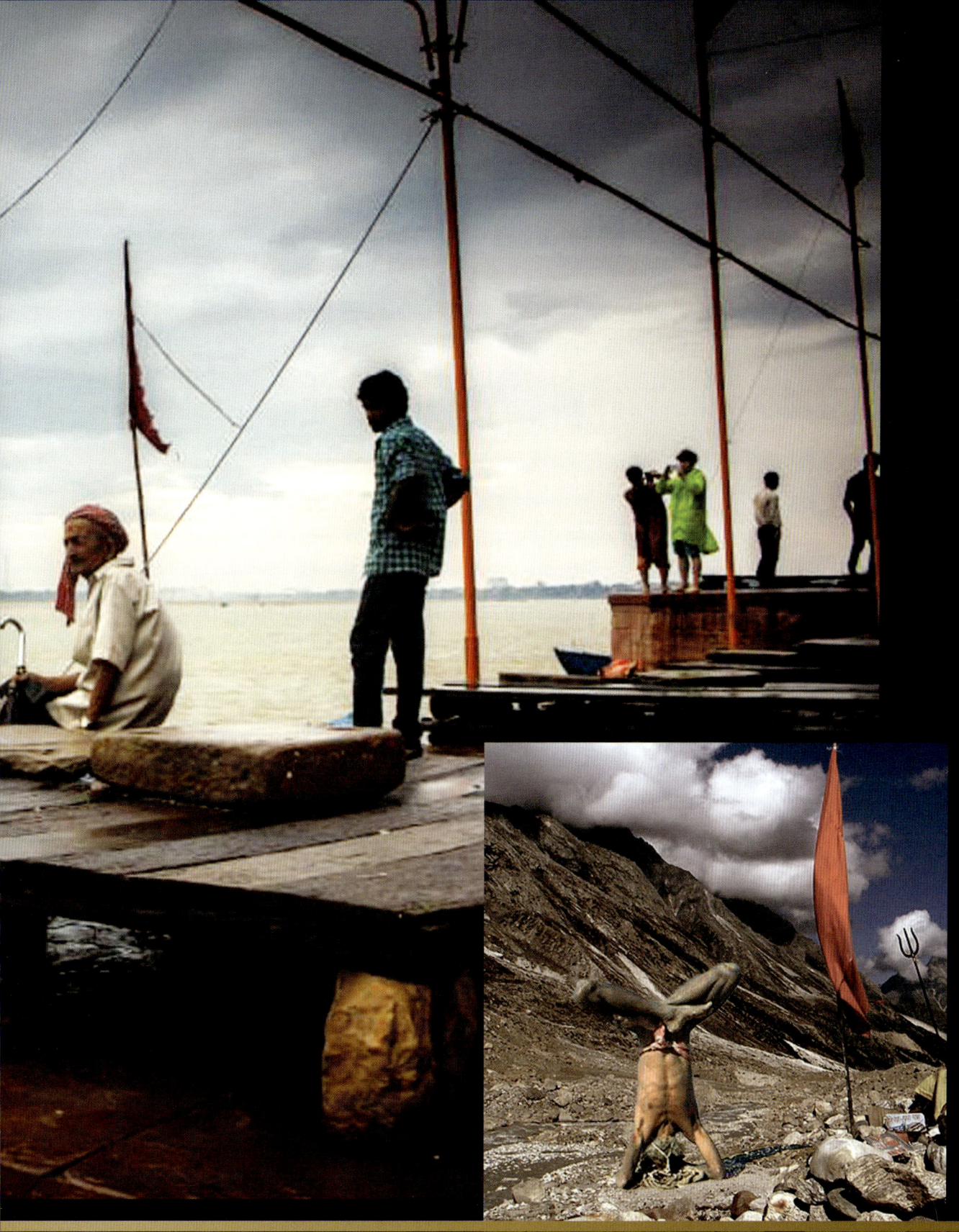

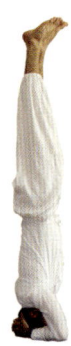

SIRSASANA OR
HEAD STAND POSE

Sirsasana is derived from a Sanskrit word 'shirsha' which means 'head'. It is a symmetrical inversion. It is the ultimate pose of all and is known to bring the most benefits. It is the King of all asanas.

1. Assume kneeling position on the floor. Bring forearms to the floor and grab elbows, ensuring they are shoulder width apart.

2. Release the elbows; interlace the fingers, while pressing forearms on the floor. Gently bring the crown of the head down to the floor. Open your palms and rest the back of the head in them. Raise your knees from the floor while inhaling. Straighten the legs and walk the feet closer to the elbows.

3. Exhale and raise one leg up and then the other. If required, bend the knees and slightly lift up with the foot so that you hop up. Turn the upper thighs inwards a little bit, and press the heels towards the ceiling. If knees are bent, straighten them now.

4. Your weight should be balanced on the forearms. While the tailbone is lifted, move shoulders away from the ears. Press up with the balls of the feet, when legs are straight and hold the pose for three minutes or more depending on your proficiency.

5. Bringing one foot down at a time, release pose and come to rest in balasana (child's pose), and hold for a few breaths.

Benefits

1. Alleviates stress and mild depression.

2. Stimulates the pineal and pituitary glands.

3. Strengthens the spine, legs and arms.

4. Tones the abdominal organs.

5. Brings fresh blood to the lower extremities and brain.

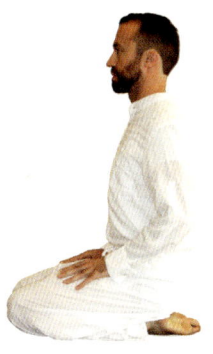

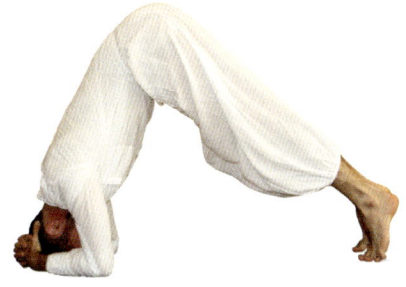

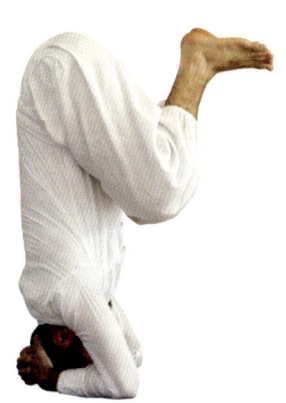

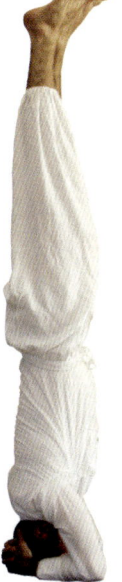

Anatomical Focus

• The erector spinae stabilizes the trunk. The rectus abdominis draws the abdomen and ribcage in.

• Scapular upward rotation occurs due to the action of the serratus anterior. Shoulder flexion and abduction involve the anterior deltoids and trapezius muscles.

• Elbow flexion takes place due to the biceps.

• Hip extension involves the hamstrings, abductor magnus and gluteus maximus. The psoas muscle balances the pelvis to keep it straight.

• Knee extension arises due to the quadriceps.

• The tibialis anterior causes ankle dorsiflexion.

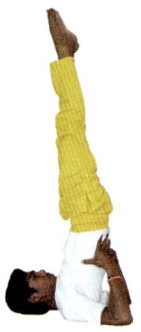

SARVANGASANA OR SHOULDER STAND POSE

Sarvangasana is derived from Sanskrit where 'sarva' means 'all-inclusive' and 'angna' means limb or body part. This pose is a restorative inversion, usually done towards the end of the practice, as a counter pose after the head stand. Sarvangasana has been nicknamed as the 'queen' or 'mother' of all asanas.

1. Lie on your back. In one move, raise your legs, buttocks and back so that you come up high on your shoulders. Support your back with your hands.

2. Move elbows closer towards each other, and move your hands along your back, creeping up towards the shoulder blades. Keep straightening the legs and spine by pressing the elbows down to the floor and hands into the back. Your weight should be on your shoulders, supported on your shoulders and upper arms, and not on your head and neck.

3. Keep legs firm. Lift your heels higher as though you intend to leave a footprint on the ceiling. Ensure that the big toes are aligned with your nose. Now point the toes up. Pay attention to your neck, do not press it into the floor. Instead keep the neck strong by tightening the neck muscles slightly. Press your sternum towards the chin. Release posture, if any strain is felt.

4. Keep breathing deeply and stay in the posture for thirty seconds up to a few minutes.

5. To release posture, lower knees to forehead. Place your hands on the floor, palms facing down. Without lifting the head, slowly bring your spine down to the floor, vertebra by vertebra. Bring legs down to the floor. Relax for a minimum of sixty seconds.

Benefits

1. Stimulates the prostrate glands and thyroid as well as abdominal organs.

2. Stretches the neck and shoulders.

3. Tones and firms the buttocks and legs.

4. Relieves symptoms of menopause.

5. Alleviates stress, fatigue and insomnia.

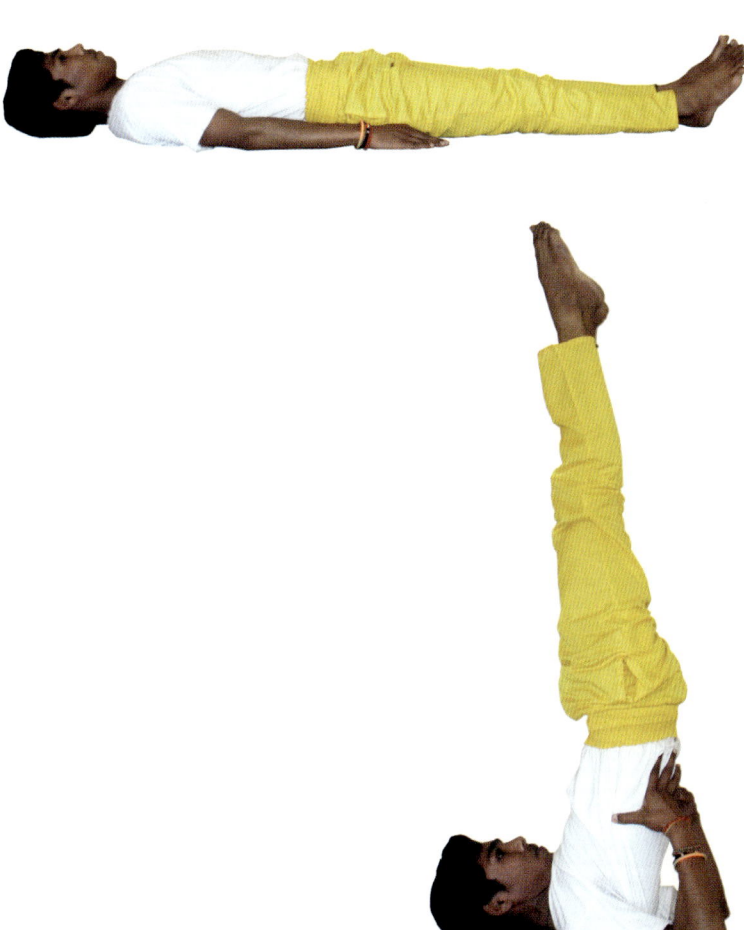

Anatomical Focus

- Cervical and upper thoracic flexion; lumbar and lower thoracic extension.

- Scapular abduction, downward rotation and elevation occur due to the rhomboids and levator scapulae.

- Shoulder extension and abduction takes place as a result of the triceps, teres major and posterior deltoid; elbow flexion occurs due to the biceps; forearm supination. The erector spinae and rectus abdominis muscles lift the trunk.

- Hip extension is activated by the gluteus maximus and psoas muscles, which support the pelvis. Abduction is activated by the adductor magnus and gracilis muscles.

- Knee extension is activated by the quadriceps.

- Ankle dorsiflexion.

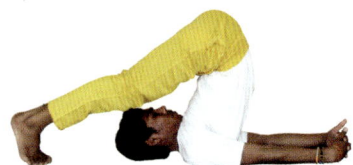

HALASANA
OR PLOW POSE

In Sanskrit, 'hala' means plow. Usually performed immediately after the shoulder stand, this pose has beneficial effects on the cardiovascular system as well as on the flow of cerebrospinal fluid.

1. Begin with the upraised posture of sarvangasana. Bend from the hip while exhaling and lower the toes to the floor above the head. Torso should remain perpendicular to the floor and legs should be extended fully.

2. While lying on your back, rest your arms by your side, with palms facing downward.

3. Inhale and raise your feet off the floor using your abdominal muscles. Legs should be raised vertically at a ninety-degree angle.

4. While breathing normally, let your hands support your hips and back as you lift them up from the ground.

5. Legs should sweep over your head in a 180-degree angle till toes touch the floor and back is perpendicular to the floor. Be slow and gentle while easing into this pose to ensure that you do not strain your neck or push it into the ground.

6. Maintain this pose and relax your body as much as you can as you take steady breaths. Release pose gently and slowly by bringing legs down while exhaling. As a beginner you will be need to release the pose after a few seconds, and about a minute after advanced practice.

Benefits

1. Stimulates the thyroid gland and abdominal organs.

2. Stretches the spine and shoulders.

3. Alleviates stress and fatigue.

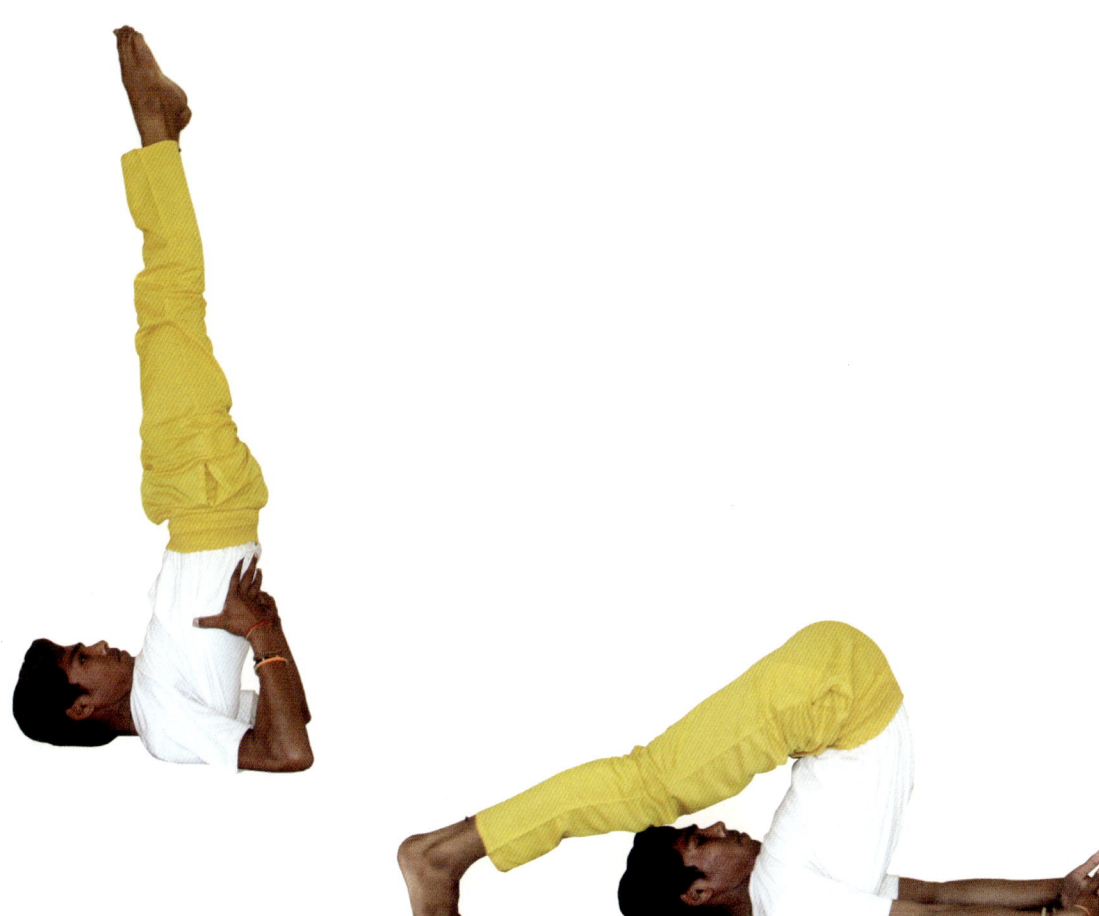

Anatomical Focus

- There is scapular abduction, downward rotation and elevation due to the rhomboids and levator scapulae.

- There is elbow flexion due to the biceps.

- Hip flexion due to the psoas and pectineus muscles, and abduction occurs due to the abductor longus and brevis.

- Knee extension occurs due to the quadriceps.

- Ankle dorsiflexion arises due to the tibilias anterior.

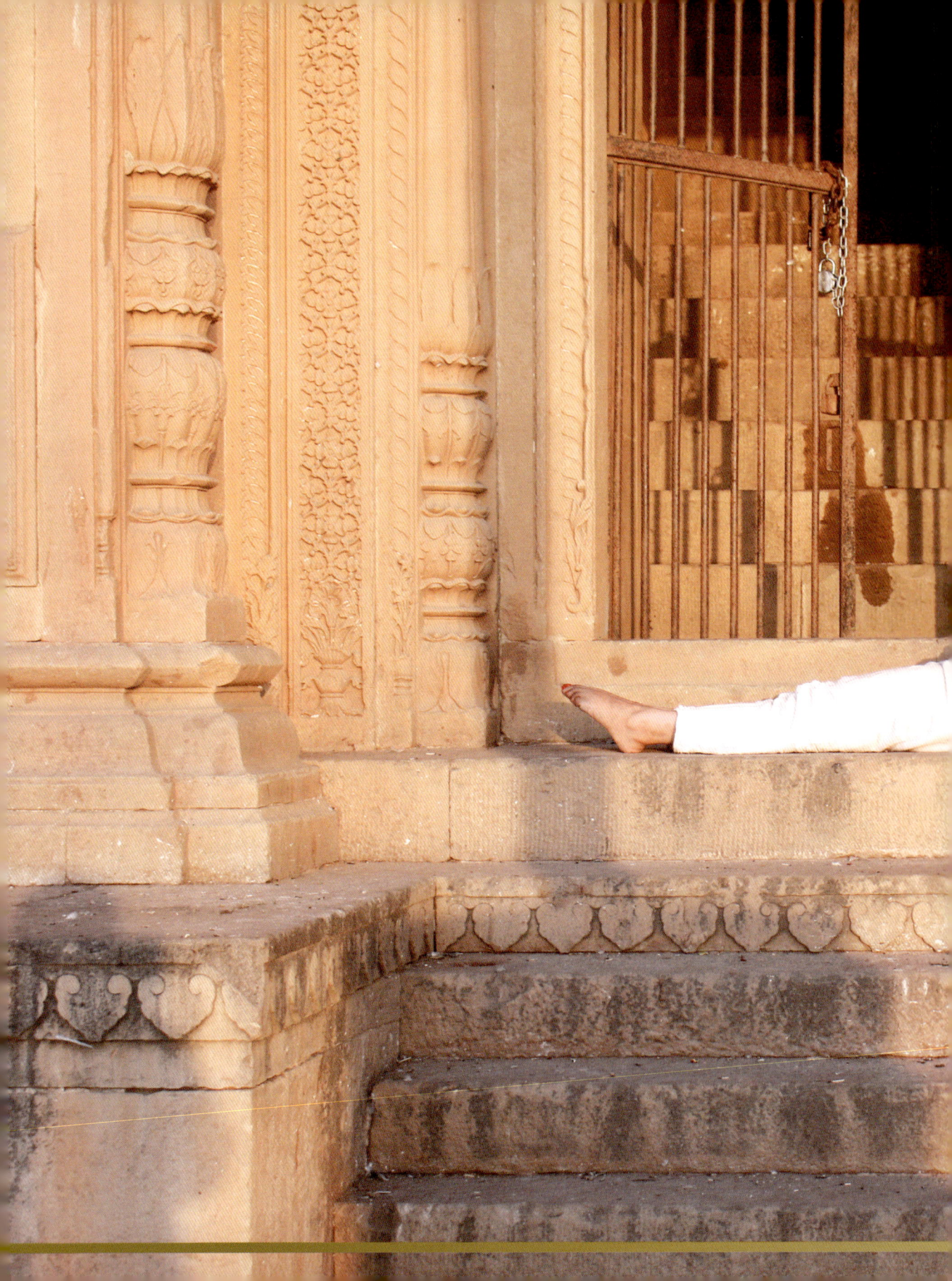

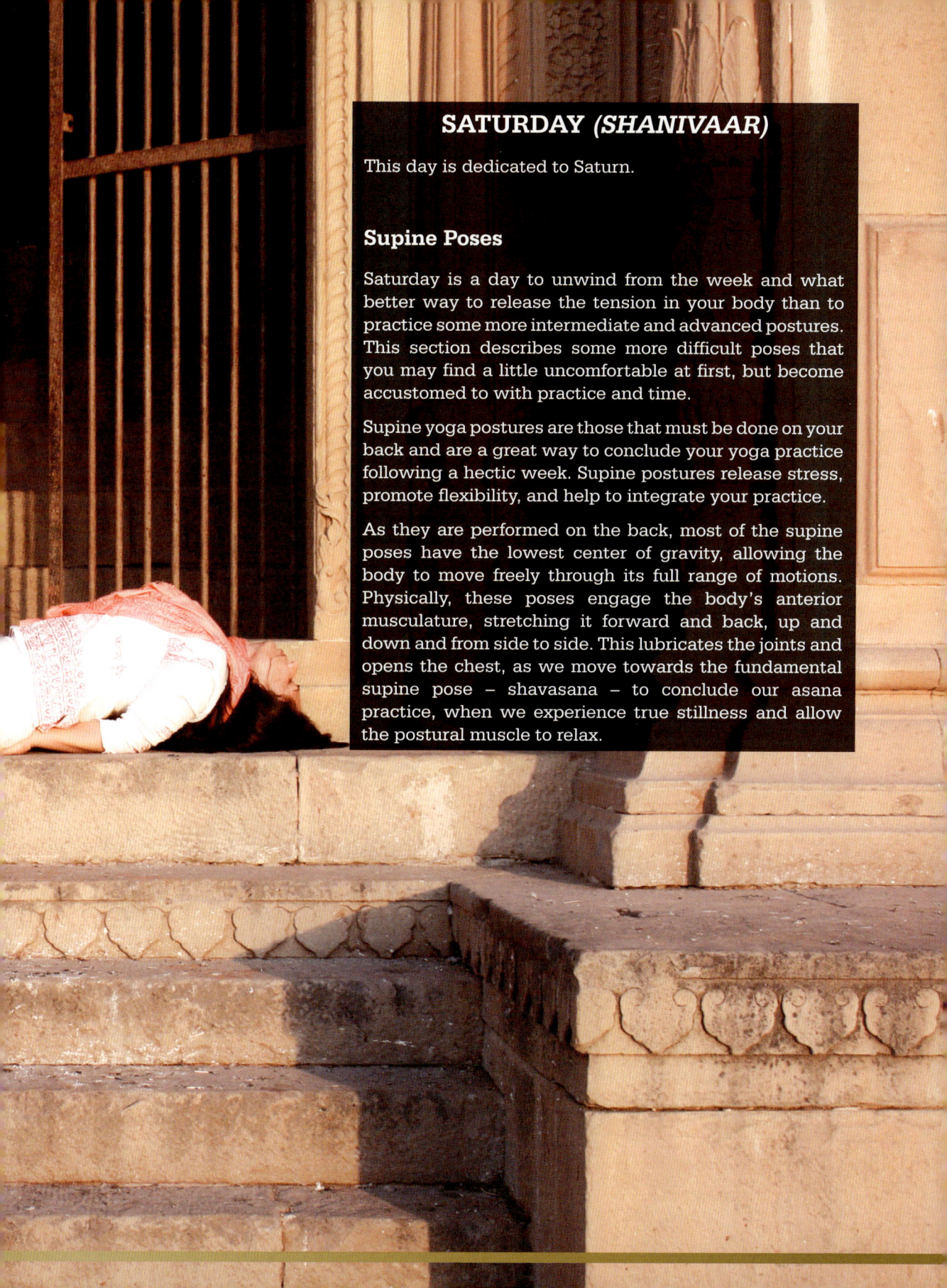

SATURDAY (SHANIVAAR)

This day is dedicated to Saturn.

Supine Poses

Saturday is a day to unwind from the week and what better way to release the tension in your body than to practice some more intermediate and advanced postures. This section describes some more difficult poses that you may find a little uncomfortable at first, but become accustomed to with practice and time.

Supine yoga postures are those that must be done on your back and are a great way to conclude your yoga practice following a hectic week. Supine postures release stress, promote flexibility, and help to integrate your practice.

As they are performed on the back, most of the supine poses have the lowest center of gravity, allowing the body to move freely through its full range of motions. Physically, these poses engage the body's anterior musculature, stretching it forward and back, up and down and from side to side. This lubricates the joints and opens the chest, as we move towards the fundamental supine pose – shavasana – to conclude our asana practice, when we experience true stillness and allow the postural muscle to relax.

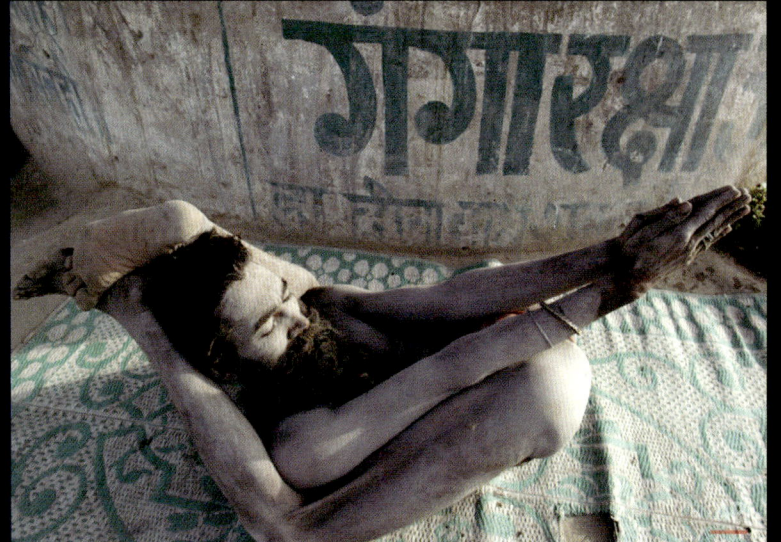
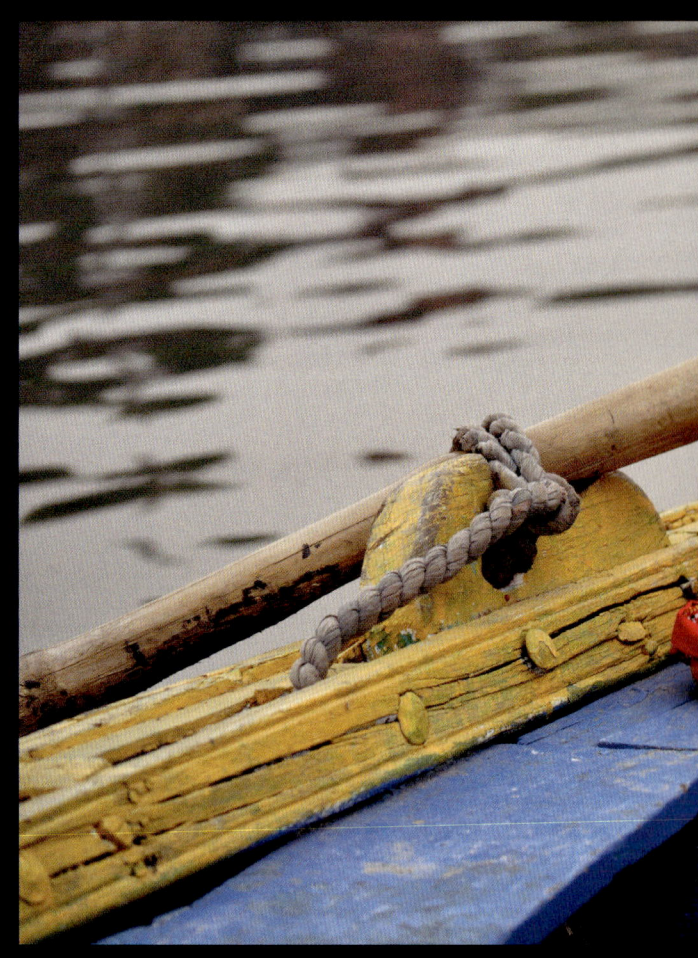

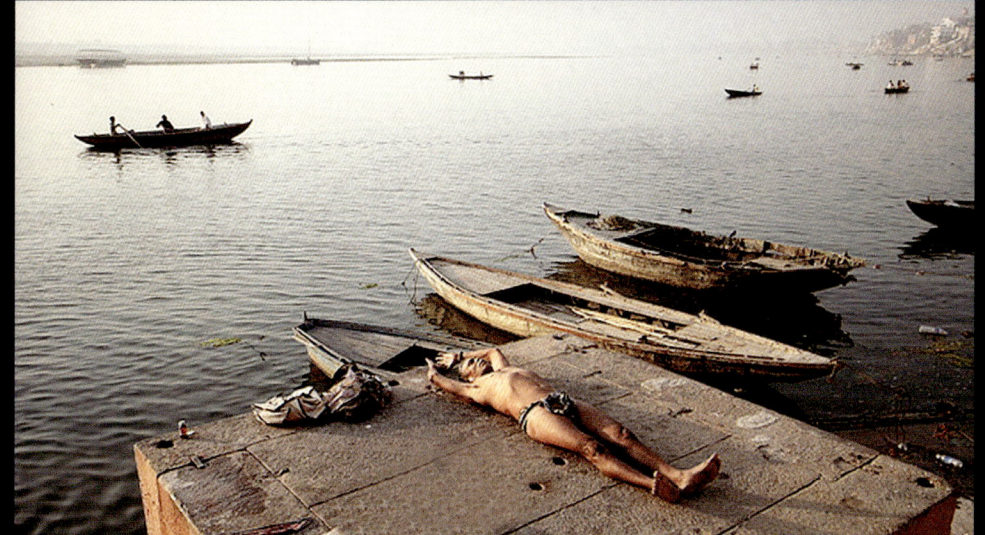
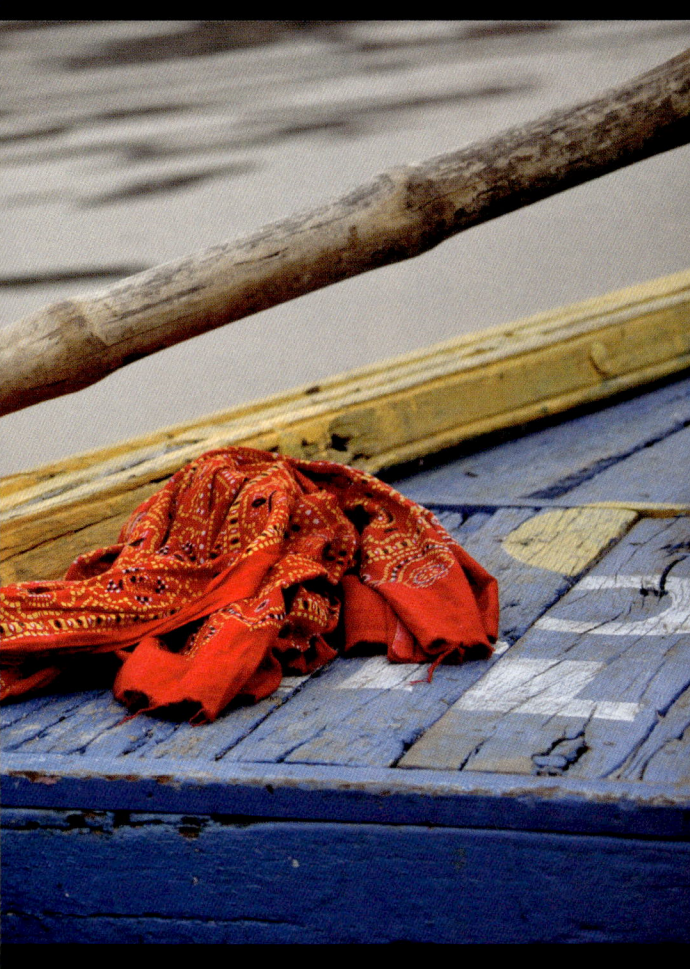

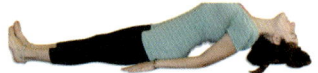

MATSYASANA
OR FISH POSE

The word 'matsya', in Sanskrit, means fish. Traditional texts state that matsyasana is the 'destroyer of all diseases'. A symmetrical supine back bending pose, the fish pose is traditionally performed with the legs positioned in padmasana, but many people practice this with legs straight and pressed against the wall.

1. Lie on your back. Your feet should be together and hands relaxed alongside the body.

2. Place the hands underneath the hips, palms facing down. Bring elbows closer to each other.

3. Breathing in, lift the head and chest up.

4. Keep the chest elevated and lower the head backward. Touch the top of your head to the floor.

5. With the head lightly touching the floor, press the elbows firmly into the ground, placing the weight on the elbow and not on the head. Lift your chest up from in-between the shoulder blades. Press the thighs and legs to the floor.

6. Hold the pose for as long as you are comfortable, taking gentle long breaths. Relax in the posture with every exhalation.

7. Raise your head and lower the chest and the head to the floor, bringing back the sides of the body and relax.

Benefits

1. Stretches the deep hip flexors (psoas) and the muscles between the ribs (intercostals).

2. Stretches and stimulates the muscles of the belly, the front of the neck and the throat muscles.

3. Strengthens the muscles of the upper back and the back of the neck.

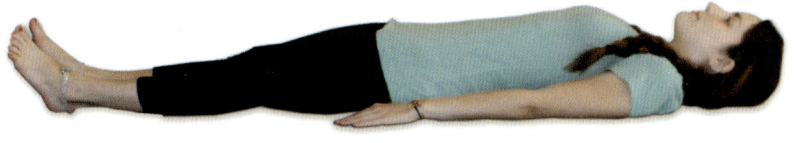

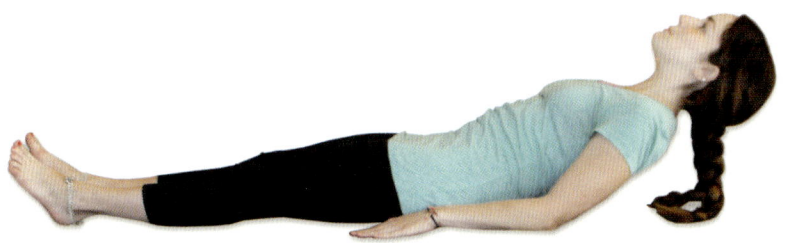

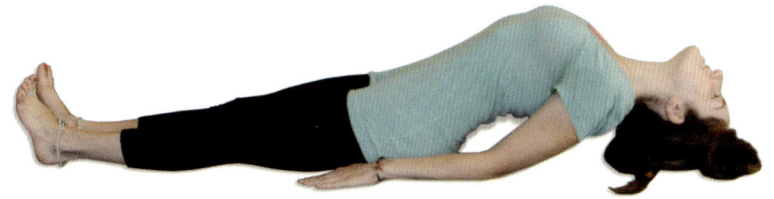

Anatomical Focus

- Spinal extension is activated by the psoas major.

- Scapular downward rotation and abduction are due to the trapezius, rhomboids and latissimus dorsi.

- Shoulder extension and abduction occur due to the triceps, elbow extension, forearm pronation.

- Hip flexion and abduction take place due to the psoas and iliacus muscles.

- Knee extension occurs due to the quadriceps.

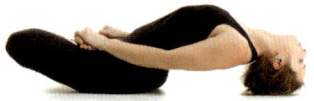

ADVANCED VARIATION OR BOUND FISH POSE

1. Lying on your back, position legs into the lotus pose with thighs pulled close together.

2. Pressing your forearms and elbows into the floor, raise yourself on the crown of head with your back arched.

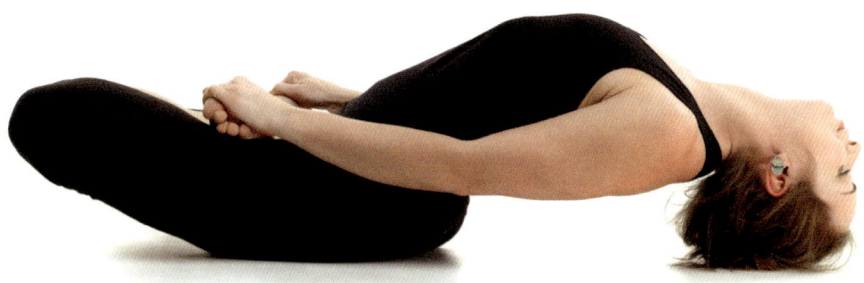

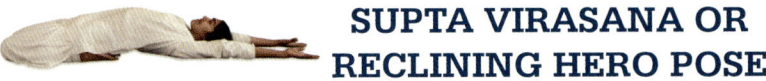

SUPTA VIRASANA OR RECLINING HERO POSE

This, in Sanskrit, means a warrior in the lying down position. This pose stretches the abdominal organs and the pelvic region and helps give relief to aching, tired legs.

1. With your knees held together, kneel on the floor. The feet should be separated so that the distance between them is wider than the hips and the seat should be on the floor.

2. With hands on the floor beside the hips, slowly begin to bring your back down towards the floor. Leaning onto the hands at first and then on the forearms and elbows, gradually release the spine and shoulders. The back of the head should be downward.

3. Lengthening the lower back, bring it down towards the floor, ensure that your arms and hands are on the floor with the palms facing up. Check that your knees are still together, as they tend to separate as you lower yourself. Inhale and raise your arms overhead, towards the floor, palms facing up. You may hold the pose like this or grab each elbow.

4. Hold the pose for thirty to sixty seconds.

5. To release, come onto the hands while pressing the forearms against the floor. Then raise yourself up with your hands.

Benefits

1. Stretches the thighs, abdomen, deep hip flexors (psoas), knees and ankles.

2. Strengthens the arches.

3. Relieves tired legs.

4. Improves digestion.

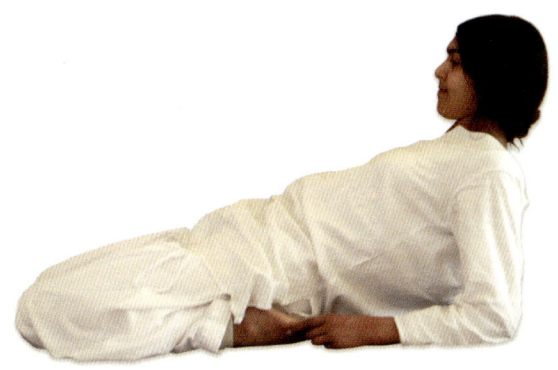

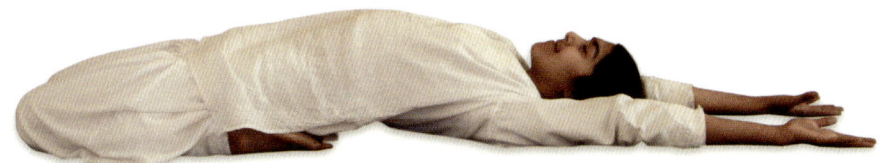

Anatomical Focus

- The deltoid muscles raise the arms over the head.

- The triceps straighten the arms.

- Hip extension occurs through action of the psoas muscles.

- Knee flexion and abduction occurs through action of the gracilis and abductor magnus.

- Ankle plantar flexion.

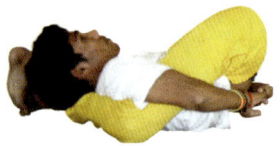

YOGA NIDRASANA
OR SLEEPING YOGI POSE

Yoga Nidrasana, in Sanskrit, means the sleeping posture of a yogi. For this pose, cross legs at the ankles behind the neck with the hands clasped behind the back.

1. Lying on the floor, flat on the back, bend both your knees and bring your legs over the head, with the knees beside the shoulders.

2. Grab the back of the ankles with each hand and lift the shoulders, using both arms to move the legs back. Place the right leg behind the back of the neck. Raise the left leg and position it behind the neck, under the right leg and cross your ankles.

3. Lift your shoulders and keep working the legs further behind the back of the neck, as you pull the arms through the legs further and clasp the hands behind the back.

4. Breathe and hold the pose for at least thirty seconds.

Benefits

1. Stretches the shoulders and the spine.

2. Stimulates abdominal organs such as the liver and kidneys, and aids digestion.

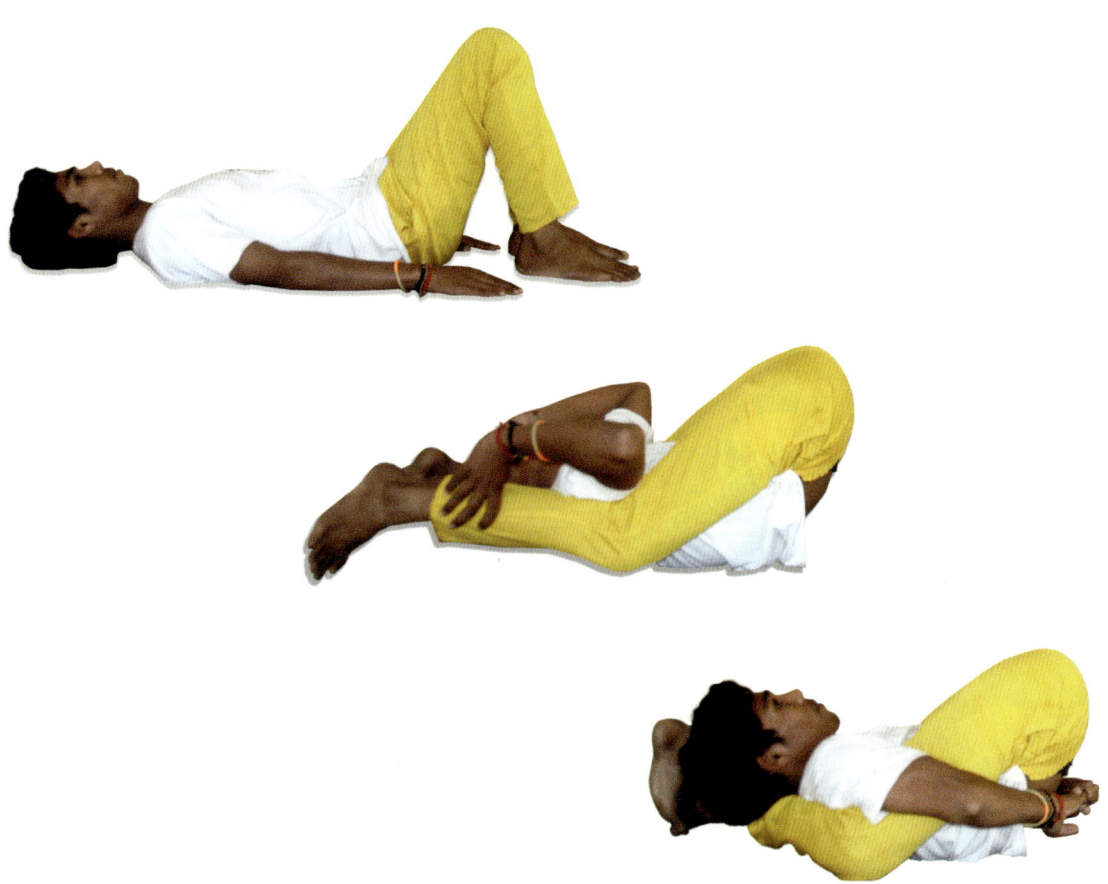

Anatomical Focus

- This allows cervical extension in the spine.

- The shoulders abduct and rotate internally to keep the legs back. The elbows are flexed due to the biceps.

- The psoas brings the hips into deep flexion. The legs are abducted and rotated internally due to the pectineus and abductor muscles.

- The knees are flexed due to the hamstrings; the ankles are in dorsiflexion.

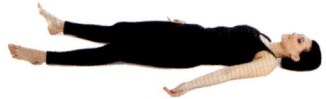

SHAVASANA
OR CORPSE POSE

Shavasana is derived from the Sanskrit word 'shava' meaning corpse. This involves conscious relaxation, invigorating and refreshing to both the body and mind. This seemingly easy pose is one of the most challenging for the yogi, as it is hard to keep the mind still while remaining motionless and fully conscious at the same time.

1. In shavasana, the body is positioned neutrally – sitting on the floor, with knees, place your feet are on the floor and lean your body back onto the forearms. Raise your pelvis a little off the floor and push it back against tailbone with your hands.

2. Return the pelvis to the floor. While inhaling, gradually stretch out and extend the right leg, then the left, and push through the heels. Gently release your legs, soften groin and make sure that the angle of the legs is evenly relative to the mid-line of the torso and the feet turn out equal. Narrowing the front pelvis, soften back but don't flatten out.

3. Using your hands, raise the base of your skull away from the back of the neck and let it come down towards the tailbone. Support neck with a folded blanket to make it easier, if required. Broadening the base of the skull, lift the crease of the neck in a diagonal position into the center of the head. The ears are equidistant from shoulders.

4. Stretch your arms towards ceiling, perpendicular to the floor. Rocking slightly from one side to the other, and pull the ribs and shoulder blades away from the spine. Lower arms to the floor, angling them relatively evenly to the mid line of torso. Turn the arms out and stretch them away from the shoulder blades. Place back of the hands on the floor as close as possible to the index finger knuckles, shoulder blades are resting on floor. Raise the lower tips of the shoulder blades diagonally into the back towards the top of the sternum and spread the collarbones.

5. Along with the physical body, the sense organs also have to be calmed and pacified in shavasana. Stay in this pose for five minutes out of the thirty minutes of the entire practice.

6. To release, begin with rolling to the right while exhaling. Take a few breaths and then with another exhalation, raise your torso, by pressing your hands against the floor and finally lift your head up slowly and gently.

Soften the base of the tongue, the nose, the channels of the inner ears, and the skin of the forehead, especially around the bridge of the nose between the eyebrows. Let the eyes sink to the back of the head, then turn them downward to gaze at the heart. Release your brain to the back of the head.

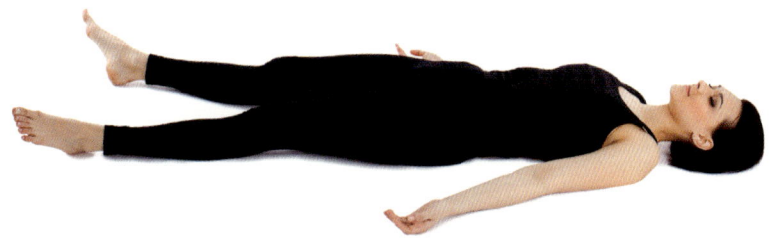

Benefits

1. In this pose, the body is completely at rest. It induces a deep conscious relaxation, which is different from sleep.

2. Shavasana energizes and refreshes the body and the mind. Steady, smooth and deep breathing is especially beneficial when the body is still as it soothes the nerves. This is the best antidote to the stress of modern life.

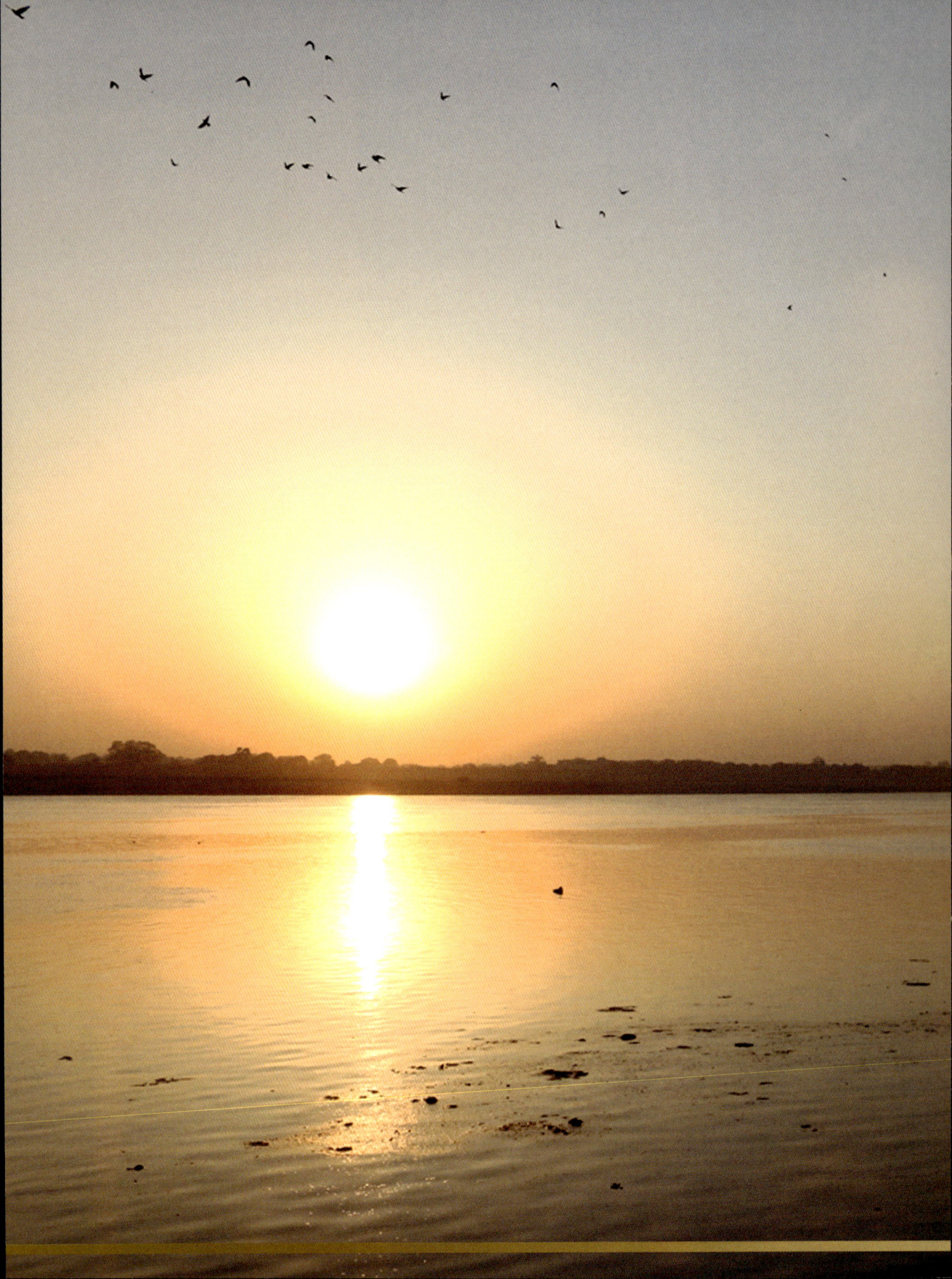

SUNDAY (RAVIVAAR)

This day is dedicated to the sun.

Surya Namaskar or Sun Salutation

Surya namaskar is a vinyasa – a sequence of asanas done without pausing between each one. There are twelve asanas in the vinyasa, each with its own name, energetic function and mantra.

To complete one round of surya namaskar, begin by practicing the twelve stages on the right side (to activate *pingala nadi*), stepping the right foot back in step four and the right foot forward in step nine, and then complete another twelve stages by stepping the left foot backwards in step four and forward in step nine. To increase concentration or for meditational purposes, the cycle can begin on the left side.

At least two rounds and as many as twelve complete rounds should precede any other asanas. This ensures that the body is fully prepared for the rest of the week.

In specific cases, 108 rounds are practiced for purification purposes.

A mantra is traditionally ascribed to each of the twelve steps of surya namaskar, and can be recited during each round.

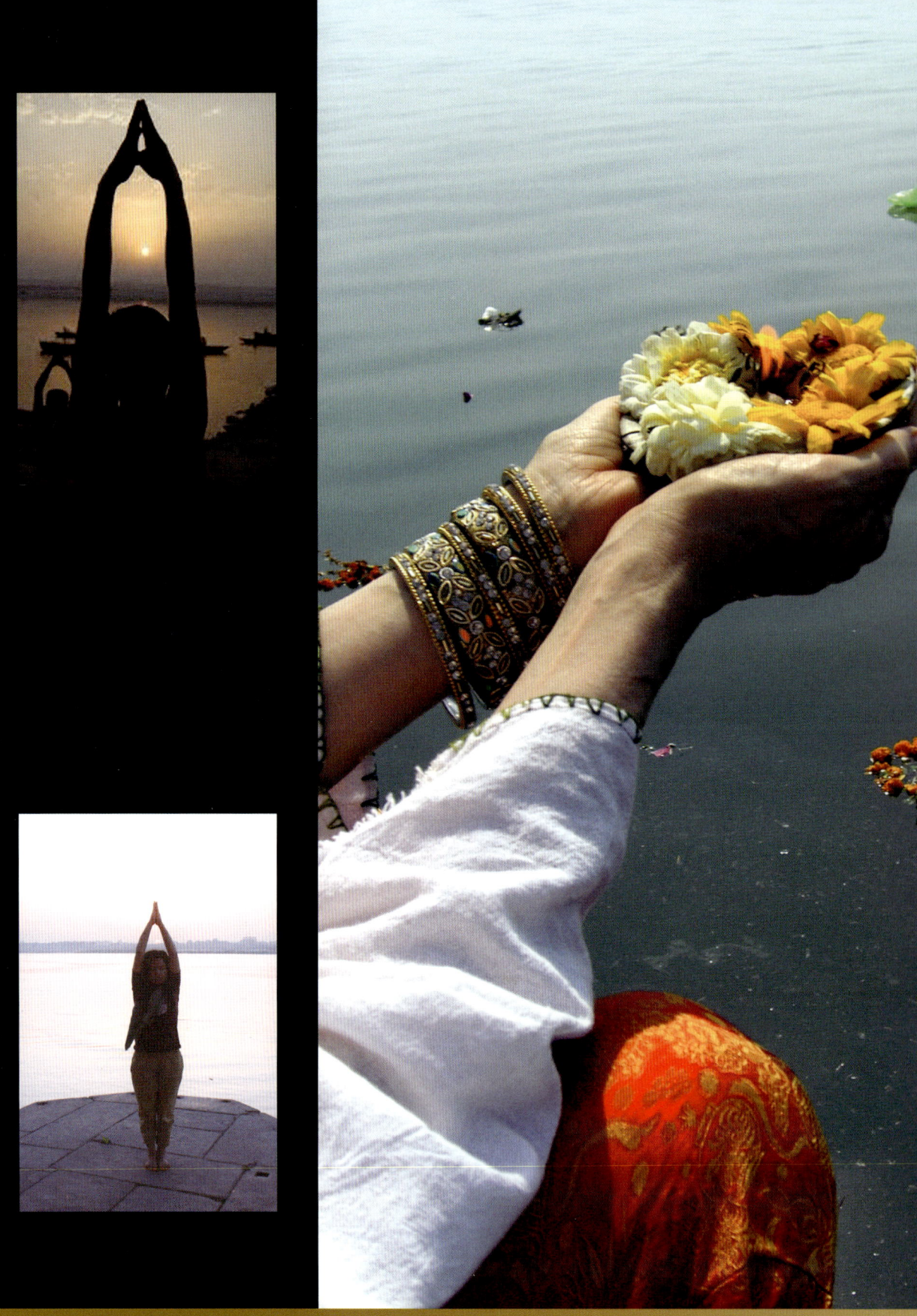

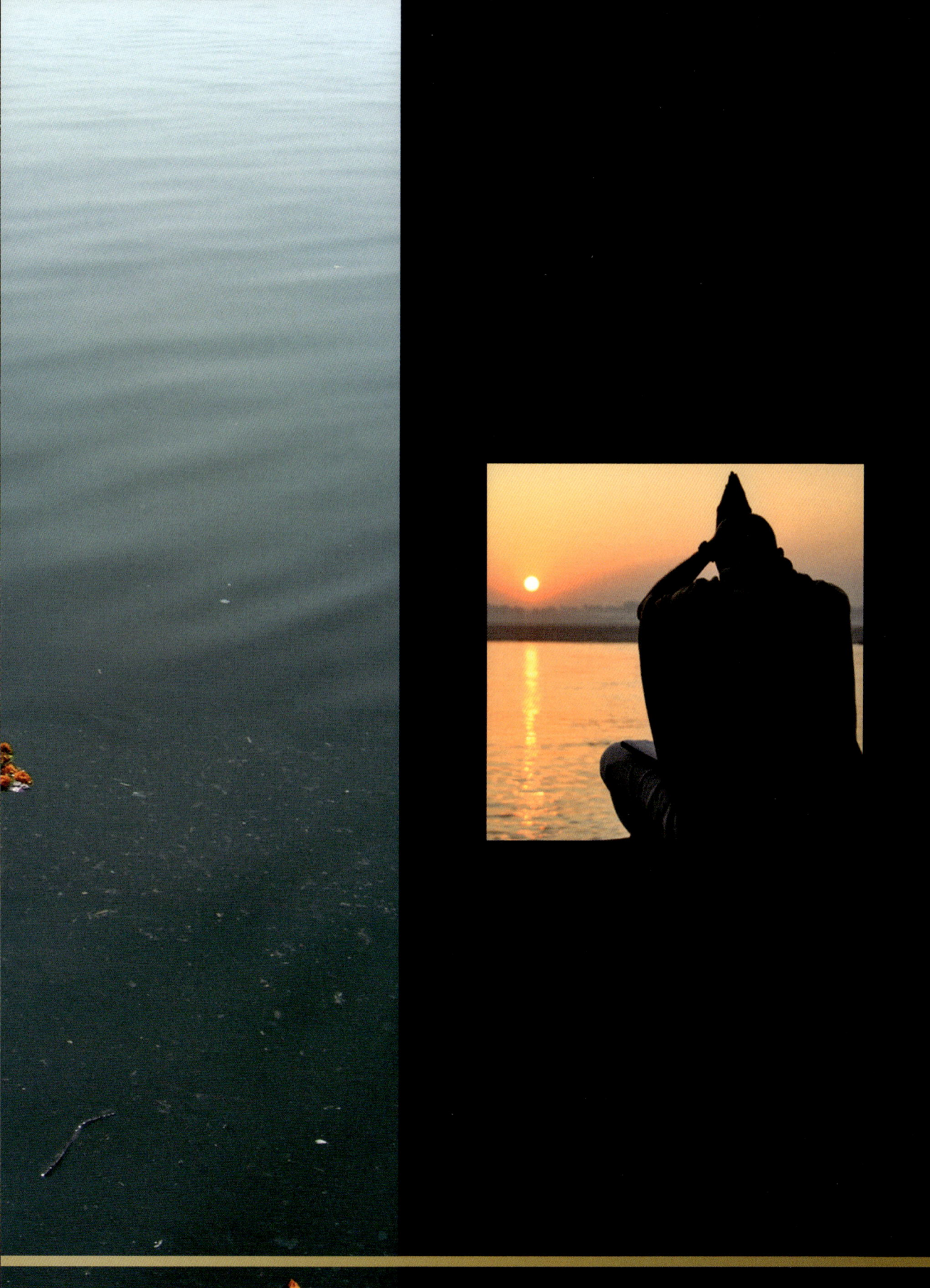

PRANAMASANA OR STANDING PRAYER POSTURE

Mantra: *Om mitraya namah* (I greet all friends)

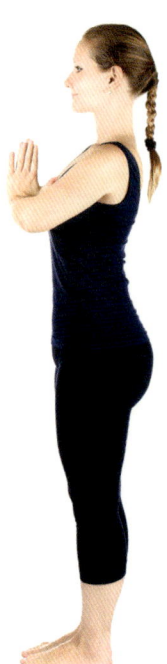

Stand with the feet together and the hands in front of the chest in pranamasana or the prayer pose. Close your eyes and focus on the right side of the heart, the center of your physical chest. This is where the spiritual heart lies.

HASTA UTTANASANA OR RAISED ARM POSTURE

Mantra: *Om ravaya namah* (I greet the Shining One)

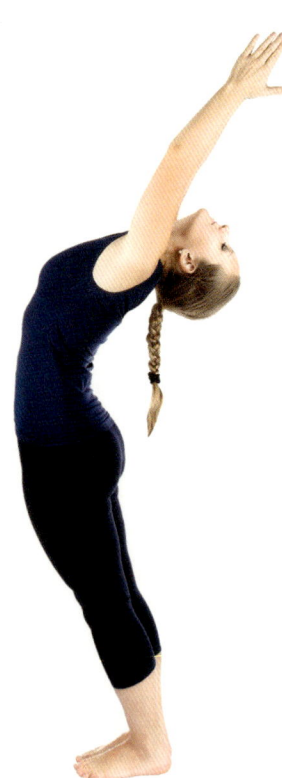

Inhale and raise the arms over the head and arch back into hasta uttanasana. Feel the front of your spine lengthening and your chest opening.

When we raise our arms and leave our heart unprotected, we signal to energy that we are ready to receive and embrace it.

PADAHASTASANA OR HAND TO FOOT POSTURE

Mantra: *Om surya namah* (I greet the Sun – initiator of all activity; the source of all energy)

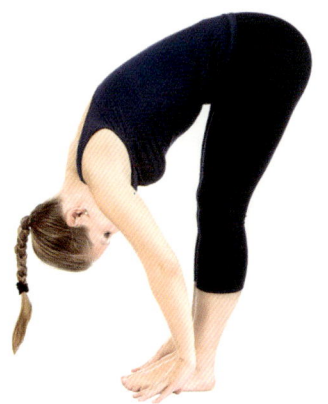

Exhale and bend forward, and bring the palms on either side of the feet and the head to the knees or shins.

Remember to keep your weight going down through your ankles and heels (not letting it come forward to your toes). If you are unable to get the heels of your hands on the floor, or allow your hands to dangle in the air, the proprioceptors (your sensitive internal sensors) get the message of instability and muscles will start to tense as they attempt to keep you upright. Once you are in the forward bend let your head go, so that its weight can stretch the long muscles of the back.

ASHVA SANCHALASANA OR HORSE POSTURE

Mantra: *Om bhavane namah* (I greet the One who illuminates all the planets of my birth)

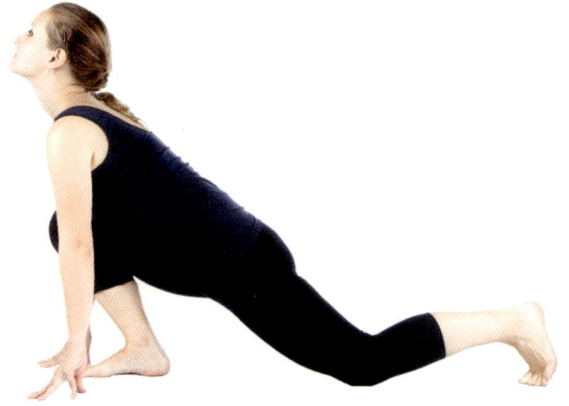

Inhale and extend the right leg back as far as possible, and bring the knee to the floor, lowering the right hip and thigh towards the floor. Lift the chest, and tilt the head back slightly.

CHATURANGA DANDASANA OR FOUR LIMBED STAFF POSTURE

Mantra: *Om khagaya namah* (I greet the One who moves across the sky)

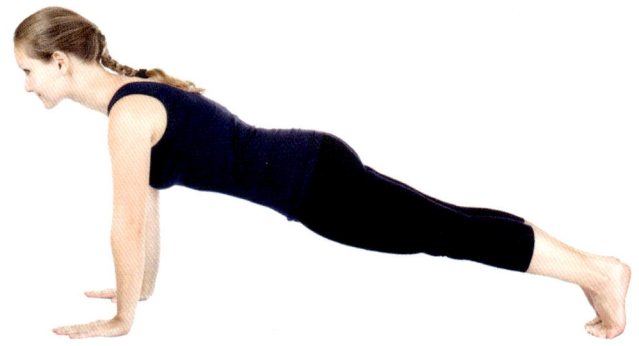

Press both palms to the floor and straighten the arms. Tuck the right toes under, lift the knee off the floor and step the left leg back to meet the right.

Be sure to drop your buttocks, to bring the entire body into a straight line.

ASHTANGA NAMASKAR OR EIGHT LIMBED SALUTATION

Mantra: *Om pushne namah* (I greet the One who cherishes and nourishes this world)

Exhale and bring the knees, chest and chin to the floor. The buttocks, hips and abdomen should be raised lifting your tailbone.

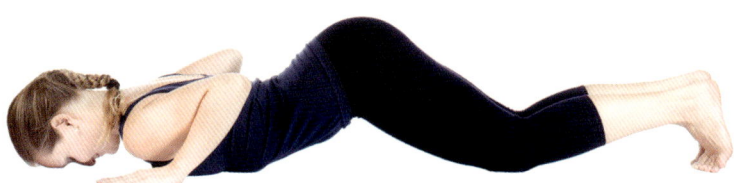

BHUJANGASANA OR COBRA POSE

Mantra: *Om hiranyagarbhaya namah* (I greet the golden embryo from which this Universe emerges)

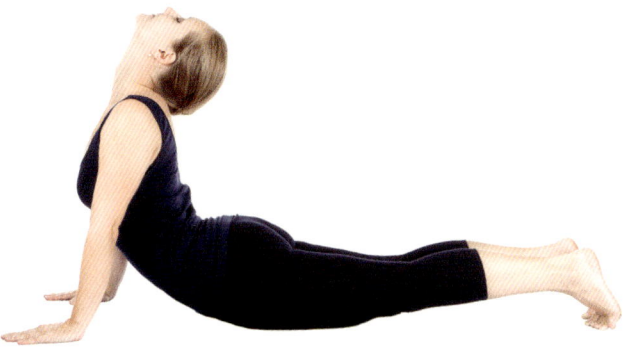

Lower the thighs and hips to the floor and inhale and lift the trunk by straightening the elbows. Arch the back as you push the chest forward into bhujangasana (cobra pose). The top of your feet should remain flat on the floor and, once you are up to your fullest stretch, you should be looking directly up with the steady gaze of a cobra.

SUMERU ASANA OR SUPREME MOUNTAIN POSTURE

Mantra: *Om marichaya namah* (I greet the Lord of the dawn)

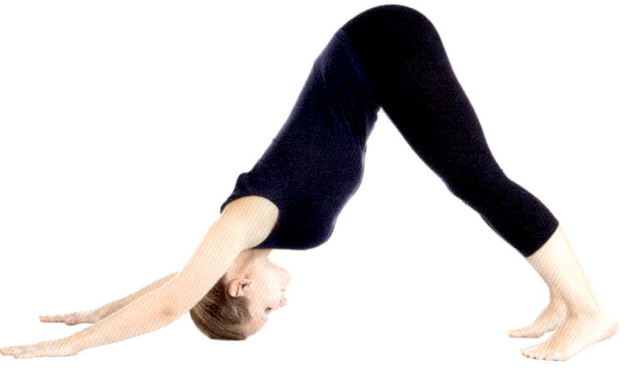

Release your body from bhujangasana and, as you exhale, take a small step forward and push up into the supreme mountain posture. The energy thrust should push up through the arms into the shoulder blades and take your buttocks back. Allow your head to release and become heavy and drop your heels down into (or towards) the floor.

ASHVA SANCHALANASA OR HORSE POSTURE

Mantra: *Om aditaya namah* (I greet the son of Aditi – sovereign of the twelve months of my natal chart)

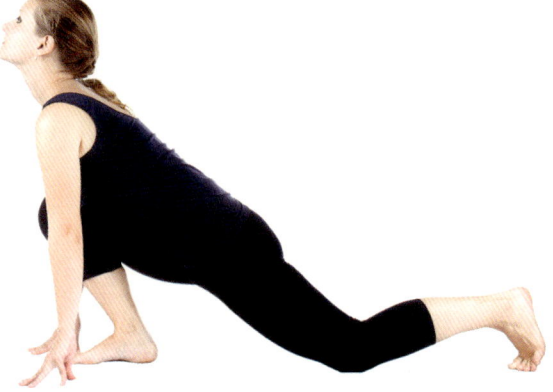

Inhale and move the right leg forward as far as possible and assume ashva aanchalasana.

PADAHASTANA OR HAND TO FOOT POSTURE

Mantra: *Om savitri namah* (I greet the Benevolent Mother of all and protector of the day)

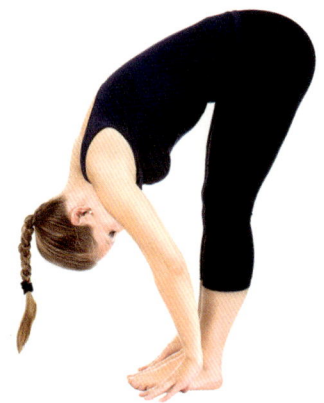

Exhale and bend forward. Bring the palms on either side of the feet and the head to the knees or shins.

HASTA UTTANASANA OR RAISED ARM POSTURE

Mantra: *Om arkaya namah* (I greet the One whose radiance arcs across the sky)

Inhale and lift the trunk. Then raise arms over the head and arch back.

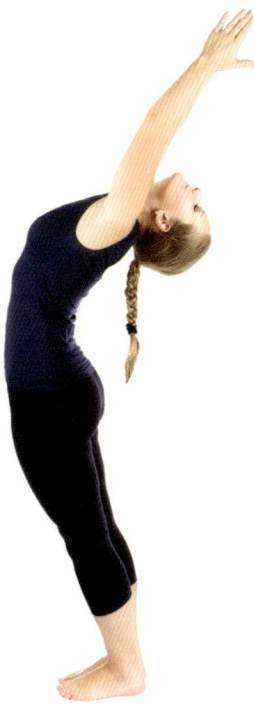

PARANAMASANA OR STANDING PRAYER POSTURE

Mantra: *Om bhaskaraya namah* (I greet the One who brings light and enlightenment)

Exhale and lower the hands into pranamasana.

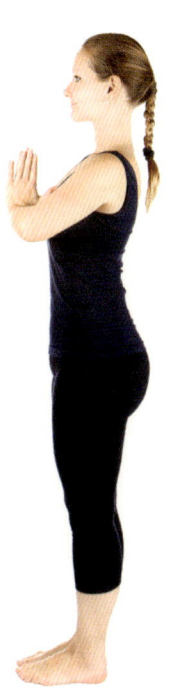

Meditation

AARTI

Aarti originates from the Sanskrit word *aratrika*, a type of meditation and chanting during which a wick soaked in camphor or purified butter is lit. It is offered to deities along with chanting.

The goal of aarti is to establish thoughts of spiritual forces in and around us. This is accomplished by the chanting of a mantra. The aarti is performed to eliminate obstacles and troubles that restrict us beginning our spiritual journey. It can also be referred to as group meditation. The benefits of aarti can be enhanced by following spiritual practices. The effects of these actions are to enable us to learn more deeply about the spiritual energy called upon by the chanting and fire, and to help purify our thoughts.

In India, aarti is performed every day in virtually all the temples, and also by the Ganges, where thousands of people gather to participate. It can be practiced all around the world – a mat and a candle is all that is needed.

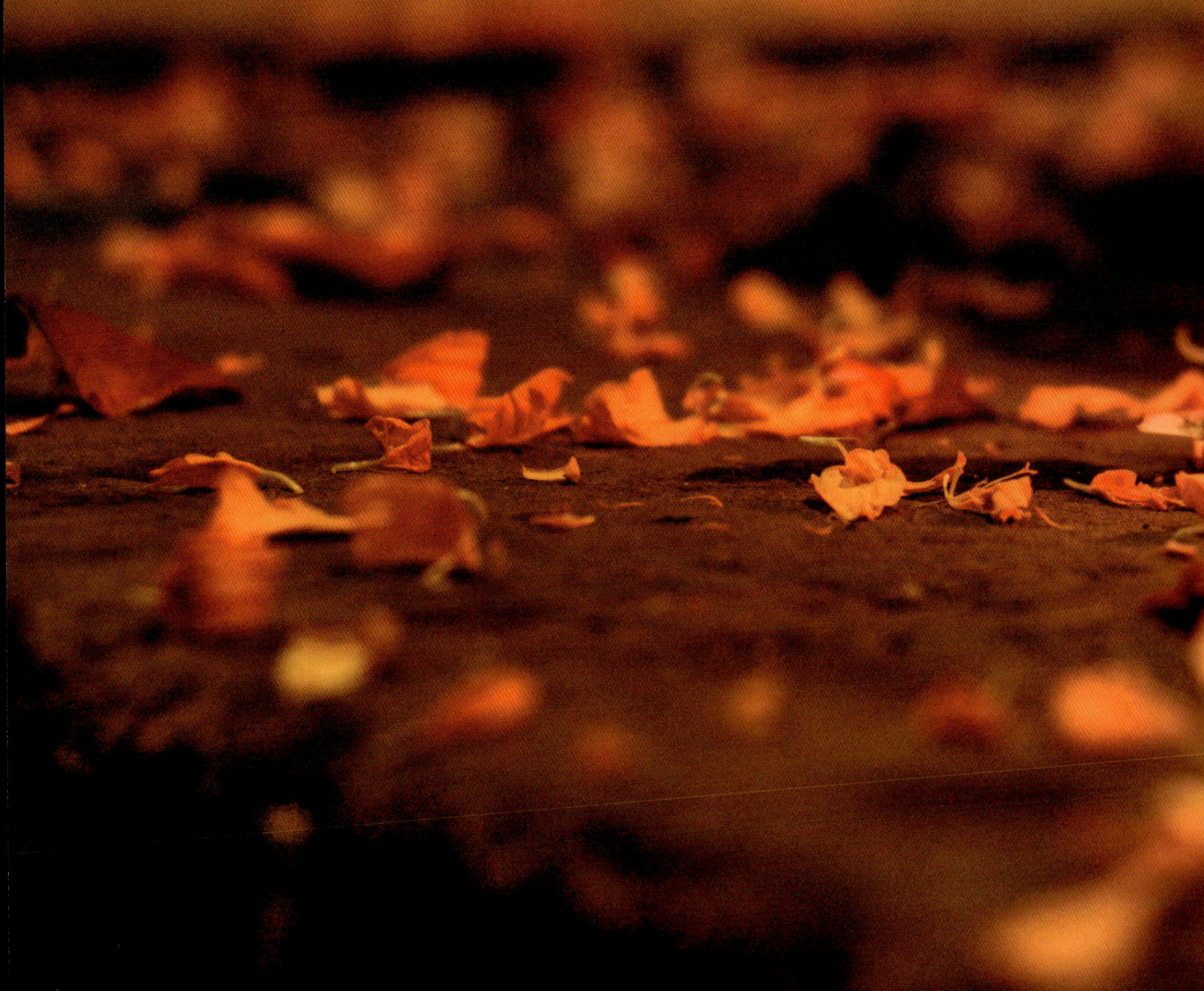

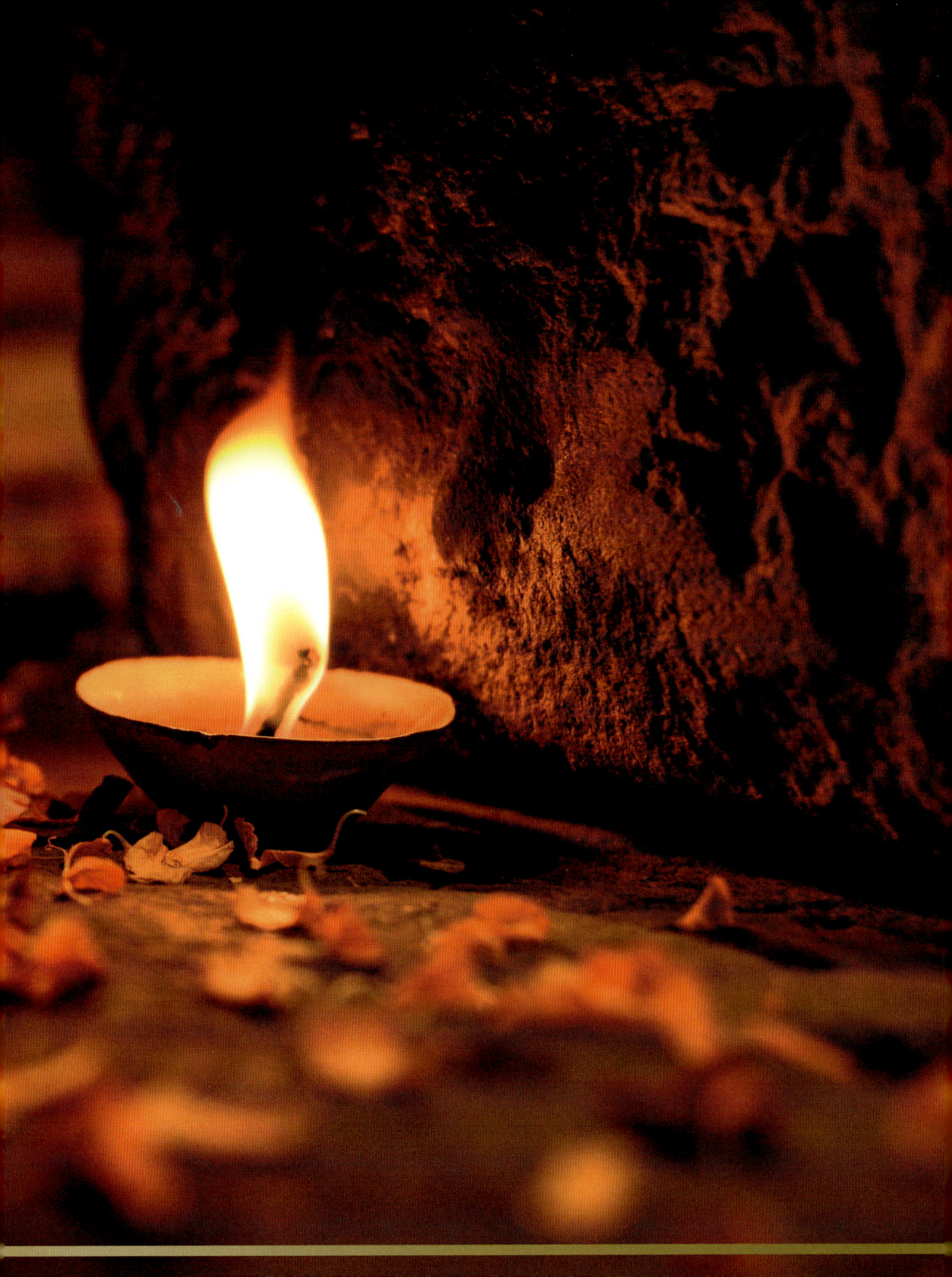

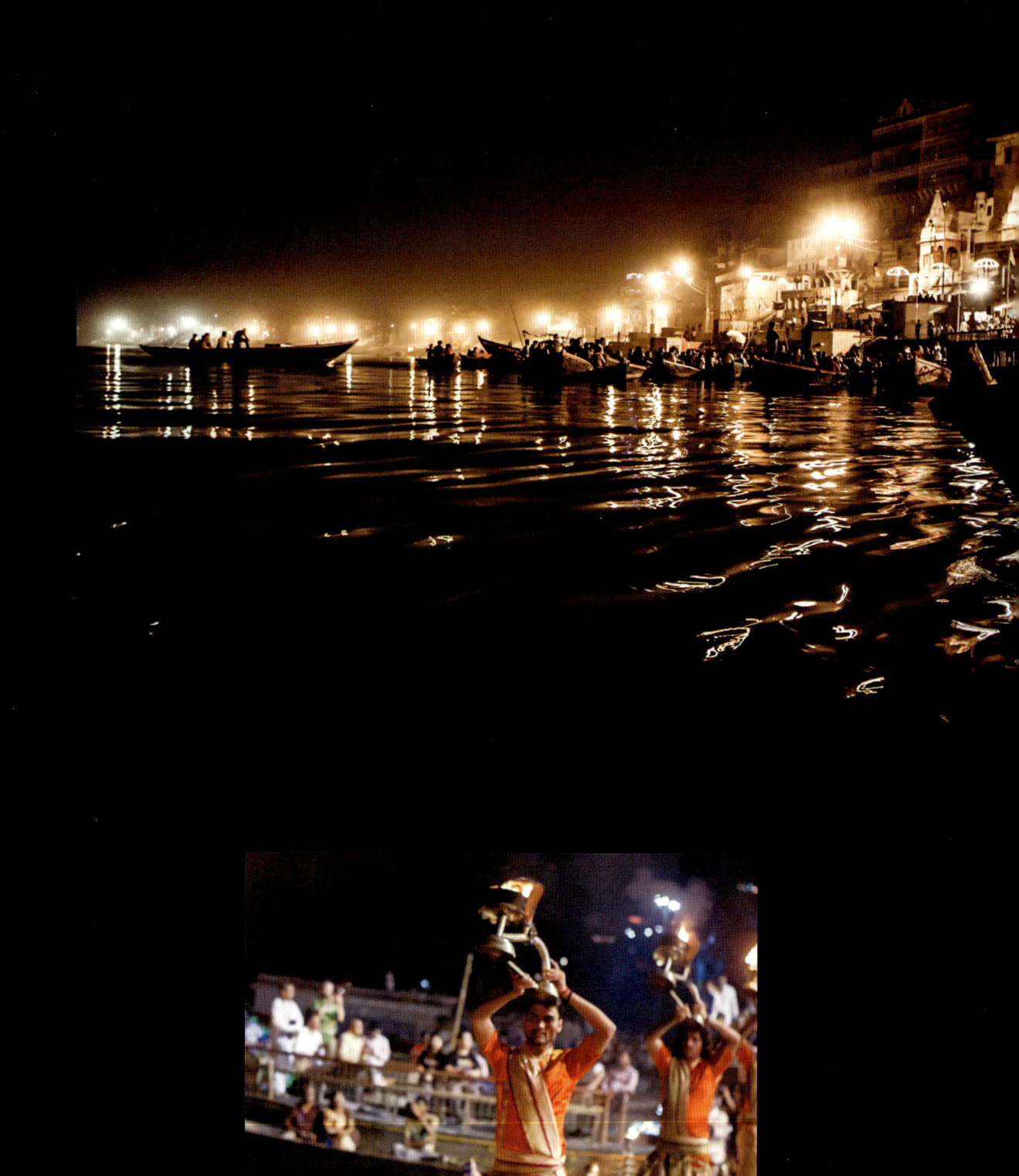

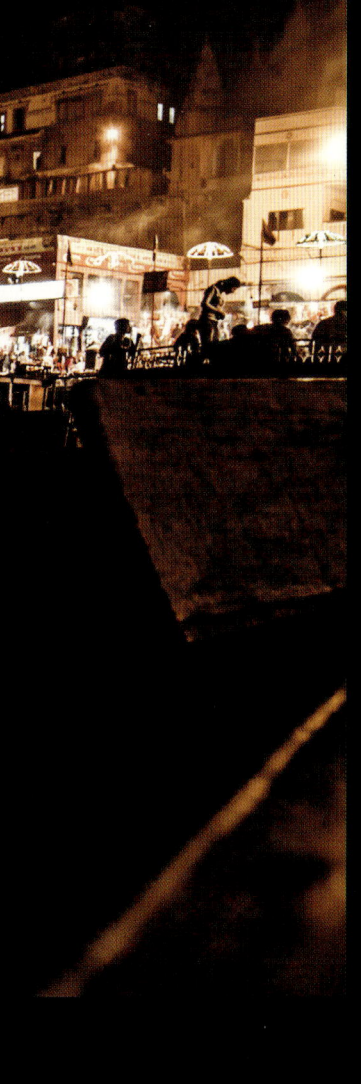
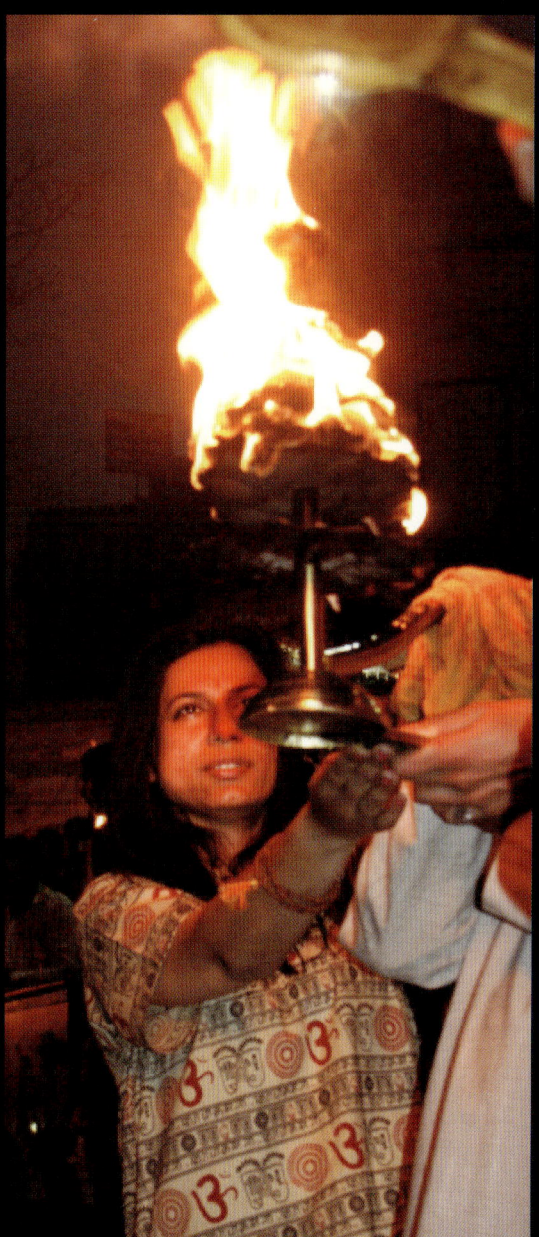

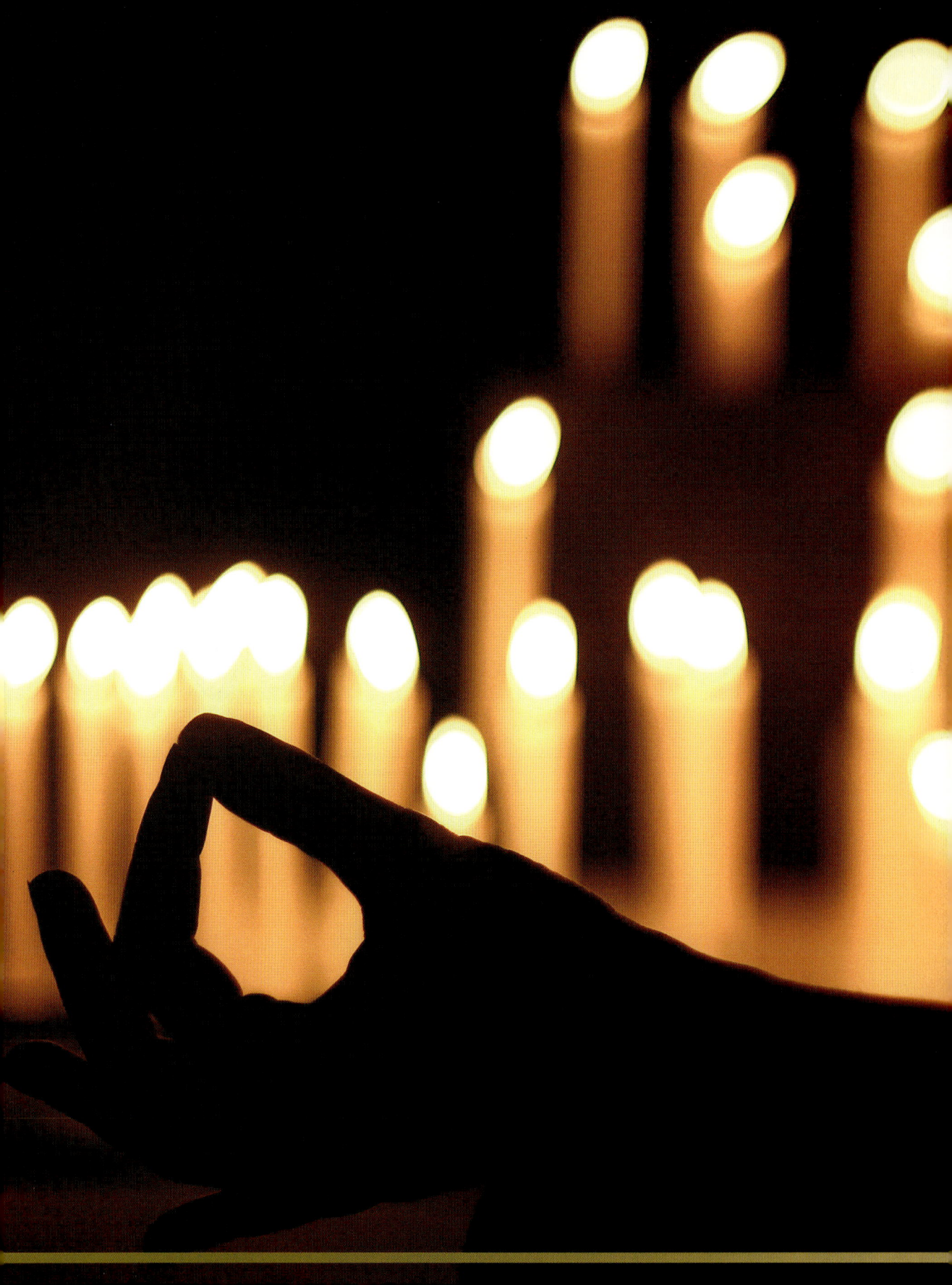

CANDLELIGHT

Awareness

Walk onto the mat or into your space. For a change, begin with your left foot to promote awareness and balance. Assume sukhasana (or kneel) with your hands in the gesture of knowledge or *gyan mudra* – join the thumb and forefinger, keeping the other fingers straight but relaxed. Breathe quietly for a few moments, sitting taller as you do so.

Gazing

You will need a candle to do this. Gazing opens the inner energy channels or *kriyas*. Light the candle and perform candle gazing or *tratakam*. Sit tall and breathe gently. Look intently at a small part of the candle flame. Blink if you need to, let your eyes water if they do, and if they feel tired, gently close them. Feel a cooling and clearing in your sinuses and clarification in your mind. Conclude and remain in pose, breathing gently.

BREATHING

Adopt a sitting position with your legs out in front of you. Begin to breathe slowly and deeply, using your abdomen only. Release your abdominal muscles a little when you breathe out. Rest after every couple of breaths. Introduce pauses or *kumbhakas* at the top and bottom of the breath. These are when the benefits occur – they will gradually become natural. Conclude and rest quietly in the pose.

Jalamdhara Bandha or Waterpipe Lock Pose

Sit in an easy pose. Sit tall and lift your head to the top of your neck, letting it tip back a little. Begin to turn down, without bending forward, as if you wanted to look at something on your chest. Feel your chest lifting as you do this and breathe in. Continue breathing by using your new abdomen technique.

To conclude, breathe gently and lift your head up and slightly back, straightening it from the chest upwards. The idea of this is to strengthen the effects of prana in your upper body.

MEDITATION

Meditate on breath, but see if you can begin to notice when your single-minded concentration or *dharana* changes into effortless contemplation or *dhyana*. In Japanese, this is known as Zen.

Relaxation

Lie quietly and breathe. Relaxation is just 'letting go', physically, mentally and emotionally. Learn to do this in your yoga and you will find that it stays with you through the rest of the day.

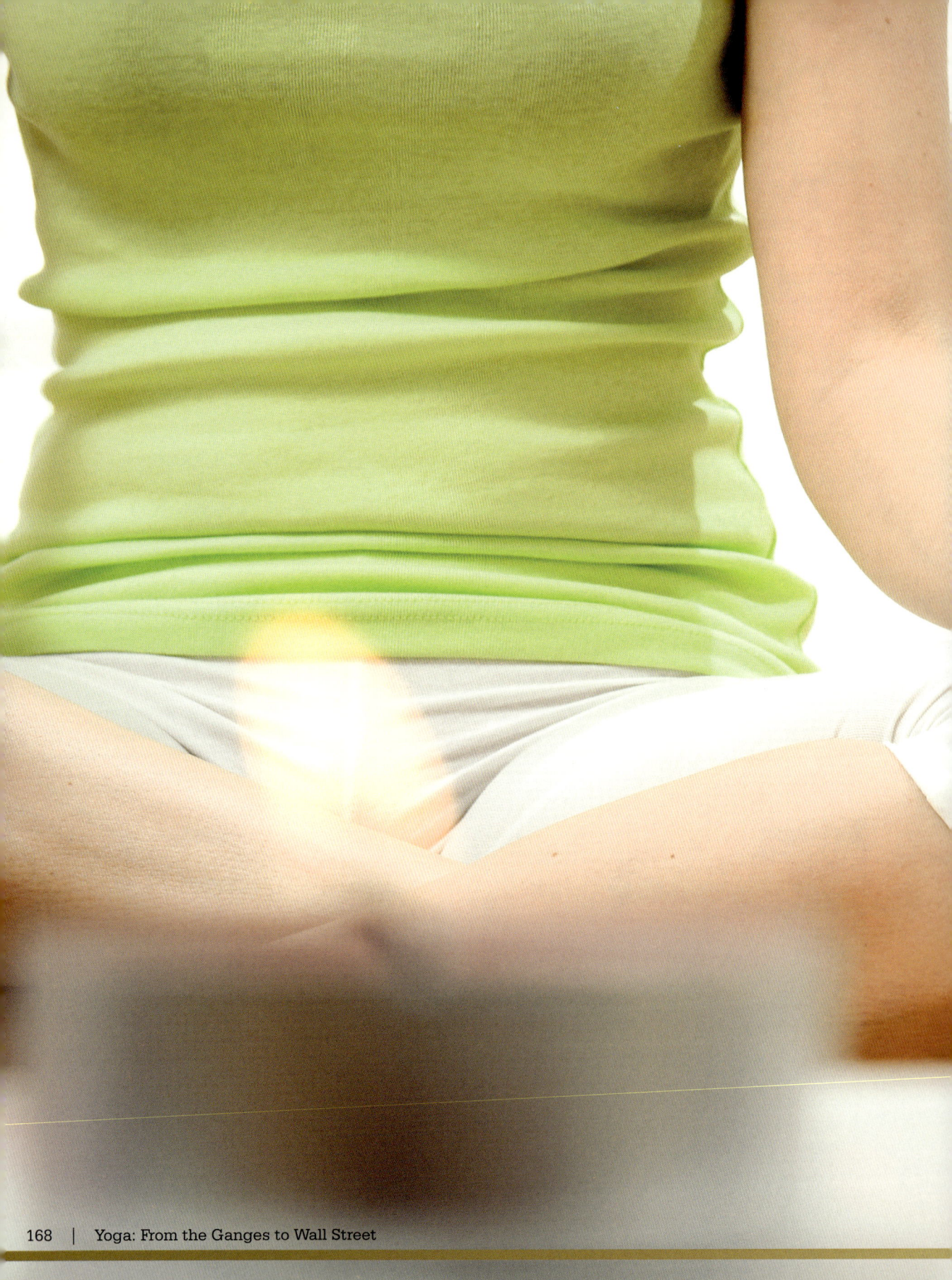

CANDLELIGHT MEDITATION

Becoming Aware

Assume the easy pose with your hands in the gesture of knowledge. Be aware and calm.

Directing Inner Energy

Sit in an easy pose with hands in any mudra.

Begin to curl your torso down so that the crown of your head gradually comes right down and touches the floor, just in front of your knees. Breathe quietly, and you should be able to settle into the pose for as long as you wish.

The devout feeling you may experience will give you a glimpse of the yoga of devotion or bhakti yoga. Curl up again, from the waist, bringing your head up last.

Meditation

Have a candle burning. Return to the easy pose, sit tall and look straight ahead, concentrating on the candle. Observe the flame closely – its size, shape, color and movement. Look at the candlestick, and make a note of everything about it. Look at any shadows cast by the candle onto the floor. Try doing this in the dark and see how effective it is.

You will probably find that you are tired after this intense concentration or dharana. Instead of looking at the candle, you are just 'seeing' it. Let this happen. Gently return to a state of concentration, blow out the candle and relax for a few moments.

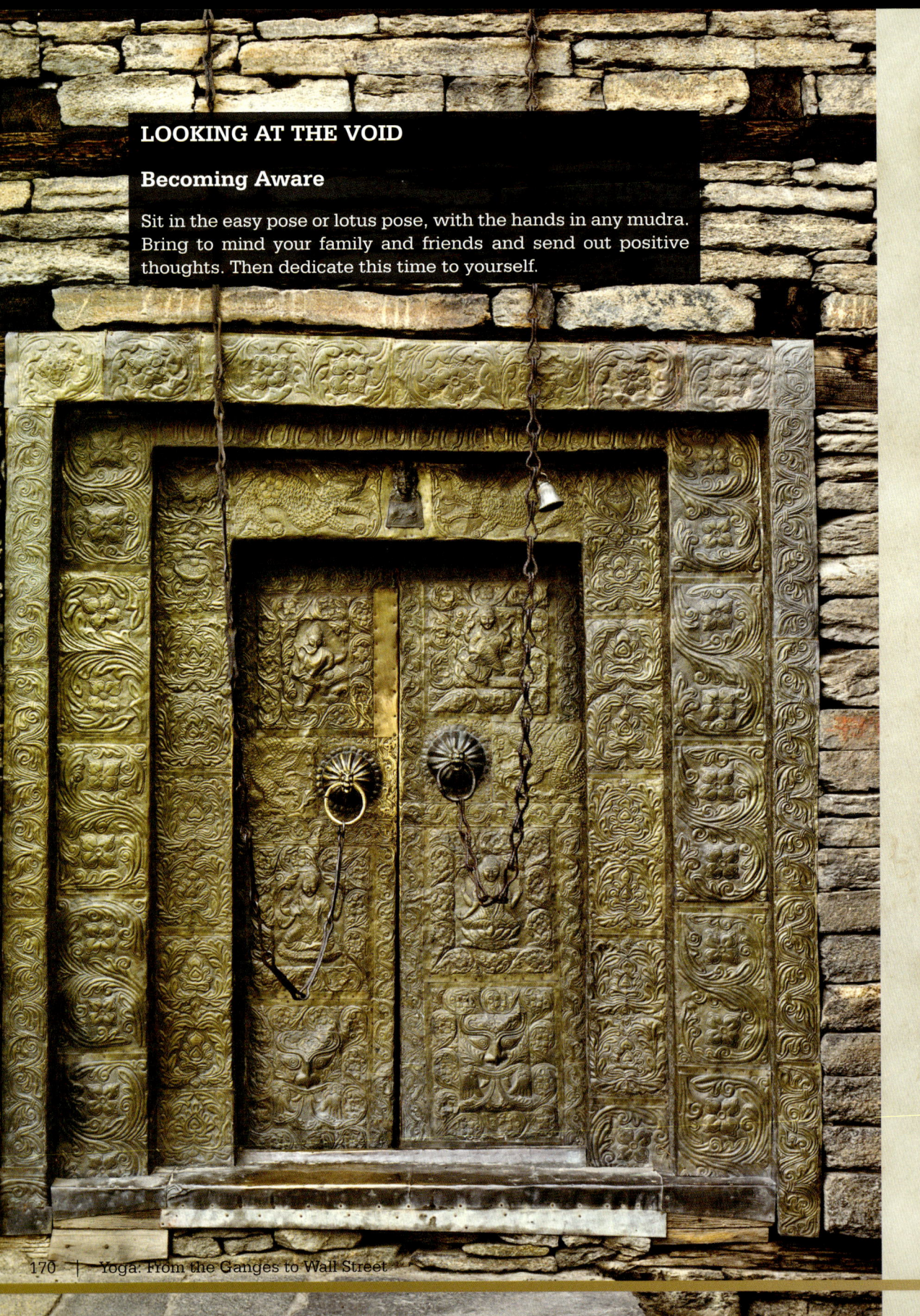

LOOKING AT THE VOID

Becoming Aware

Sit in the easy pose or lotus pose, with the hands in any mudra. Bring to mind your family and friends and send out positive thoughts. Then dedicate this time to yourself.

Opening Energy Channels

Stay in the pose of the expert, with the gesture of consciousness, and perform the shining skull breathing technique. Make the abdomen movements as small as you can, without losing the rhythm or the style. Try to make little punchy tugs of the muscles around your navel with exhalations, with little automatic inhalations between them. If the movements are small, you can make them quicker – aim for about two a second.

Breathing

Sit comfortably with your eyes closed. Take a couple of minutes to relax. Pay attention to what is being experienced in the moment – sounds, physical sensations, emotions, without attempting to make a move. Proceed like this for a short time, allowing yourself to settle down.

Focus on your breath. Just notice how it moves in and out smoothly the breath as it moves in and out as the body breathes in and breathes out. Try not to attempt to control it. Notice all the subtle elements of the experience of breathing – the inclination of the air moving all through the nose, the way the body moves as it inhales, and so on.

Predictably, the wandering mind will be uncontrollable, which is perfectly fine. This is why meditation is needed! When you see that you are no longer focusing on your breath, bring your attention back to it.

Directing Inner Energy

We are going to practice the *boochari mudra*, also called the seal of the void or looking at the void. Sit tall and breathe gently throughout. Place your right thumbnail on the tip of your nose and lift your little finger so you can focus on it. Spend a few moments getting this right. Blink when you need to, but you will probably find that as you get used to it, you won't need to.

Put your hand back on your thigh, in the gesture of consciousness, and continue looking at the space where your little finger was. Close your eyes when they get tired or your focus changes to normal and perform the exercise again. The prana behind your eyes is stimulated and your subtle awareness is heightened. It actually works best if you sit facing a blank wall.

Meditation

Sit tall in the pose of the expert and concentrate on your candle. Let contemplation gradually affect you and maybe you will feel the deep joy that is the sign of yogic bliss or *samadhi*. Most of the yoga that we do is meant to 'put us back together', but there is a further, more important stage when we begin to be less aware of 'us' and start to 'float away on the universal ocean'. Remember that your meditation is not over until you have passed back through the three stages – yogic bliss, contemplation and concentration.

Relaxation

Lie on your back and lift your left knee (right knee first next time) to your chest, breathing gently. Put it down again. Repeat with the right knee. Finally, raise both the knees. Do this again if you wish: you can perform this up to three or four times if you are not in a hurry.

Yoga for Professionals

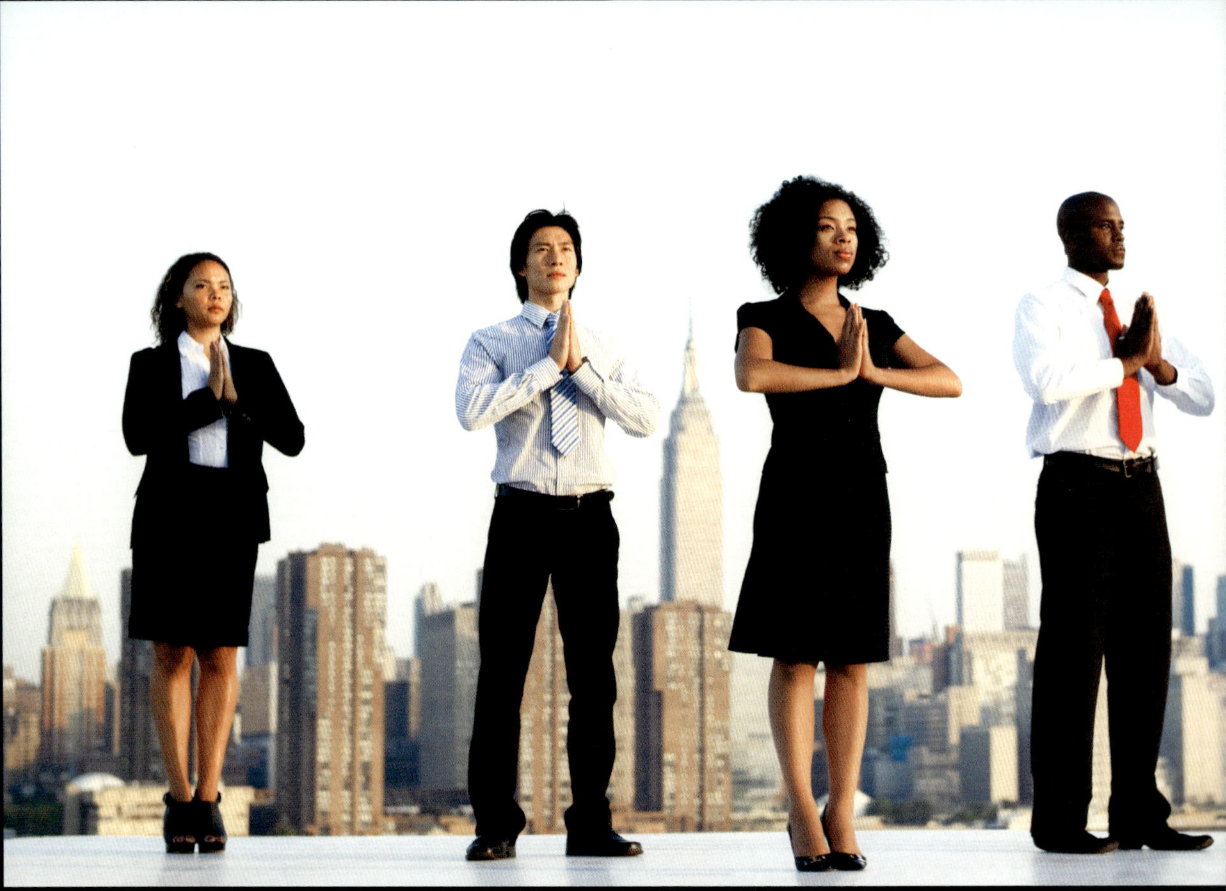

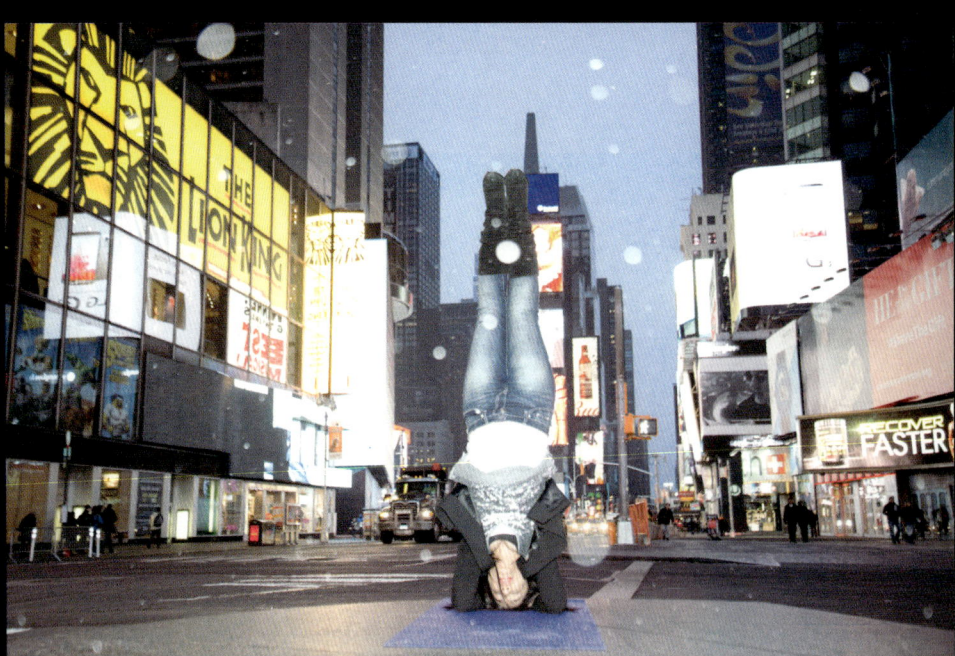

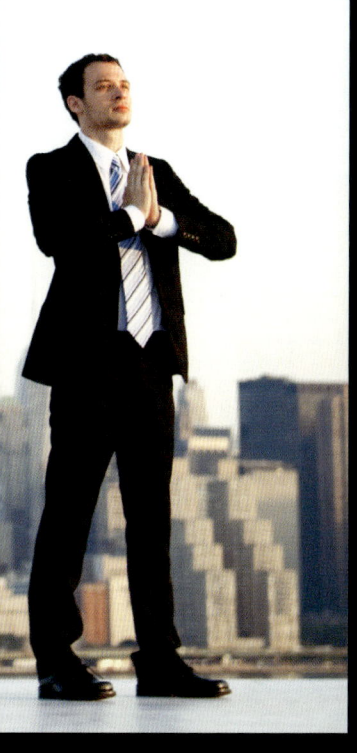

Anyone can practice yoga. There are numerous benefits of practicing yoga. It aids with stress relief and offers a rare sense of complete relaxation.

All you need to practice yoga is a small amount of space and a genuine desire to live a healthier, more mindful, and more fulfilling lifestyle. You can reap the benefits of yoga with regular practice. For each of the poses explained here, you only need to set aside a two to five minute break in your busy schedule. Once you make the time for yoga and get accustomed to practicing it, doing yoga becomes a habit just like brushing your teeth, making coffee, or any other part of your morning routine. If your schedule is so busy that you do not think you have the time to practice these exercises even for a few minutes each day, that is a sign that you are someone who would benefit the most from doing yoga.

Energy is vital to health. In yoga, this energy is known as prana - the vital force. Prana enters the body every single time you breathe, and all exercises you do in yoga focus on your breathing patterns.

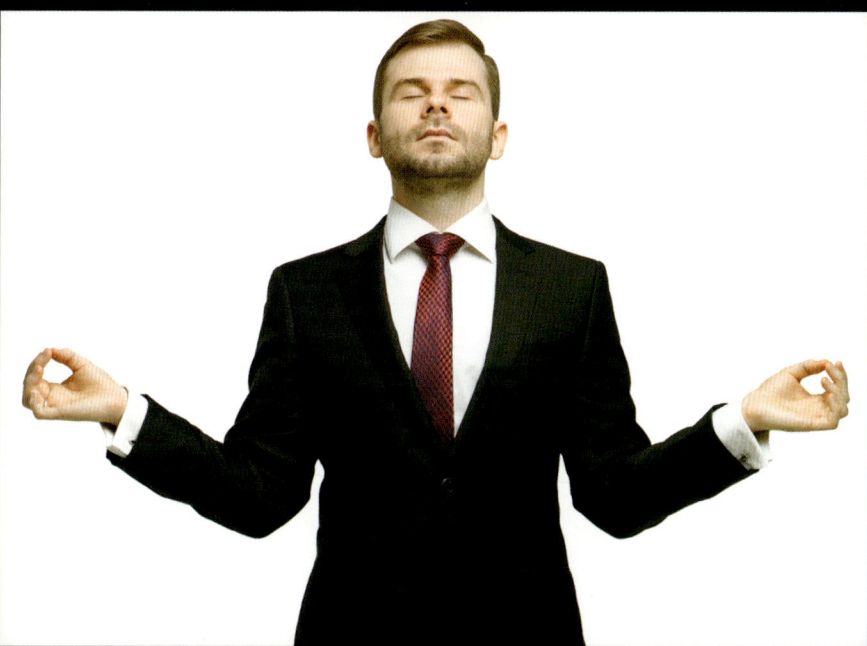

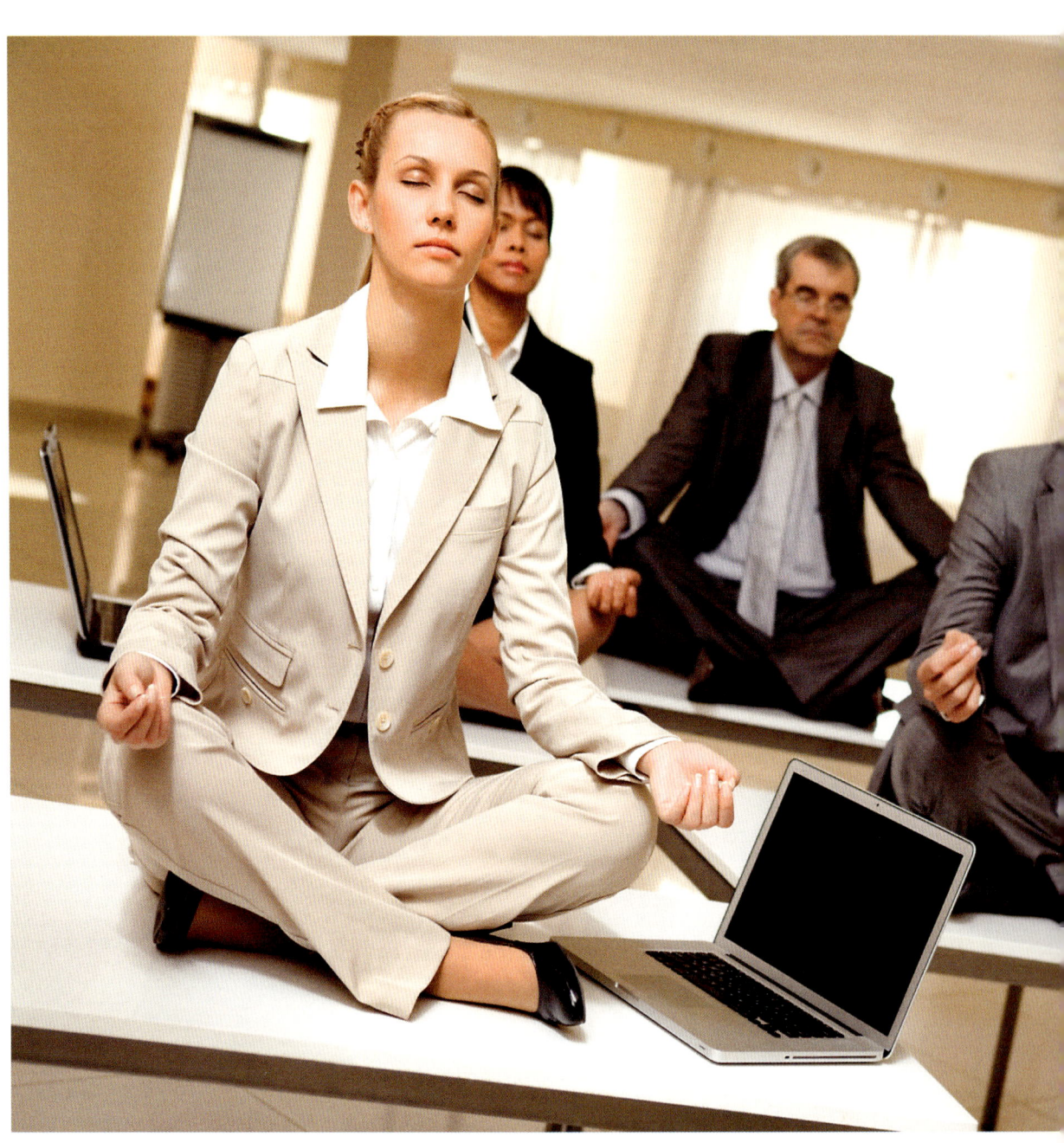

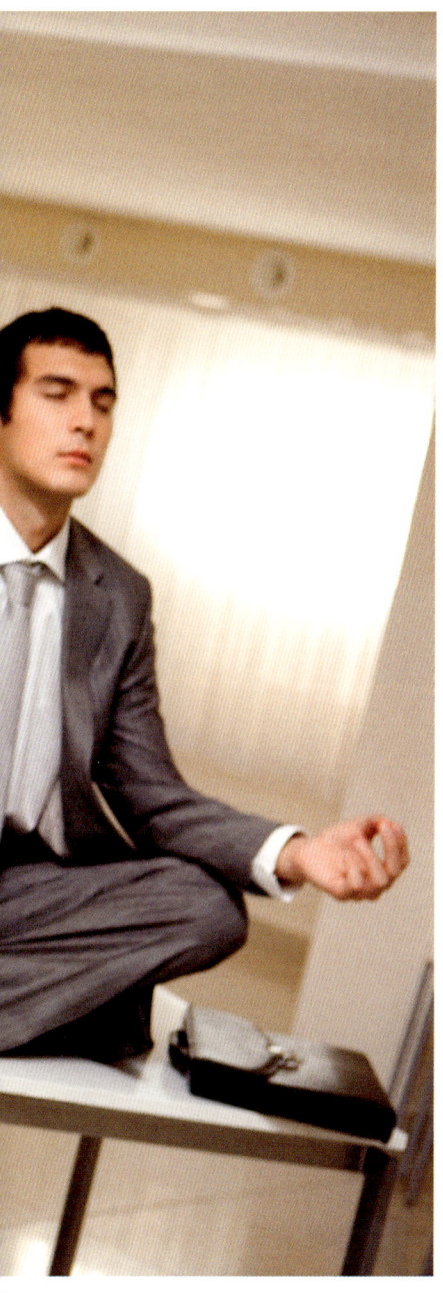

Eye Defender

In the office, people often complain of eye problems such as eyestrain, itchy eyes, headaches, fatigue, dry eyes and difficulty in focusing after long periods of computer use. These symptoms stem from a health issue called Computer Vision Syndrome (CVS). There are many different causes for eyestrain symptoms. When the muscle inside the eye that controls the eye's focus is overworked, eyestrain symptoms can occur. In many cases, these symptoms will not show up immediately, but rather, will arise after a few hours of working on the computer. When the muscle in the eye becomes fatigued, eye discomfort may result. A mild headache also may occur as the strain on the eye worsens. In some cases, the muscle within the eye can become so fatigued that it is unable to fully stop focusing. This leads to blurred distance vision.

Here are some basic exercises that you can easily practice while sitting on your chair. These exercises will serve to relax your eyes and prevent issues such as headaches, eyestrain, dry eyes and difficulty in focusing. They will keep you fresh and improve the quality of your work in the office.

EYE ROLL EXERCISE

Time duration: One minute

Like any other muscle in the body, eye muscles require exercise to be healthy and strong.

Benefits

The eye roll will strengthen the eye muscles, prevent eyestrain and improve eyesight.

Method

- Look up and look down. Repeat twice.
- Look as far right and then as far left as possible. Repeat twice.
- Look to the top right corner and look to the bottom left corner. Repeat five times.
- Look to the top left and look to bottom right corner. Repeat twice.
- Look up and rotate your eyes clockwise. Repeat twice. Do the same thing counter-clockwise twice.
- Look at your thumb, then the wall, then back.
- Have an imaginary orbit around your head.

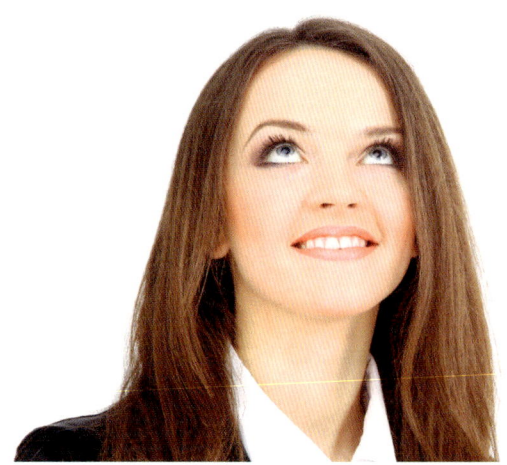

PALMING

Time duration: Thirty seconds to one minute

After completing the eye roll exercises, do palming to relax the eye muscles.

Palming is an ancient yoga relaxation technique and is similar to meditation in many ways.

Benefits

Natural vision improvement is primarily about relaxing the vision system and releasing mental strain. Palming is an effective means of achieving relaxation.

Method

- Rub your hands together vigorously until you feel warmth in your palms.
- Place your palms and fingers over your closed eyes.
- The darkness and heat generated by rubbing the hands will relax and soothe your eyes.

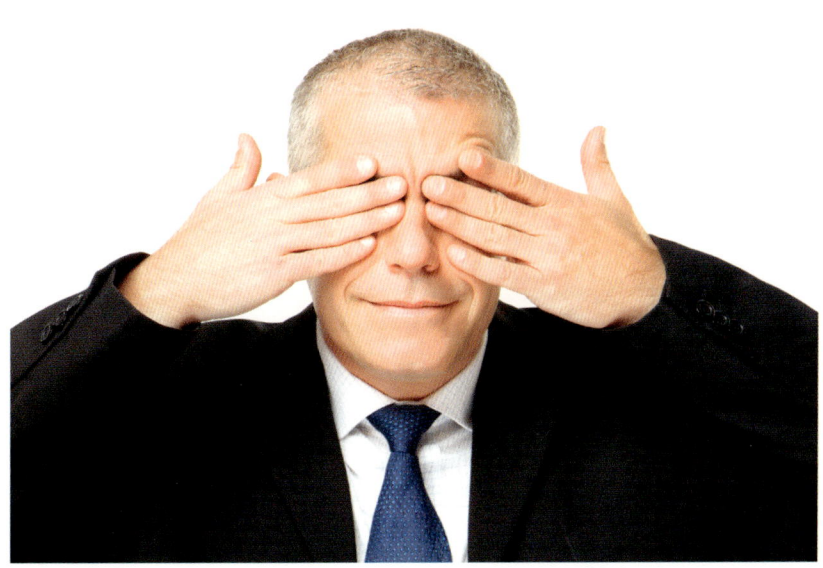

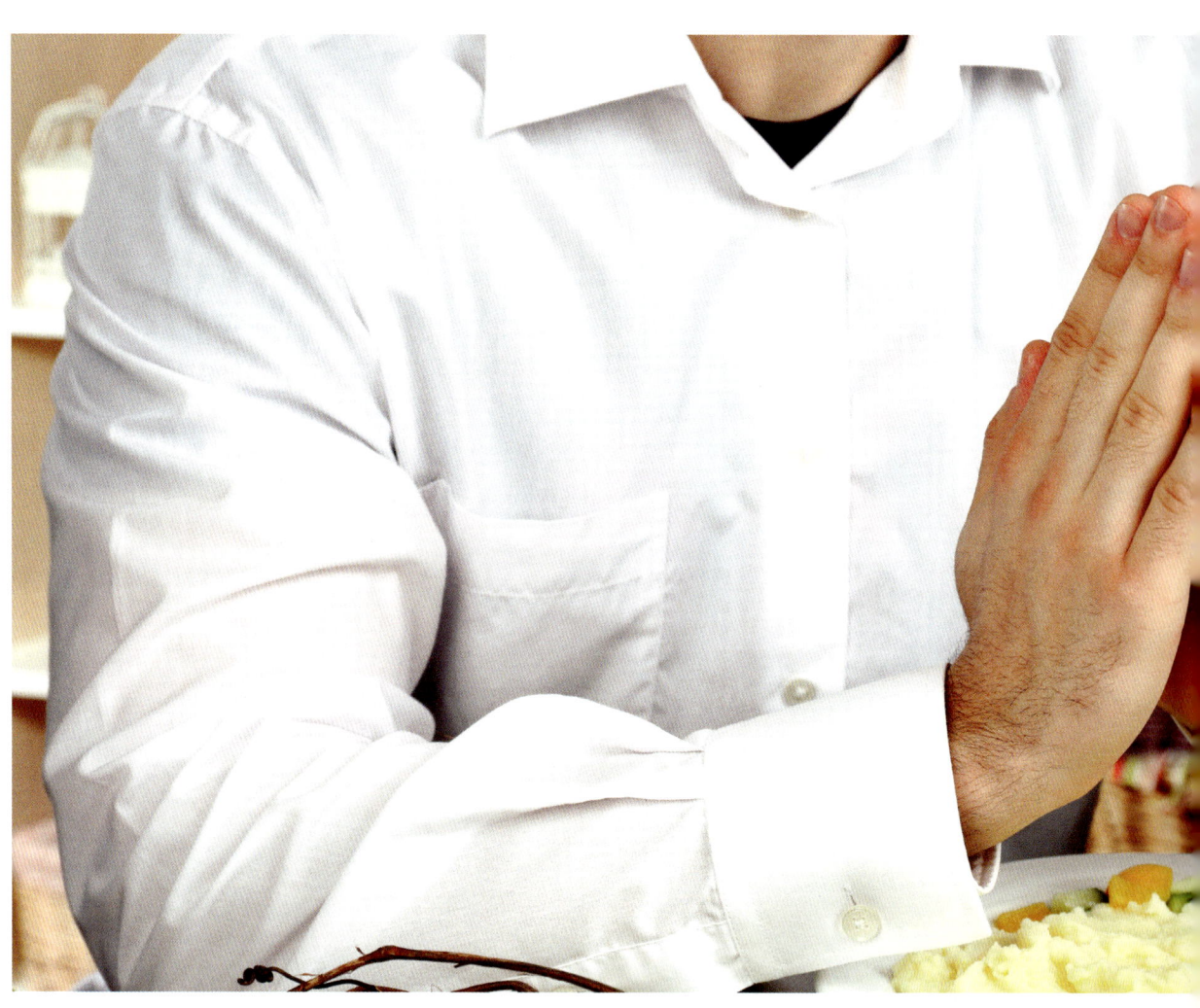

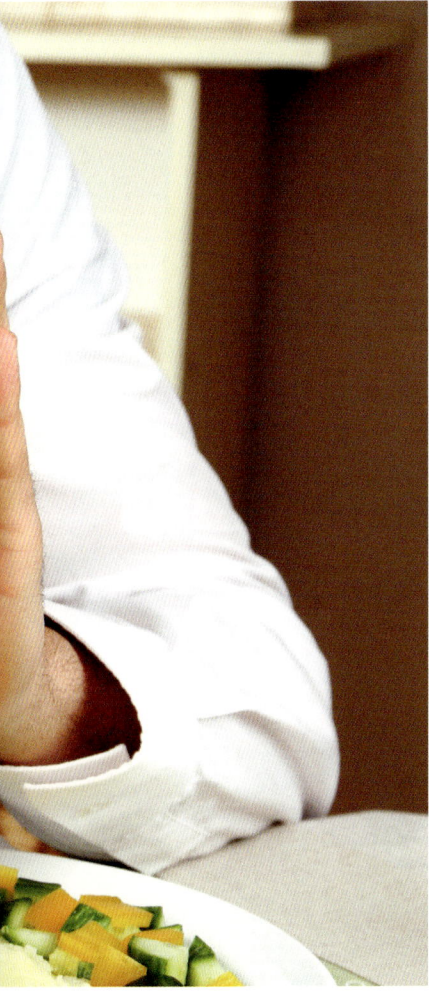

Eat to Live

Due to our busy schedules, we barely get enough time to relax and eat proper meals. Sometimes we end up eating at our desks at work, lacking sufficient time to even think about the digestion of our food. Studies have proven that our stomach behaves very differently when we rush our meals as opposed to when we eat our food in peace. Eating food under stressful conditions leads to poor health, even if the food is healthy. Here are some exercises that make you feel the good kind of hunger and then help you with the digestive process.

"Practice conscious eating. Your digestion is affected by the conversations at the table, your environment, and your mood when you eat. If you're having an argument or watching a violent TV show, your stomach will knot and your digestion will be disturbed. To extract the most nourishment from your food, never eat when you feel upset. Create a settled, peaceful atmosphere for your meals, eat only when you're hungry, and choose fresh, organic food whenever possible."

— Dr Deepak Chopra

RIGHT NOSTRIL BREATHING: BEFORE MEALS

Time duration: One to two minutes

Before you eat your meal, check the flow of your breath in the nostrils. We typically breathe from one nostril at a time, with the flow of our 'breathing' changing at specific intervals. According to yogic principles, the right nostril is connected to the left hemisphere of the brain, which controls the physical actions of the body, including digestion. The left nostril's breathing is an indicator of bad physical health. Eating food when you are breathing from the left nostril can result in impaired digestion. Eat at a time when the right nostril is active.

You can practice this at the table or at any location where you plan to eat your meal.

Benefits

It improves digestion, and good digestion helps with weight control.

Method

- With your food in front of you, sit comfortably and shut your eyes.

- Use your finger to close your left nostril.

- Breathe abdominally from your right nostril until it opens up (around a minute and a half).

- Shut your eyes and inhale and exhale in a natural manner several times.

- Imagine yourself having a healthy meal. Imagine yourself starving.

- Open your eyes.

- Eat your food.

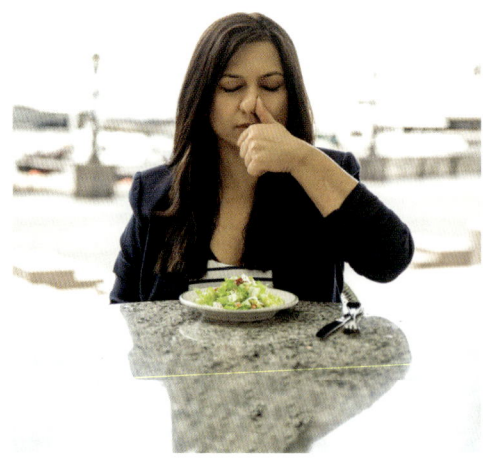

THUNDERBOLT POSE OR VAJRASANA: AFTER MEALS

Time duration: Two minutes

You can practice this pose at the office, or at home. All this pose requires is a sitting place on the floor and two minutes of your time.

Digestion is the key of food consumption, and the best way to digest properly is to walk. However, since we are often busy with work and many other things, an alternative option is a two-minute vajarasana. Two minutes of this pose is equivalent to a thirty-minute stroll.

Benefits

This asana alters blood flow and nervous impulses in the pelvic region as well as strengthening the pelvic muscles. The entire digestive system gets a boost of efficiency by relieving stomach issues such as hyperacidity and peptic ulcer.

Method

- Kneel on the floor.

- Bring your big toes together and separate the heels, forming a 'V' shape with the feet.

- Sit on your heels.

- Place your hands on your knees with your palms down.

- The back and the head should be completely straight.

- Close your eyes, then relax your arms and your whole body.

- Breathe normally and focus your attention on the flow of air traveling in and out of your nostrils.

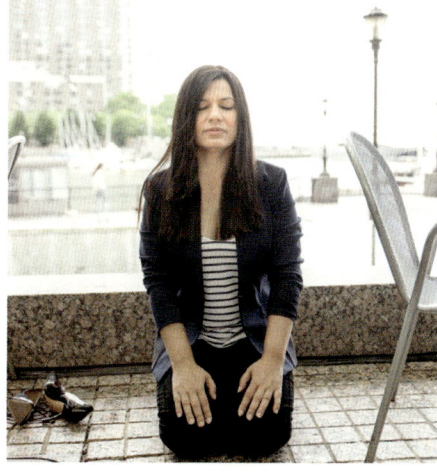

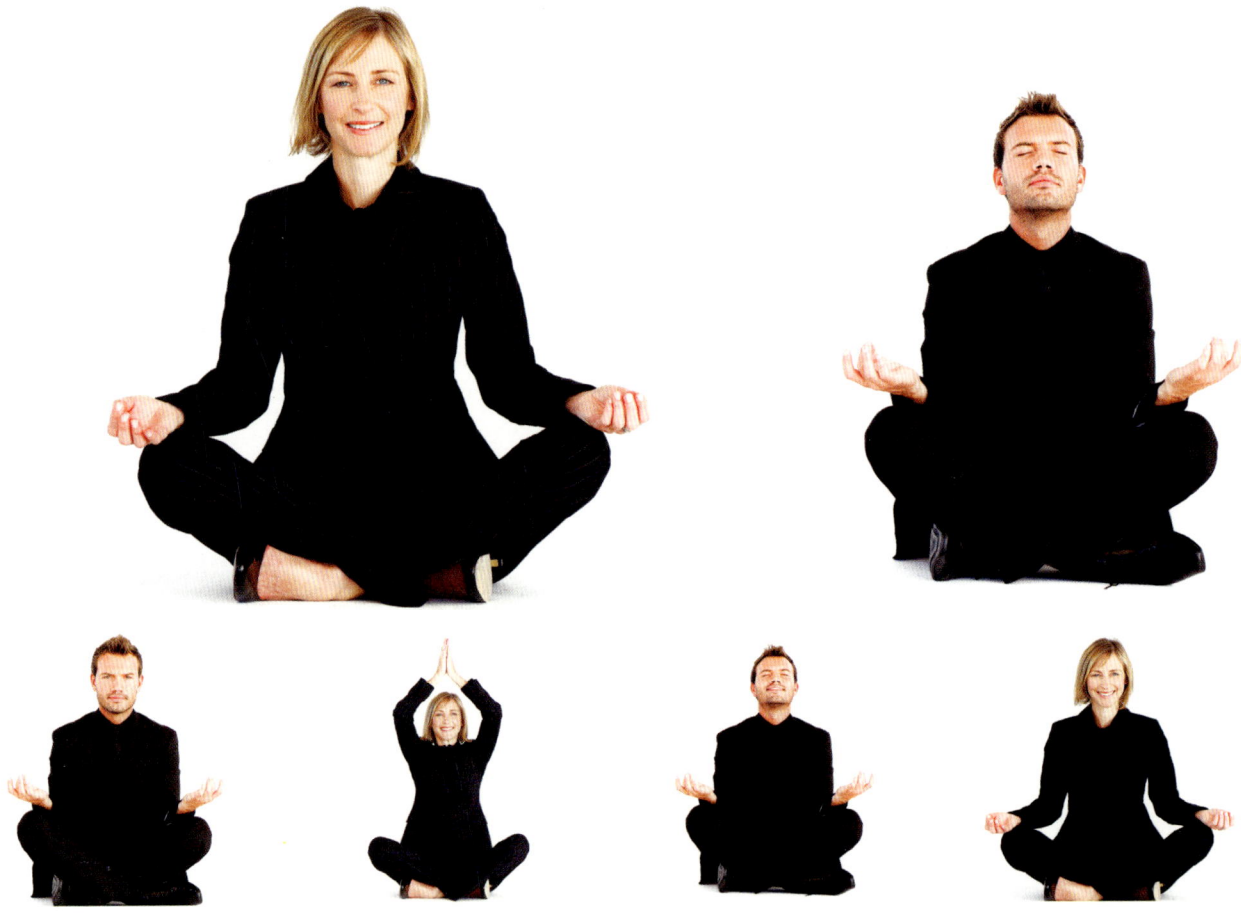

Effective Meetings

In the professional world, attending meetings is part of the job. There are several kinds of meetings, however at most of them the participants are expected to solve problems and discuss new ideas. A stressed mind can result in an unsuccessful performance and poor input at meetings. This is because stress prevents the mind from achieving full productivity. A balanced and relaxed mind is always significantly more successful and productive than an agitated mind. Nervousness not only damages your mood and negatively impacts your work, but is also the root of health issues such as palpitation, a dry mouth and a churning stomach.

Stress is inevitable in the workplace, but controlling our stress levels is up to us. To defeat the symptoms of stress, breathing exercises are highly effective. These exercises can be performed anywhere at any time.

The best way to achieve relaxation and balance the mind before a meeting is to practice this asana.

ALTERNATE NOSTRIL BREATHING OR *ANULOM VILOM*

Time duration: Two to three minutes

Anulom vilom harmonizes the left and right sides of the brain, allowing logical and creative thoughts to come together. It keeps you balanced and focused. Also, the increased oxygen flow in the body turns negative thoughts into positive ones. Before going into a meeting that you are perhaps nervous about, sit in a chair with your spine straight and practice Anulom Vilom for two or three minutes.

Benefits

Alternate nostril breathing balances your mind and body. It keeps your energy from being drained and helps you achieve stillness of the mind. It also helps you improve your sense of personal boundaries and stops you from worrying about other people's emotions and energy.

Method

Sit comfortably in your office chair with your hands in a meditative position. Take a few deep breaths for about thirty seconds.

After taking a few deep breaths, sit with your right hand in Vishnu mudra – press the middle finger and the right index finger against the palm, extending the thumb and the other two fingers. The left hand can relax on the knee.

Round 1

- Inhale through the left nostril, closing your nostril with the right thumb, and count to four in your mind.
- Closing both nostrils, hold your breath to the count of sixteen.
- Exhale through the right nostril, closing the left nostril with the little and the ring finger and count to eight in your mind.
- Inhale through the right nostril, left nostril should be kept closed with the little fingers, and count four.
- Hold your breath, closing both nostrils, to the count of sixteen.
- Exhale through the left nostril, while your right nostril is closed with the thumb, and count eight.

Repeat Round 1 two to three times.

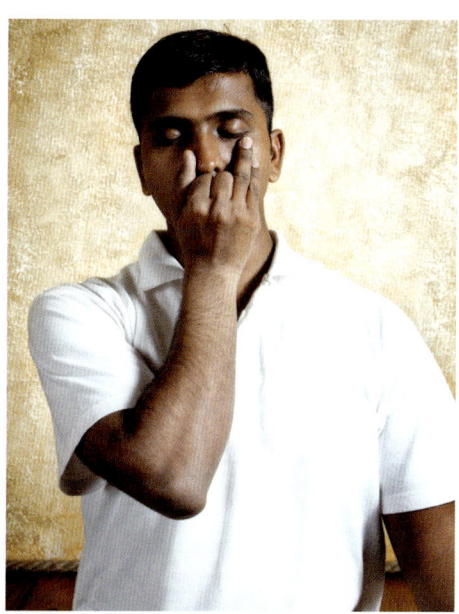

1. Breathe in through the left nostril and count four.
2. Hold the breath and close both nostrils and count sixteen.
3. Breathe out through the right nostril and count eight.
4. Breathe in through the right nostril and count four.
5. Hold the breath and close both nostrils and count sixteen.
6. Breathe out through the left nostril and count eight.

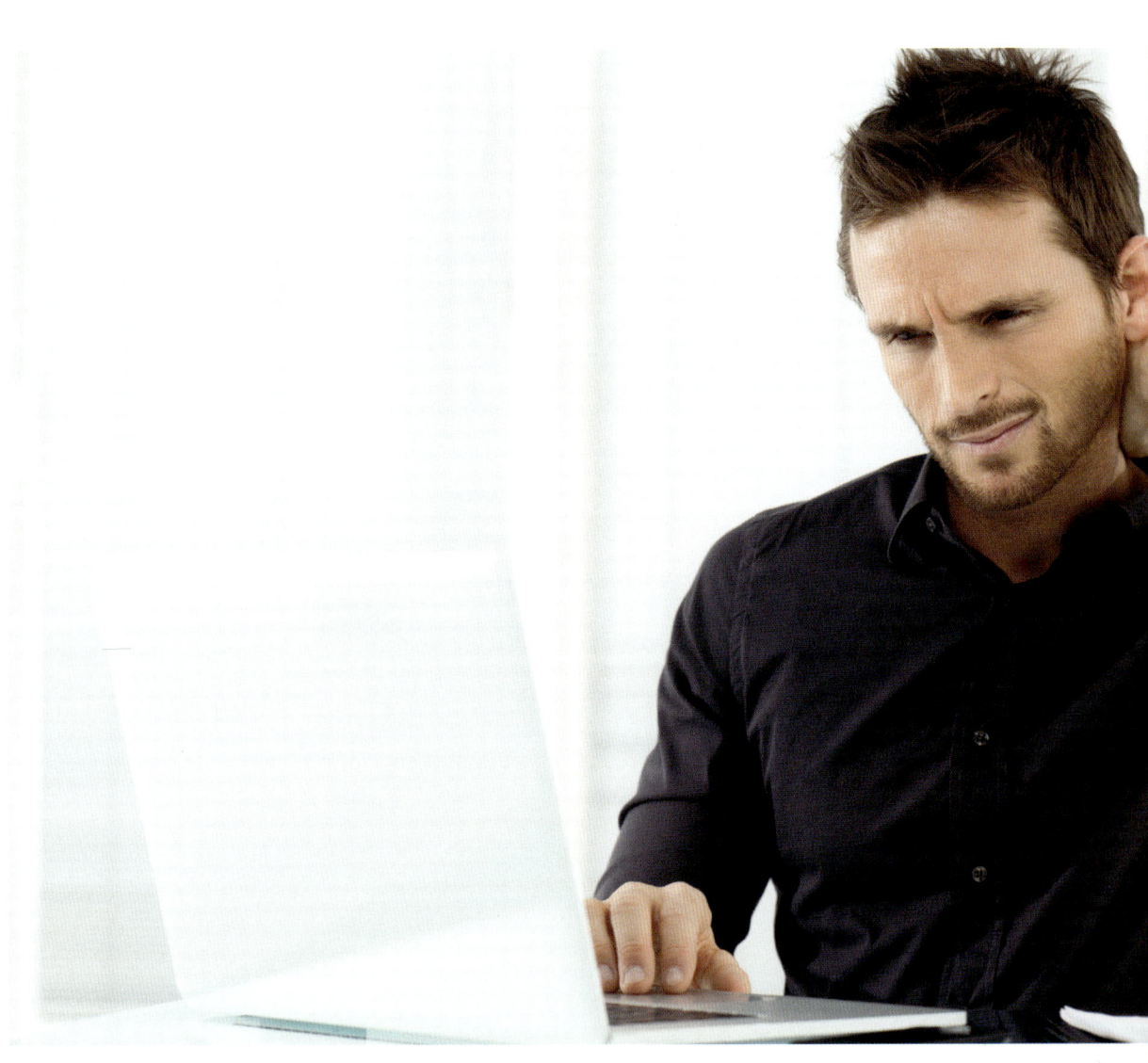

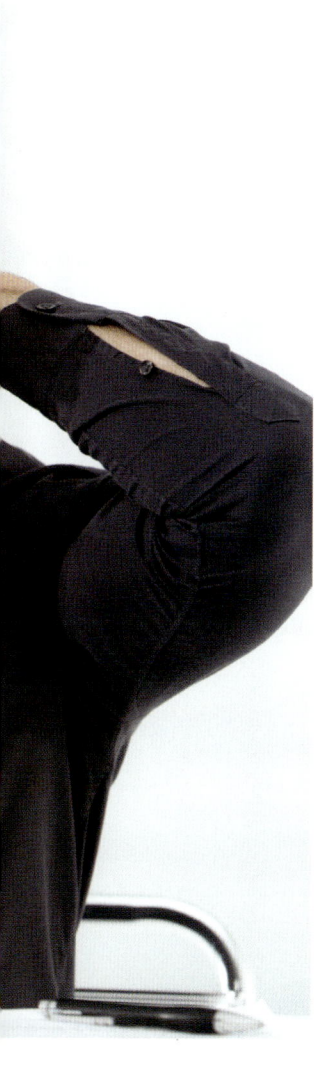

Pain in the Neck

Unpleasant situations can create tension in the neck muscles and cause neck pain, hence the idiom 'pain in the neck'. In our day-to-day lives, we come across many people and situations that are unpleasant. This can result in tension in our neck muscles and can lead to neck pain. This tension is worsened when we sit for long hours in a chair without getting up and moving. This could jeopardize your health, as it adversely affects the muscles in the torso, neck and shoulders. These parts of the body are somewhat immobile when you are sitting, the blood vessels are squeezed, and there is a reduction in the blood supply in these places, resulting in fatigue. In turn, this can cause overall exhaustion and stiffness. Moreover, this can lead to the spinal nerves being impinged and cause the electric impulses moving to and fro from the brain to all parts of the body to be disturbed. Malfunction of the glands and the organs can follow.

To prevent these conditions, it is essential to release the tension in the back regularly. If you are one of those people who sit at a desk all day long, here are some simple steps that you can follow to improve your posture and to maintain your overall health and well-being.

NECK AND SHOULDER ROLL

Time duration: One minute

Most of our tension is concentrated in our neck, shoulders and lower back, causing stiffness, bad posture and tension headaches. Repeating these exercises a couple of times while at work will help reduce the pain in your neck. Sitting on your office chair, clasp your arms around your knees, making sure you maintain an erect spine and that your head and body are completely straight.

Benefits

These neck exercises will aid in releasing blocked energy, easing pain, melting away tension knots and alleviating stiffness.

Step 1

- Head back.
- Head forward.
- Chin to chest.
- Repeat twice.

Step 2

- Right ear to right shoulder.
- Left ear to left shoulder.
- Repeat twice.

Step 3

- Neck circles.
- Head forward.
- Chin to chest.
- Right ear to right shoulder.
- Left ear to left shoulder.
- Repeat twice.
- Then opposite.
- Repeat twice.

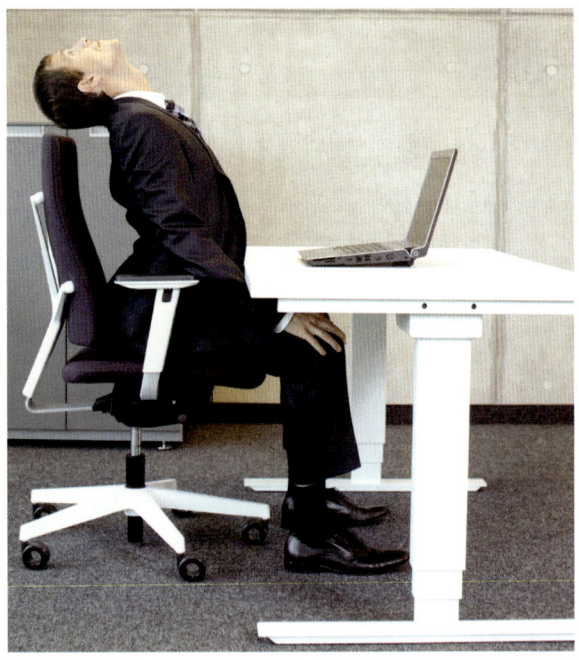

Step 4

- Right shoulder up; then down.
- Left shoulder up; then down.
- Repeat twice.

Step 5

- Both shoulders up.
- Both shoulders down.
- Repeat twice.

RESTORATION

Time duration: One minute

Before returning to work after completing the shoulder and neck exercises, give yourself a few seconds to relax. This relaxing pose is very simple, yet extremely effective in reducing stress in your facial muscles and preventing fatigue.

Benefits

Restoration helps in reducing stress.

Method

- Cross your arms and put them on the surface in front of you. Then rest your head on your crossed arms.

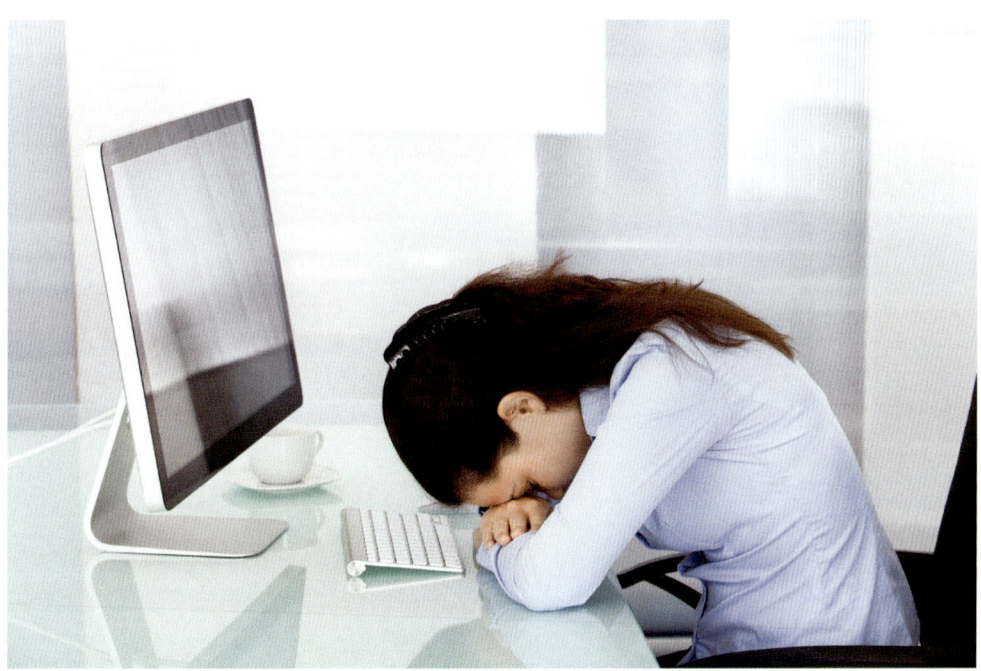

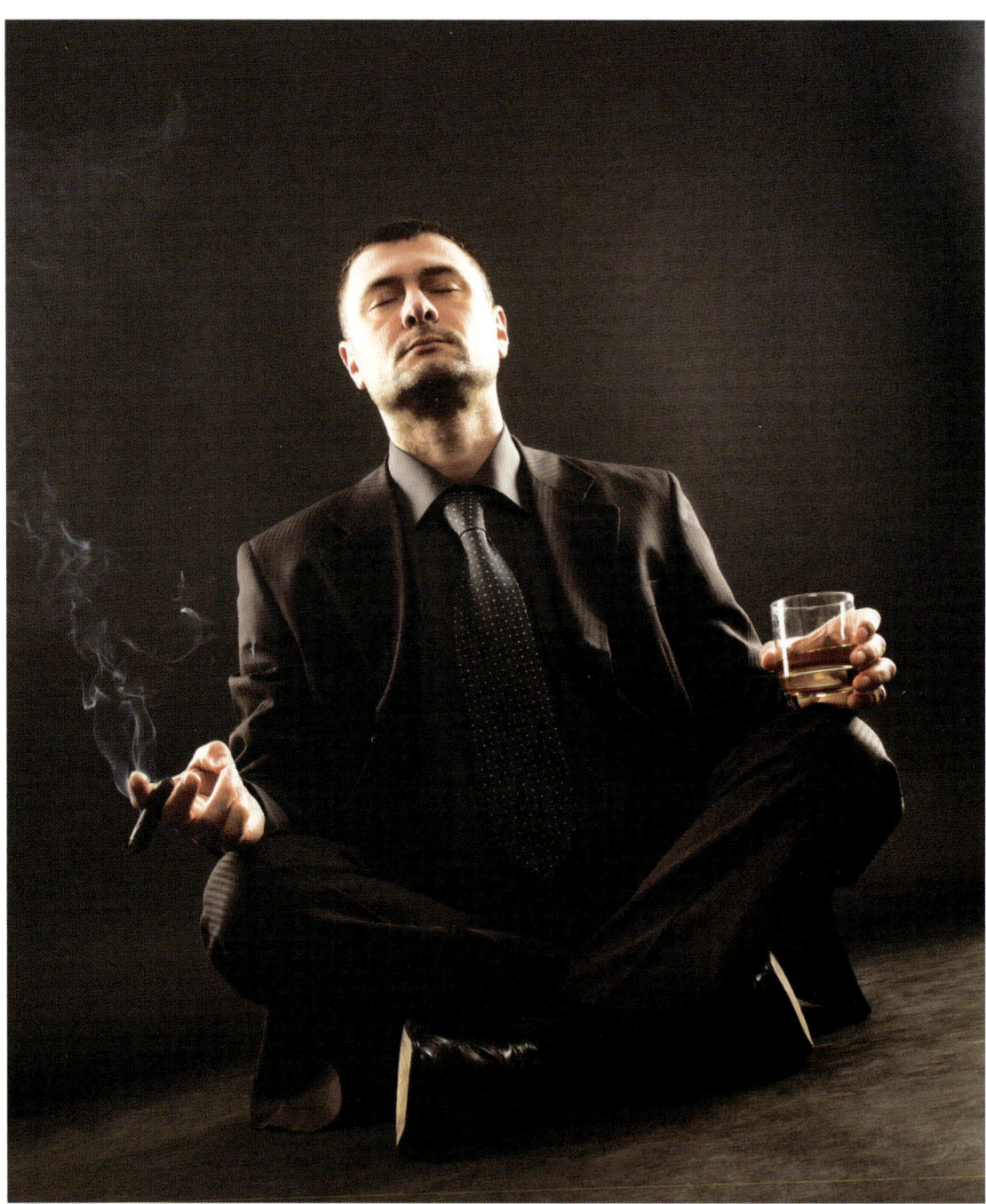

Happy Hour

Working in a stressful environment can sometimes result in a bad mood. We need entertainment to de-stress so we end up going out to the bars on the weekends, which is an effortless way of feeling happy. Alcohol may make you feel fresh and lively momentarily, but in excess, it can destroy your body completely. Alcohol weakens the liver, which is our powerhouse of energy.

Therefore, it is best to find alternatives that make you feel fresh, relaxed and happy. Fatigue is common after work because work saps the level of oxygen in our body, resulting in shallow breathing. Consequently, there is an improper intake of oxygen. Carbon dioxide starts accumulating in our body, which causes our body to feel tired and lethargic. This stale air must be effectively eliminated from the body. We need to breathe properly, engaging our lungs as fully as possible, so that our blood is again oxygenated enough to give us energy.

AGNISAR PRANAYAMA

Time duration: One to two minutes

The Sanskrit word *agni* means 'fire', *sara* means 'essence', and *kriya* means 'action'. There is no fire in the stomach, but the essence or nature of fire is comparable to the digestive process. It cures sleepiness and is important for the circulation of inner energy. In other words, the process of vital energy needs to be kindled and aroused to stimulate the most powerful digestive effects. *Agnisar kriya* or source of internal energy does just this.

Benefits

It makes the digestive fire blaze, causing the energy level to go up.

Method

- Sit in vajrasana.
- Move your knees apart and put your hands on your knees.
- Drop your chin towards your chest.
- Lift up your shoulders and stick your tongue out.
- Breathe heavily and quickly. Repeat twenty times.

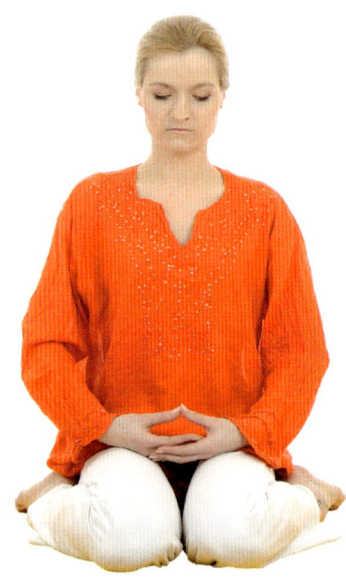

FRONTAL BRAIN PURIFICATION OR *KAPALBHATI*

Time duration: One to two minutes

The aggressive inhalation helps to freshen you up. It is equivalent to three cups of coffee. The forced exhalation eliminates stale air from the lower lungs, making room for a fresh intake of oxygen-rich air and cleansing the whole respiratory system. This is a wonderfully invigorating exercise and the perfect way to start your evening. Kapalbhati increases oxygen levels in the body. Its helps clear the mind and improve concentration. It consists of exhalations and inhalations, followed by the retention of breath. To exhale, you must contract your abdominal muscles sharply, raising the diaphragm and forcing air out of your lungs. To inhale, you must relax your muscles, allowing the lungs to fill up with air. The exhalation should be brief, active, and audible, while the inhalation is longer, passive, and silent.

Benefits

The repeated up and down movement of the diaphragm is good for the face, stomach, heart, and liver. It increases the lung capacity. Since Kapalbhati creates good movement in the diaphragm and all the respiratory organs, it makes the practice of other poses much easier. It also rejuvenates tired cells and facial nerves, keeping your face youthful-looking and wrinkle-free. It could serve as a natural replacement for Botox.

Method

- Sit in a comfortable, meditative pose, and make sure your spine is completely erect.
- Place your hands in gyan mudra.
- Close your eyes and breathe normally for thirty seconds.
- Once composed, take a deep breath.
- Exercise the diaphragm by exhaling suddenly and quickly through both nostrils. This will produce a puffing sound.
- The air will leave the lungs with a sudden, vigorous stroke while simultaneously drawing the abdominal muscles inward.
- The breath should be expelled completely.
- Don't focus on inhalation. It should be automatic and passive.
- The abdominal muscles will relax automatically.

This exercise should be done for three rounds, with each round consisting of eleven strokes (for the beginner). Each round should take about a minute. A little rest can be taken in between the rounds based on individual needs.

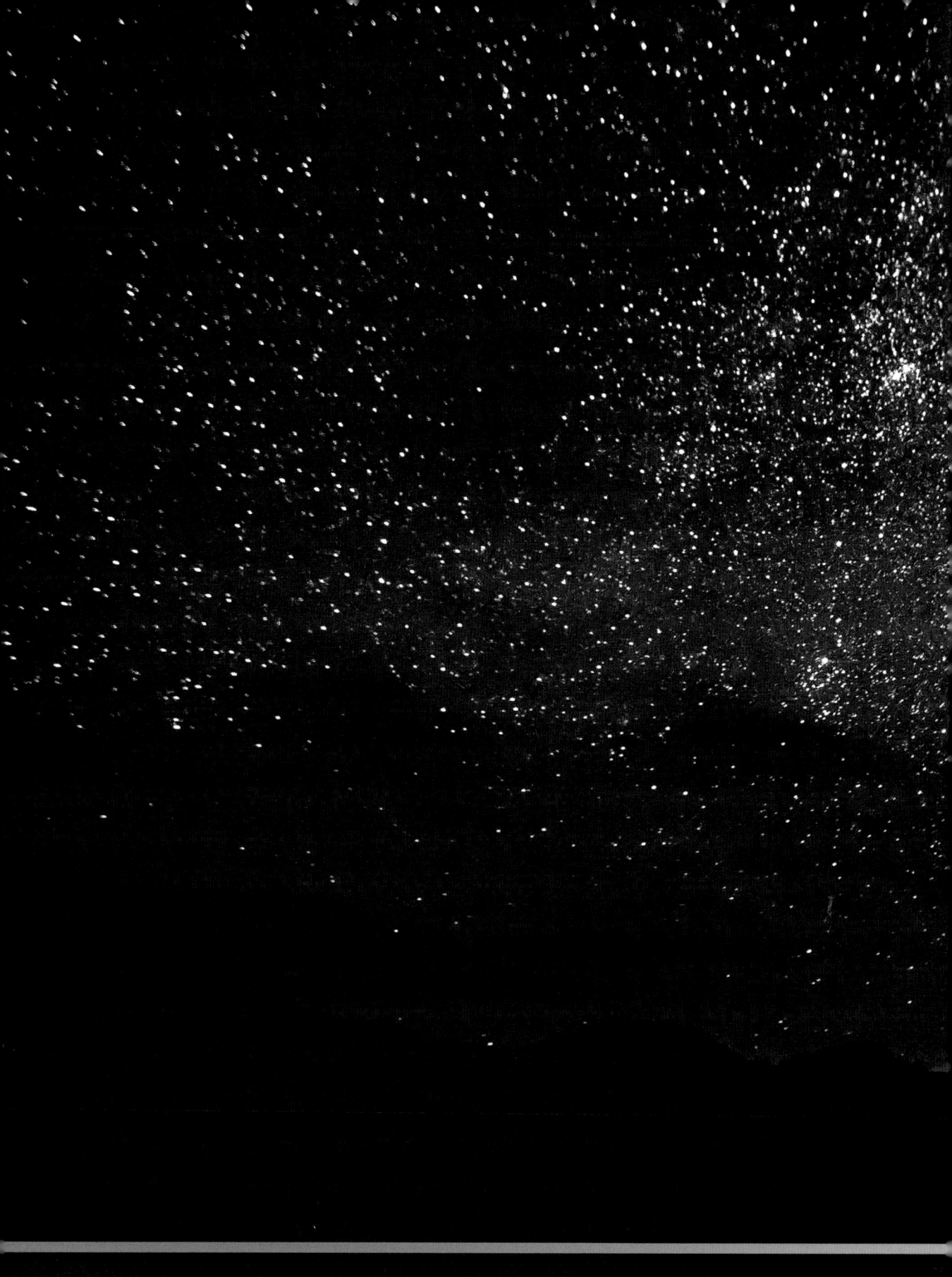

Re-pose or Yog nidra

Time duration: Ten to twenty minutes

Sleep is the most essential part of our lives. Seven to eight hours of sound sleep keeps us balanced and happy, as well as bringing us good dreams.

Most of us think that relaxation is attained by merely closing our eyes or sleeping when we feel tired. However, this will not free us from muscular, emotional and mental tension. In order to sleep soundly, we must release all our worries. This complete state of relaxation and deep sleep is obtained through a process called *yog nidra*.

Method

- Turn off the lights.
- Turn on some relaxing instrumental music.
- Lie on your bed in shavasana.

Step 1

Breathing (Pranayama)

Take twelve deep breaths while mentally saying:

- I am inhaling: twelve times
- I am exhaling: twelve times

Repeat until you reach Step 1.

Breathe naturally and mentally repeat 'relax' after each exhalation.

Practice for three to four minutes.

Step 2

Relax all parts of your body while lying still.

Imagine individual parts of your body being relaxed. Do not move *said* body parts.

Begin by focusing on the right side and repeat the process with the left side.

'I am relaxing my brain — my brain is relaxed.'

'I am relaxing my face — my face is relaxed.'

'I am relaxing my neck — my neck is relaxed.'

'I am relaxing my shoulders — my shoulders are relaxed.'

'I am relaxing my arms — my arms are relaxed.'

'I am relaxing my liver, kidneys, spleen, and intestines — my liver, kidneys, spleen, and intestines are relaxed.'

'I am relaxing my legs — my legs are relaxed.'

'I am relaxing my feet — my feet are relaxed.'

At the end of this process, utter some short, positive sentences:

'I will attain and maintain perfect health.'

or

'I am perfectly healthy in body and mind.'

VISIT TO PARADISE

Imagine a beautiful location. Picture yourself standing near it and taking in the beauty of everything there. It should be a very relaxing experience.

Visualize the following symbols: a night sky full of stars, a rising sun, a setting sun, a blue sky, different colored flowers, a rainbow, a candle flame, a full moon, etc.

Again, mentally, repeat your resolution three times.

Benefits

With this exercise, you can certainly doze off, if sound sleep is your intention. Otherwise, open your eyes and stretch your body. Yog nidra is a powerful technique to program your subconscious mind, which is a condition that accepts the full truth.

Whatever you listen to or say to yourself in your subconscious mind, you accept it as the truth, without any contradictions. Therefore, if you want to change your life or heal your body and your mind following emotional and physical trauma, this is an effective technique. It can also be used for stabilizing your emotions or calming your body. Yog nidra helps you to ground yourself and to stabilize your emotions.

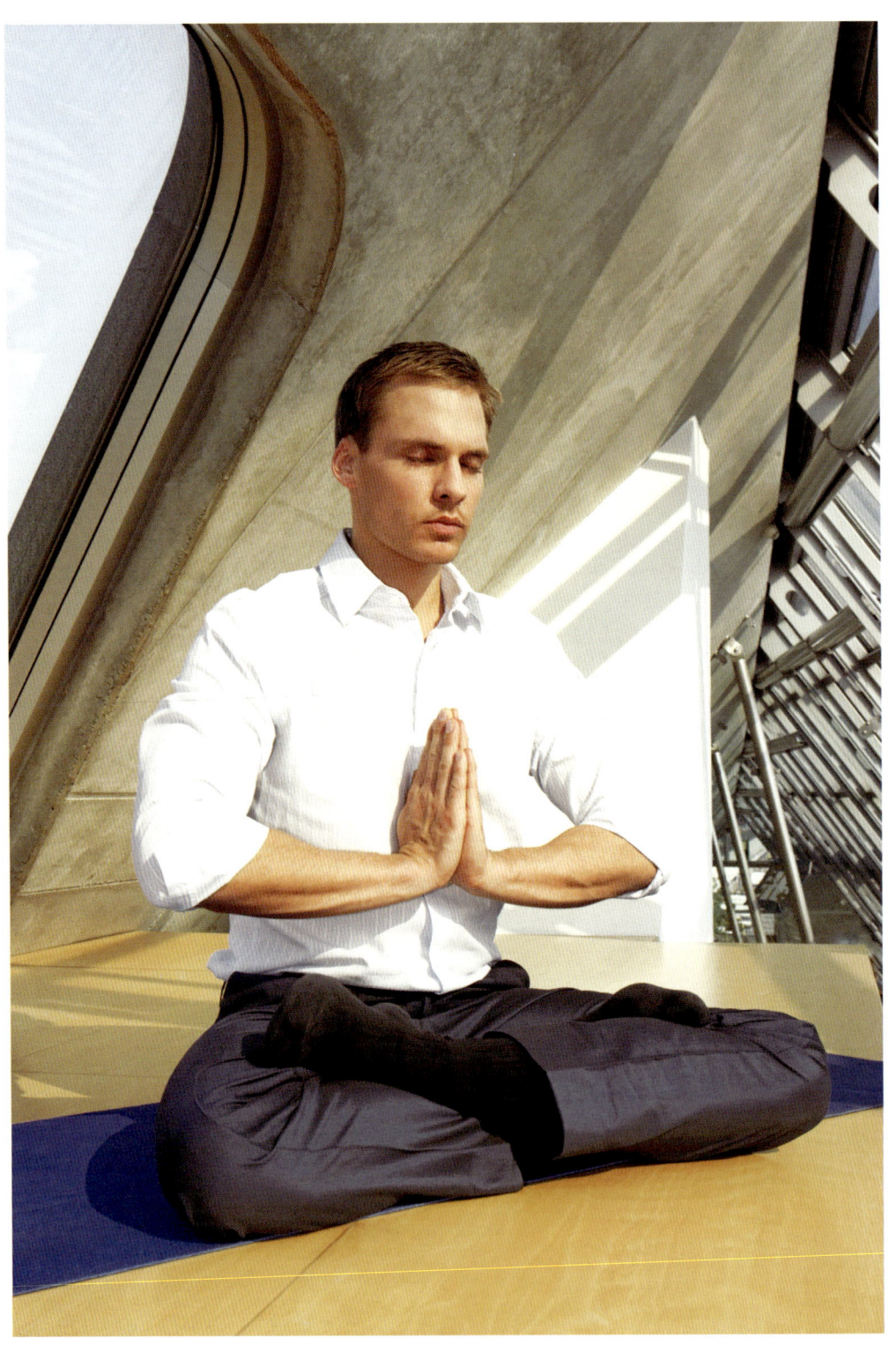

Frequent Flyers

Traveling requires you to be seated continuously for several hours. This means that your hands and legs experience very little movement and become inactive. As a result, blood circulation slows down. We end up feeling extremely fatigued by the time we land at our destination. Sometimes this can lead to serious issues when a person is travelling for many hours, can suddenly develop a stasis in the blood vessels that can lead to a clot formation. In rare cases this clot can travel to the heart and cause a sudden cardiac arrest. Getting up and walking up and down the aisle is an effective way of exercising your legs and improving blood flow. We also have these exercises that will improve circulation even while remaining seated.

Here are two poses that you can practice in your plane seat.

KNEE TO CHEST OR *APANASANA*

Time duration: Thirty seconds to one minute

This is a flexibility exercise, in which stretching contributes to abdominal strengthening. Abdominal muscle strength stabilizes your back, which is the best way to stretch out your body and take pressure and stress off your spine in the cramped seats of an aircraft. It will surely make you less fatigued when you land at your destination.

Benefits

This releases stress from the spine and helps keep your body fresh.

Method

- Bend slightly forward.

- Fold your hands together around your knees and pull the knees as close to your chest as possible. Make sure your body is relaxed.

- Hold this position for fifteen seconds and allow your knee to drop lowly.

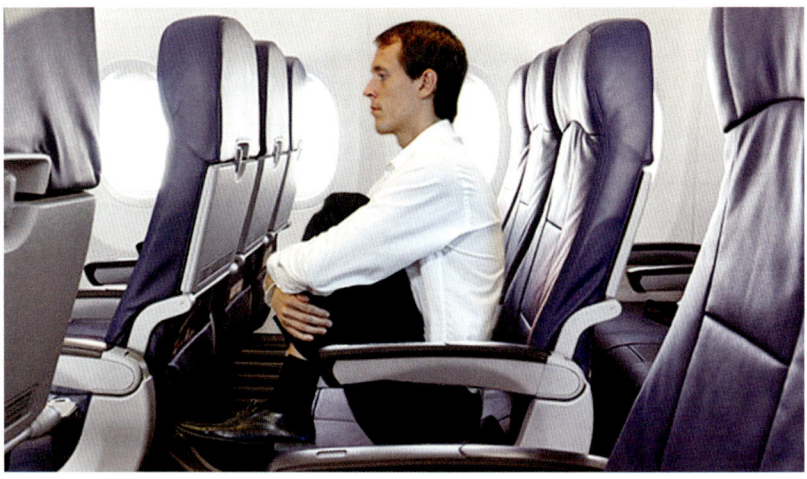

ANKLE EXERCISE

Time duration: One to two minutes

When you sit for a long period of time, whether on a long car trip or an airline flight, your risk of developing a blood clot becomes greater.

Clots form when clumps of blood, tissue, fat, or air bubbles get stuck in your arteries.

By doing these exercises, you will provide sufficient blood circulation to the body to avoid clotting.

Benefits

These exercises prevent the formation of blood clots.

Method

- Do this while you are sitting in your seat.
- Lift both feet off the ground.
- Rotate your feet in opposite directions - clockwise with one foot and counterclockwise with the other foot.

After fifteen seconds, reverse the directions of your feet.

- Place the tips of your toes on the ground.
- Thrust your heels as high as possible.
- You should feel a stretch in the upper surface of your foot by contracting your calf muscles.
- Hold for two seconds and release the contraction.
- Repeat immediately to create a pumping motion.
- Stretch your muscles and move your ankles by rolling your foot in a circular motion or from side to side as often as possible.

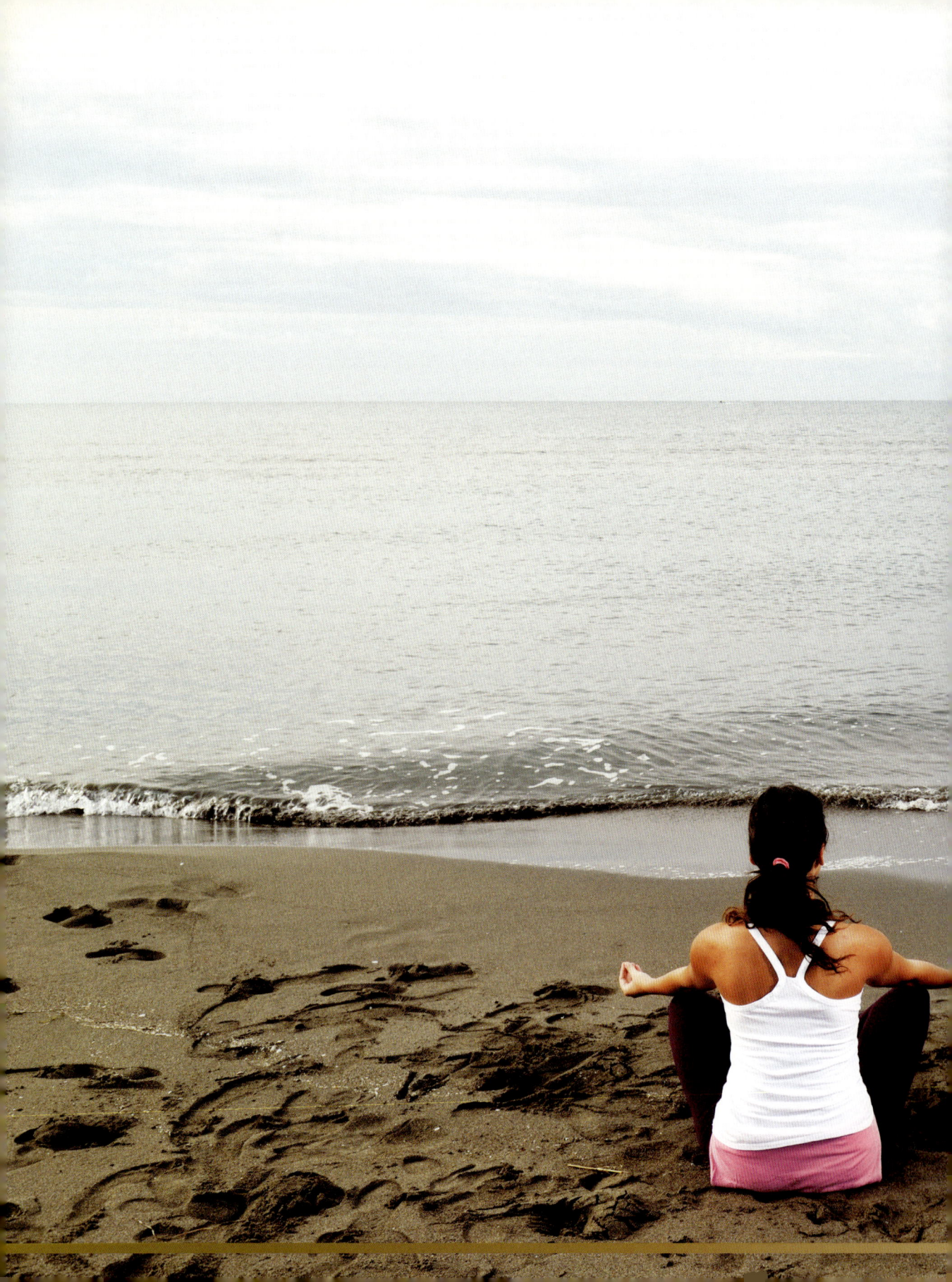

Happy Ending

Do you find it difficult to unwind when you get home from work?

Sex has been proven as one of the best stress relievers, but sometimes stress can start to harm your love life. When stress is ignored, the body can react to stress by releasing cortisol and adrenaline. Chronic stress can negatively interfere with your body's hormone levels, which can result in a low libido. One may feel very detached from the present, thus making sex boring or unemotional. Some yoga poses can improve your mind-body connection so you can enjoy sex without worrying or thinking about anything else in the world during sex.

Starting outside the bedroom and moving in, here are some yoga poses that will help you reap the benefits of sex.

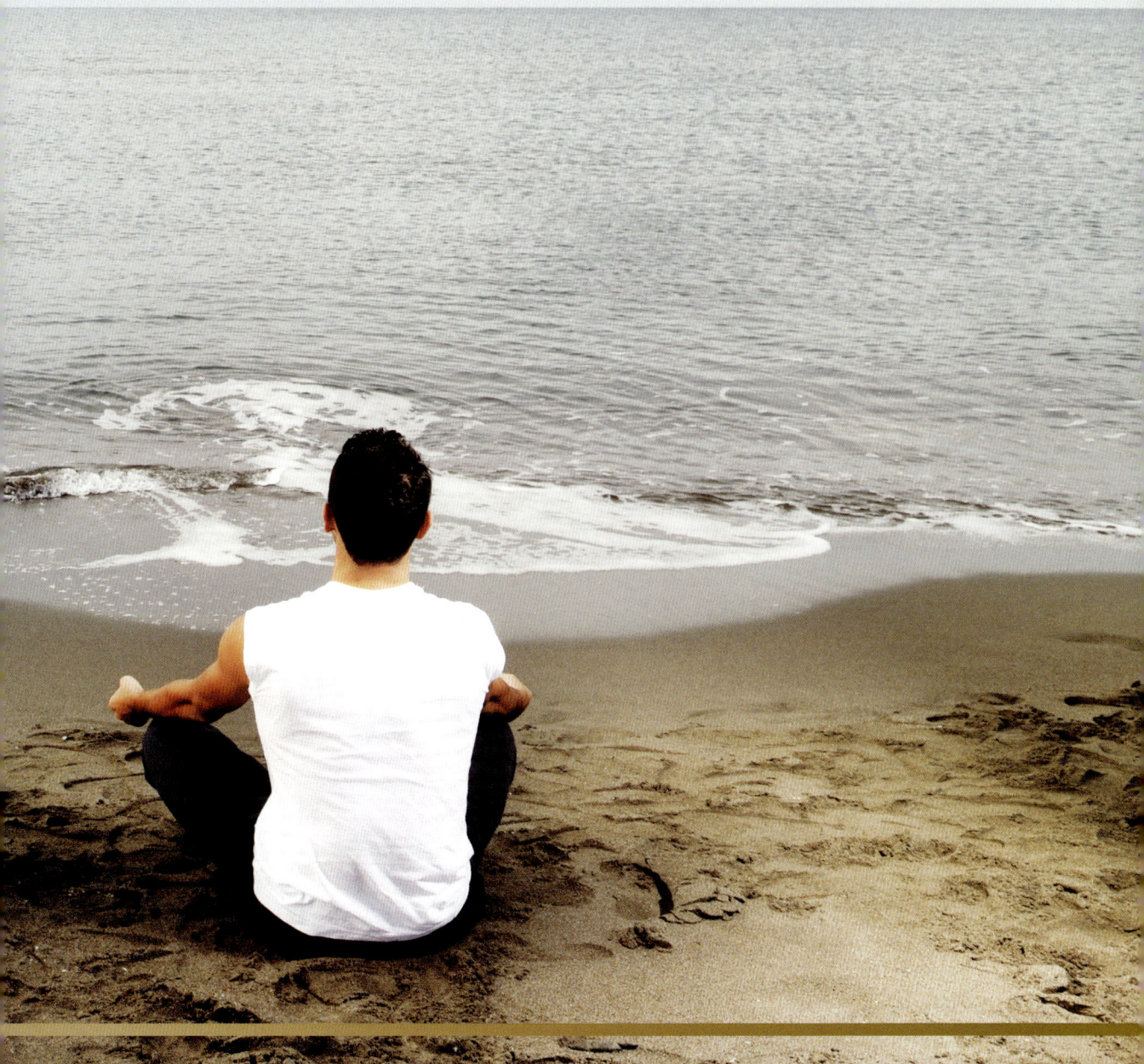

PIGEON POSE OR *SALAMBA KAPOTASANA*

Time duration: One to two minutes

This is a hip-opening pose. These muscles are stretched and extended in salamba kapotasana. The pigeon pose is an effective way to release deep tension in the hips and to get the mind into a relaxed state. Most men have a tendency of storing tension in their shoulders, whereas women tend to hold it in their hips.

Benefits

It relieves tightness and restores flexibility.

Method

- Begin on all fours in a squared table pose.
- Slide the right knee forward toward your right hand.
- Angle your right knee at two o'clock.
- Slide your left leg back as far as your hips will allow it to go.
- Keep your hips square to the floor. If your hips are not square, there will be unnecessary force on your back. Consequently, you will be unable to open your hips to their fullest.
- Your right thigh should have an external rotation, and your left thigh should have a slight internal rotation.
- This keeps pressure off your kneecap.
- Stay in this position anywhere from ten breaths to five minutes.

Knee at 2 o'clock position

Hips square

Slide as far as you can

Hands can rest.

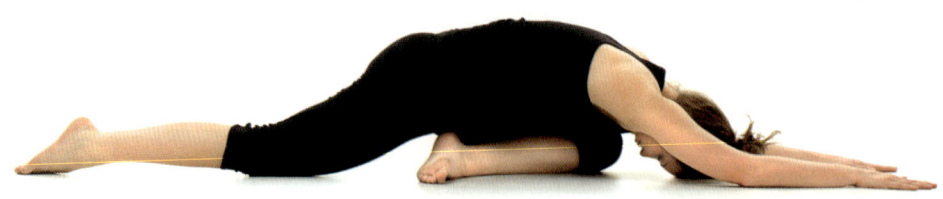

WIDE-LEGGED STRADDLE OR *UPAVISTHA KONASANA*

Time duration: Two minutes

This pose addresses the issue of low libido. It improves blood flow to the pelvic area. Circulation is closely linked to arousal.

Benefits

Kegel exercises while you are in this pose will strengthen your pelvic muscles and will improve circulation. It can prevent reproductive health related issues and can have a positive effect on your sexual responsiveness, including an intensified female orgasm.

Method

- Sit with your legs open at a ninety degree angle with your pelvis as center.

- Hold your feet with your hands to keep yourself in the position.

- Flex your feet to align the knees, with toes pointing up to the sky. If you feel your pelvis rocking back, or you feel a loss of the curve on your lower back, sit up to allow the pelvis to tilt forward.

- Inhale, drawing up the sides of the body. This will create space in the spine.

- Draw the muscles of your pelvic floor gently upward with Kegel exercises.

- To do Kegels, tighten the muscles around your vagina as though you are trying to stop the flow of urinating midstream.

- Exhale as you begin to walk your hands out in front of you.

- Slowly, using your breath as a guide, keep your spine long. Lead with your heart.

- Stop when you have reached a challenging but sustainable position.

- Instead of trying to get closer to the earth, imagine growing longer through the spine.

- Breathe comfortably as you hold this forward bend.

- To exit the pose, exhale and reconnect with your core muscle support. Slowly walk your hands back towards your body.

- Gently bend your knees and bring your legs back.

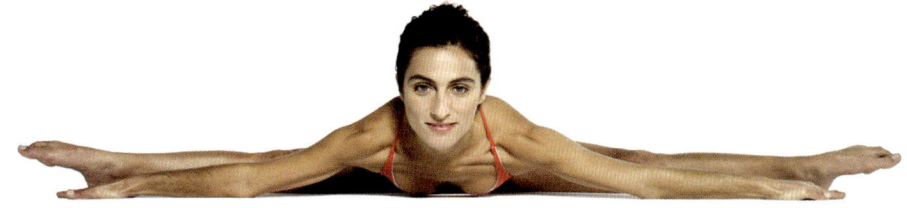

SHOULDER STAND OR *SARVANGASANA*

Time duration: Two to three minutes

Sagging skin is not the only adverse effect of the earth's downward pull. The lower half of your body is more likely to suffer from slow circulation because as blood returns to your heart, it faces an uphill climb. Beat gravity by turning upside down. This pose will also help you achieve a healthy sex drive.

Benefits

It alleviates fatigue, calms the mind, reduces symptoms of depression and anxiety, and lessens digestive problems.

Position 1

- Lie down on the floor with your legs together.
- Keep your hands, with palms down, by your sides.
- Inhaling, push down on your hands and raise your legs straight up above you.

Position 2

- Lift your hips off the floor and bring your head at an angle of above forty-five degrees.

Position 3

- Exhaling, bend your arms and support your body.
- Hold as close to the shoulders as possible, with your thumbs around the front of the body and your fingers around the back.
- Push your back up.
- Lift your legs.

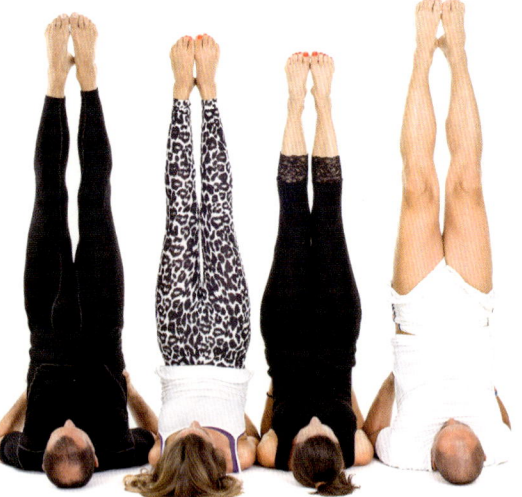

Position 4

- Straighten your spine and bring your legs up to a vertical position.
- Press your chin firmly into the base of your throat.
- Breathe slowly and deeply into the pose.
- Keep your feet relaxed.

Shoulder stand roll-out

To come down from the pose, lower your legs to an angle of forty-five degrees over your head. Then place your hands with the palms down behind you and slowly roll out of it, much like the way you came up.

BABY POSE (BALASANA)

Time duration: 1-2 minutes

A child's pose is very soothing and can really tune the mind to the body. The gravitational pull of '*Balasana*' is sure to induce a great sense of physical, mental, and emotional relief in you.

Benefits

It is the best way to get connected with your body, to release all emotional stress and to enjoy sex thereafter.

Method

- Come onto your knees and bring your heels together.
- Widen your knees and exhale.
- Bring your torso down between your thighs, lengthening your spine.
- Place your forehead on the ground, and allow your shoulders to fall forwards.
- You can stretch your arms in front of you (as in the picture)

  Or

- You can have your hands by your sides.

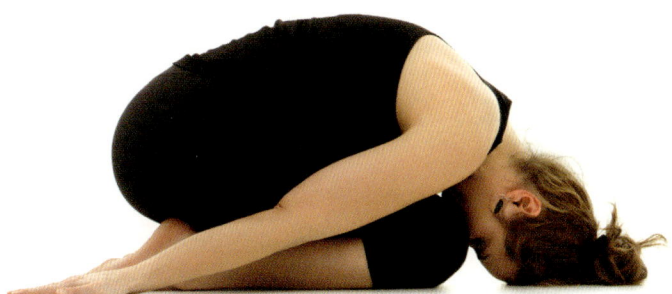

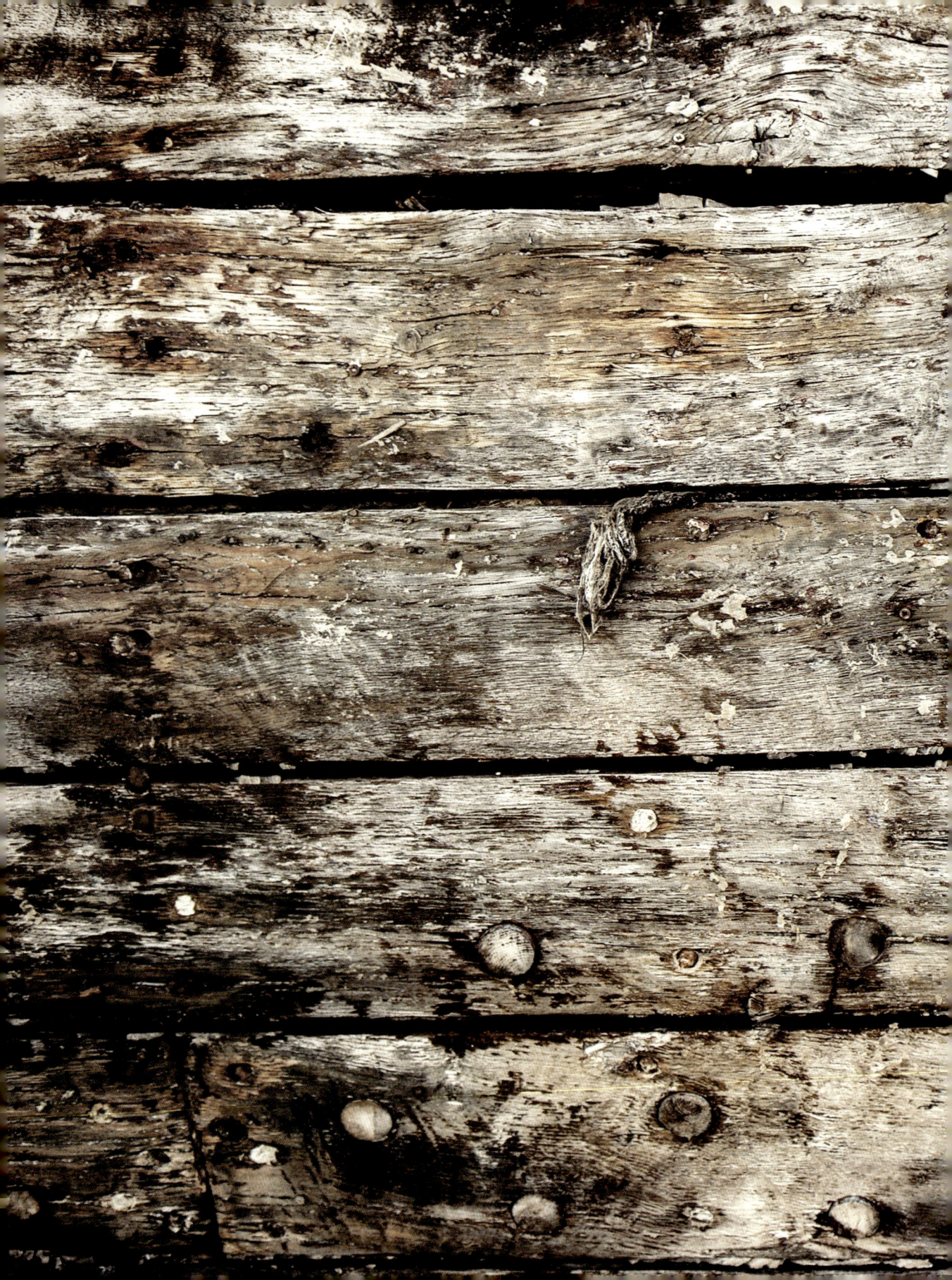

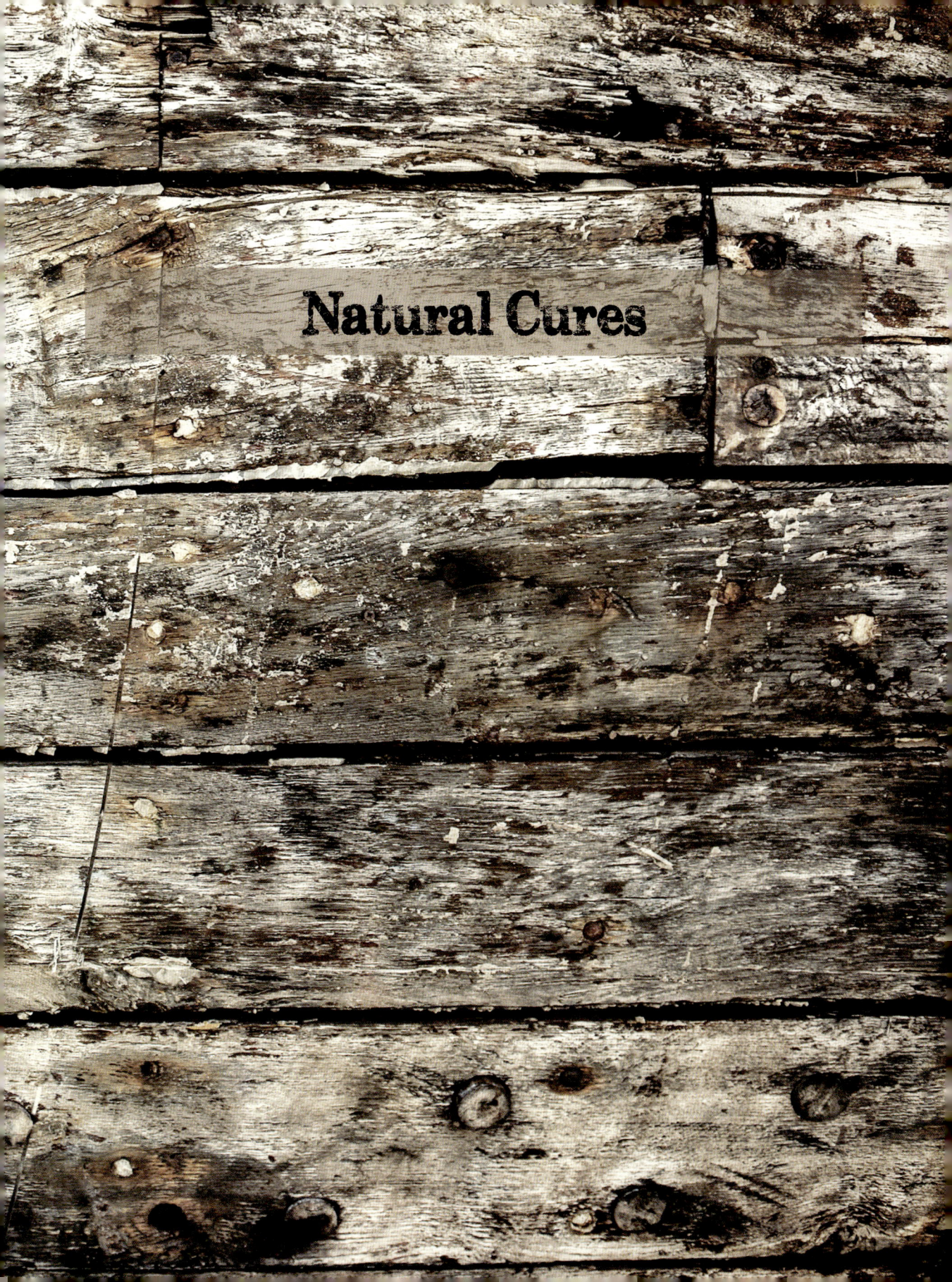

Natural Cures

Yoga is incomplete without naturopathy. Many traditions of natural medicine are several centuries old. Over this time, an impressive amount of practical knowledge has accumulated.

Yoga is a healing system in which we practice a combination of breathing exercises, physical postures, meditation, healthy eating and holistic lifestyle. It is a complete union of our cleansed mind and body. Healthy is the most natural state of the human body. The origins of the word 'health' are associated with wholeness and healing, as well as a complete sense of harmony. The achievement of true health is the primary aim of natural healing systems. It is vital to note the holistic approach of natural healing systems like yoga, aromatherapy and naturopathy in contrast with the reductionist perspective that prevails in conventional modern medicine.

When we talk about aromatherapy or naturopathy, the first thing that comes to our mind is holistic approach. Anything we give to our body in a natural and calming way that unites us and heals us is yoga. In the last few years, interest in natural remedies has revived as people have begun to appreciate their tremendous value. Natural therapies are a breath of fresh air compared to allopathic medicine, with its side effects and impersonal approaches. In this chapter, we will discuss how natural therapies can be used at home. If in doubt about any medical issues, do seek professional medical advice.

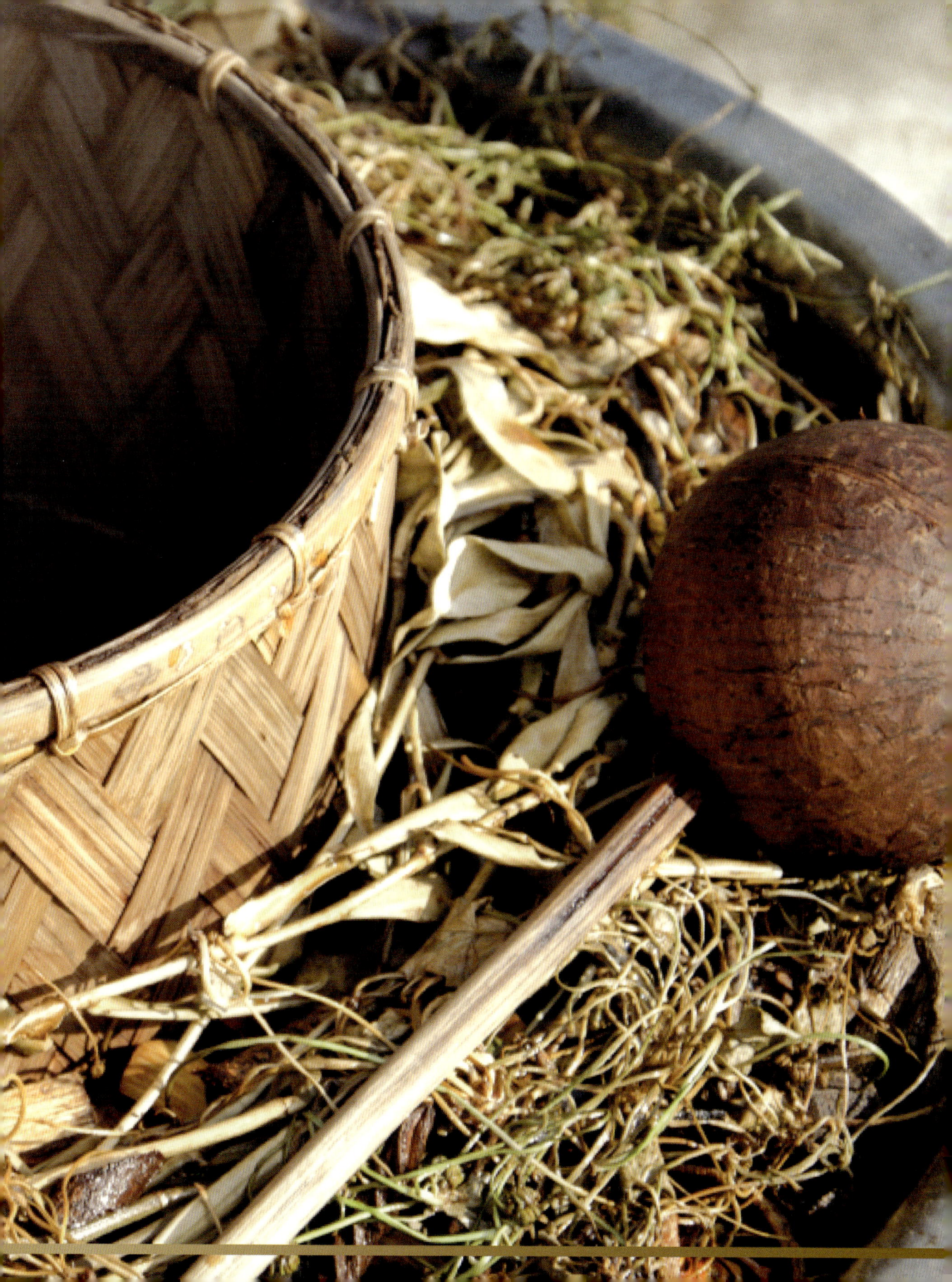

THE NERVOUS SYSTEM

The nervous system is a vast network that controls nearly every aspect of the human body. Our ability to move, breathe, digest, sense and feel are all products of the complex functions of the nervous system.

A key principle of natural therapy is its holistic approach. It takes into account the physical, mental, emotional and spiritual well-being of a person in the assessment of health and is thus useful in the treatment of nervous disorders. Both physical and emotional symptoms suggest a problem in the functioning of your body.

Therefore, when trying to treat disease, it is essential to consider all potential causes for the discomfort. Your headache may be due to an alcohol binge the previous night, your anxiety may stem from your nerves about tomorrow's interview; and your insomnia might be caused by the four cups of coffee you had in the evening. Identifying the cause may not be enough to solve the problem, but it will help you to take preventive measures. In many instances, of course, the causes are not as obvious. For persistent or recurring problems, professional help is needed.

Aside from the natural therapies described here, there are several sources of help for nerve related conditions. Since stress is a major factor in many health issues nowadays, most forms of alternative therapy take stress into account in their approaches. These approaches might range from counseling and hypnotherapy to acupuncture and cranial osteopathy. These approaches will not only help you, but also empower you to help yourself.

Depression

Sadness is a normal reaction to the trials and tribulations we face in life. Many people describe their feelings of sadness using the word 'depression', but depression is not just sadness.

Depressed people often think they 'live in a black hole', and they experience nagging feeling of impending doom. However, some people with depression don't feel sad at all. Rather, they may feel completely lifeless, apathetic and empty. Men in particular may even experience feelings of anger, aggression and restlessness.

Regardless of what symptoms manifest themselves, depression is entirely different from normal sadness in that it takes over your day-to-day life and interferes with your ability to live a normal life. The helplessness and worthlessness associated with depression is relentless and intense.

Conditions like constipation, headaches, insomnia and loss of appetite are all associated with depression, and in continuing instances of depression, professional help is necessary. This is especially important when there is no obvious reason for the feelings, a condition generally known as endogenous depression.

Aromatherapy

Many oils can have profound effects on one's moods, and it may be essential to change the oil used as symptoms vary. Aromatherapy massage with diluted essential oils is a useful way to treat someone with depression.

Bergamot: Bergamot is a plant that produces a certain type of citrus fruit. Oil is taken from the peel of the fruit, and this oil can also be used to make medicine. Additionally, this oil is one of the most refreshing, with a citrus fragrance that is appealing to men and women alike. This oil gives the Earl Grey tea its distinctive aroma.

Clary Sage: Clary sage or *salvia sclarea* is an essential oil that has natural phytoestrogens. This oil has a mellow and warm scent, and has relaxing effects. It is a good oil to use when chronic tension has led to depression or exhaustion.

Geranium: Geranium essential oil has a sweet, floral fragrance that is calming and relaxing for both the body and mind. This oil is traditionally used to support the circulatory and nervous systems' functions, and a great deal of its strength stems from its capacity to revitalize body tissues. It originates from varieties of scented pelargonium and has a stimulating effect on the adrenal cortex, which regulates stress hormone production.

Neroli: Neroli is an oil that comes from the blossom of the bitter orange. It is very concentrated (and expensive!), so a little can go a long way. This oil relaxes and soothes the muscles, and also provides relief for muscle spasms. It also counters the irritability that often accompany depression.

Anxiety

Everyone gets nervous or anxious from time to time. For some people, however, anxiety completely takes over their lives.

How can you tell if your anxiety has crossed the line and morphed into a full-blown disorder? It's not easy. Anxiety comes in many different forms, and the line between an official diagnosis and everyday anxiety is often blurry.

In many situations, some amount of anxiety is a perfectly normal, natural response to stress. It only becomes a problem when the amount of anxiety is disproportionate to the situation, or when there is no external cause for the anxiety. Symptoms of anxiety might include constant feelings of tension, sweating, palpitations, hyperventilating and lack of sleep.

Aromatherapy

Many oils have a relaxing, calming effect on the nervous system. The best way to use them is in the bath, because warm water aids the absorption of the oils.

Clary Sage: Clary sage has a relaxing, warming and almost euphoric effect. It is especially useful in situations where anxiety leads to exhaustion.

Lavender: Lavender is a calming oil that helps to balance the mind and emotions. It is also one of the gentlest oils to use.

Headaches

There are numerous causes for headaches. Some common causes include eyestrain, fatigue, nasal congestion, sinusitis or tension. However, the vast majority of headaches are caused by stress, with muscle spasms in the neck turning into head pains. These headaches are exacerbated by poor posture as well as the spatial problems created by many jobs — for instance, computer operators strain their eyes and suffer from stiff shoulders or neck muscles, which result in headaches.

Aromatherapy

Numerous essential oils have analgesic properties. The best way to use oils for headaches is as a cold compress, which you apply to the temples and forehead. Pour five drops in a bowl of cold water, wring out a cloth, and place it on the affected area. An alternative method is gently massaging a couple of drops onto the temples.

Lavender: Lavender is relaxing and warming with analgesic properties. It is an extremely gentle oil that is very useful for neck tension. Apply a hot compress to the upper back and neck at the same time (using the same proportions listed above for cold compresses).

Peppermint: Peppermint has a cooling effect and is also an effective way of relieving catarrh and nasal congestion symptoms. Peppermint has stimulating properties and can be used in equal amounts with lavender, as described above, on the forehead and temples.

Rosemary: Rosemary provides even more stimulation to the central nervous system. This oil is excellent for headaches caused by mental strain and exhaustion, and is also useful for clearing the sinuses.

Severe Headaches

High blood pressure, meningitis or brain tumors are much rarer causes of headaches. These causes require professional medical treatment, and severe headaches that are persistent and unexplained should be carefully looked into. However, most headaches can be cured at home using natural remedies. After an accident, it makes sense to seek the services of a therapist such as a chiropractor or an osteopath.

Migraine

Migraines are pulsating headaches that often take place on one side of the head. Exercise may exacerbate the pain of migraines, but symptoms of migraines can vary. Anyone who has experienced a migraine knows that it is more than a severe headache. Migraines generally involve acute pains, often over one eye, and even disturbed vision or flashing lights. Migraines can also cause nausea and sensitivity to bright light.

Aromatherapy

Since migraines heighten the sense of smell, aromatherapy is best used between attacks. Use aromatherapy in the earliest stage of a migraine only if the smell is tolerable. A central element of the holistic approach to migraines is the distinguishing between a 'hot' migraine, where the blood vessels are dilated, and a 'cold' migraine, where the blood vessels are constricted. For hot migraines, a cold or cool compress across the forehead will offer relief, as well as peppermint or lavender oils. For cold migraines, a hot compress on the forehead or back of the neck may help.

Naturopathy

The naturopathic approach looks at prevention. It considers lifestyle changes that can reduce the occurrence of headaches. Eating a nutritious diet of whole foods, reducing consumption of alcohol and caffeine, and getting more physical activity and fresh air are all likely to help lower the number of headaches you get. Drinking plenty of fluids is essential as dehydration can be a cause of headaches, especially for people exposed to hot environments or after the consumption of alcohol. It is important to avoid dramatic changes in your eating habits because such changes can upset blood sugar levels and contribute to the occurrence of headaches. For hot congested headaches, use cold compress on the forehead and perhaps combine them with a hot footbath, which will help improve circulation.

Diet needs to be carefully assessed. Try to avoid the following items as much as possible: tea, coffee, alcohol, red meat, cheese, chocolate, tomatoes and eggs. Eat plenty of fresh, raw salads and drink lots of fluids, as dehydration can be a factor in migraines. In between attacks, exercise regularly to relieve tension in the neck and shoulders, and massage those areas.

Stress

Modern life is replete with hassles, deadlines, frustrations and demands. For many people, stress is so commonplace that 'stressed out' is their natural state. Stress isn't always bad. In small doses, stress can help you perform under pressure. However, when you're constantly running in emergency mode, your mind and body will pay the price. You can protect yourself from these negative impacts by recognizing the signs and symptoms of stress and taking proactive steps to reduce its harmful effects.

Stress is one of those vague terms that is difficult to precisely define. While stress is not in itself harmful, and a certain amount can be necessary to motivate us, too much stress is a problem. Human beings have an impressive capacity to adapt to and cope with various sources of stress, but when they get overloaded with stress to the point that nervous or adrenal exhaustion sets in, they can become seriously ill.

Aromatherapy

Many oils can help reduce the impact of stress. The best way of utilizing these oils is diluting them in a vegetable oil and using them for a massage. If you do not have someone to help you with massaging, then use the oils in a bath. For better effects, choose from the following oils: bergamot, clary sage, geranium or rosemary. For relaxing effects, use lavender or marjoram. Three luxurious (although expensive) oils with excellent de-stressing properties and wonderful scents are rose, jasmine and neroli (or orange blossom).

Rose: Use rose sparingly as this oil is very concentrated. It is calming and relaxing.

Jasmine: This is relaxing and almost euphoric.

Neroli: This oil is an antidepressant and is refreshing.

Naturopathy

Look at the basics, especially the diet. Cut out all the stimulants such as coffee, tea and cola drinks, which only increase your exhaustion when their effects wear off. In small amounts, alcohol may help you relax. However, since it can easily become a dangerous habit and has depressive effects, it is vital to reduce alcohol consumption. Try to get some exercise, which will not only help you use up excess adrenaline, but will also build up your physical and mental stamina. Make sure you breathe deeply, as this will supply more oxygen to the brain. It may be helpful to incorporate a multivitamin and mineral supplement to your diet for a while, as the body uses up nutrients faster when under stress.

Insomnia

Insomnia is a persistent disorder that makes it difficult to fall asleep, stay asleep, or both. People with insomnia do not wake up feeling refreshed, which affects their ability to function during the day. Insomnia can reduce not only your energy level and mood but also your health, work performance and quality of life.

It is essential to understand the difference between regular sleeplessness and a temporary sleep issue caused by stress. It is also important not to grow overly concerned with sleeping for a certain number of hours every night because not everyone needs a full eight hours of sleep each night. Quality is more important than quantity when it comes to sleep. In general, humans require fewer hours of sleep as they get older.

Aromatherapy

Essential oils are a pleasant and effective means of unwinding and aiding restful sleep. Try using these oils in the bath or putting two to three drops onto a paper tissue under your pillow at night. Choose from the following oils, using a single oil or a blend of oils. Do not use the same oil for more than two weeks, because you will find that it becomes less effective over time.

Chamomile: Chamomile has calming and relaxing effects. It is a good oil to use in cases where indigestion contributes to broken sleep.

Clary Sage: Clary sage has a sedating and almost euphoric effect. Do not use if you have consumed alcohol as you can quickly get drunk and experience nightmares or the feeling of having hangover later on.

Lavender: Lavender has soothing effects and analgesic properties. If aches or pains contribute to your insomnia, lavender is probably the best remedy.

Marjoram: Marjoram is relaxing and warming. In large amounts, this oil is quite sedating. It can leave you feeling a little thickheaded the next morning, so do not overdo your use of marjoram.

Naturopathy

In order to have enough energy during the day, it is helpful to get a lot of exercise and fresh air. Waking up early can also help maintain a good balance of energy. Do not sleep in a stuffy room, and avoid consumption of caffeine at night. At bedtime, drink a warm herbal tea.

THE CIRCULATORY SYSTEM

The circulatory system transports nutrients, water and oxygen throughout the entire body, to billions of cells. It also carries away wastes such as the carbon dioxide produced by the cells. This system is an impressive highway traveling throughout the body and connecting with all its cells.

The circulatory system is divided into three major parts:

- The heart
- The blood
- The blood vessels

Without good circulation, we are unable to be in good health. In cooler climates, many people suffer from poor circulation, which results in weak immune systems. Circulation disorders can occur in the heart or in the blood vessels. Such disorders should not be self-treated, and for any prolonged or serious circulatory problems, professional treatment is recommended.

For example, angina is a cramping of the heart muscles caused by the narrowing or obstruction of the coronary arteries. When the supply of oxygen to the cardiac muscles is unable to meet any extra demand, the characteristic cramps and pains of angina can take place for a short while. Resting can ease the pain after a few minutes. Infusions of lime blossom or *tilia europaea* can offer some relief from angina, but professional medical opinion is necessary to determine individual causes as well as the overall health of the heart.

Poor Circulation

Poor circulation to the extremities is rather common in cooler climates, especially among elderly people or those who get little exercise. It should not be neglected as this can lead to the development of more serious conditions such as phlebitis or thrombosis. If in doubt, professional medical help should be sought.

Aromatherapy

Perform a massage on the hands or feet using diluted oils such as black pepper, lavender, marjoram or rosemary. These oils can be added to a warm footbath for a short-term treatment that is highly effective. Use a maximum of ten drops in total, and try a blend of two or three of these oils. Avoid these oils if the skin is broken, and instead, get professional medical advice first.

Hand Massage: Put some base oil in a bowl, with essential oils added as recommended. Massage into the palms of your hands with a steady circular movement. Squeeze down your fingers to stretch and loosen them, pushing towards the palm. Repeat these two steps numerous times.

Foot Massage: To stretch your feet, place your hands with your thumbs on top of the foot, maintaining a firm grip with both of your hands. Move your thumbs outward, as if you are breaking a piece of bread. Repeat this movement numerous times.

THE RESPIRATORY SYSTEM

The respiratory system consists of the organs in our body that help us breathe. The goal of breathing is to deliver oxygen to the body and to remove carbon dioxide.

In order to prevent respiratory problems, or to help solve these problems more quickly, it is essential to adopt a holistic view of health. If you live in a relatively mild, damp climate, you will be more prone to respiratory infections. The increase in air pollution over the past century adds significantly to the burden. However, internal factors, such as diet, exercise and general health, also affect our resistance to infections. The more we pay attention to these internal factors, the healthier we will be. Breathing is a bodily function that occurs automatically, but can also be controlled consciously. Our breathing can serve as a good illustration of the effects of stress and anxiety on our body, as shallow or over-rapid breathing, nervous coughs and even bronchial spasms can occur in an agitated state. Poor posture, lack of exercise, lack of fresh air, smoking, and exposure to smoke are all factors that can contribute to an inadequate intake of oxygen and, consequently, respiratory problems.

Colds

Since there are more than one hundred strains of the cold virus, it is not surprising that a cure is yet to be found. Prevention is far better than treatment because once a cold has developed, it generally has to run its course. However, treatments can provide relief and also stop the cold from becoming a persistent or deeper infection.

Aromatherapy

The two most appropriate methods for using oils to combat symptoms of cold and prevent complications are steam inhalations and baths. In the early stages, if the cold is accompanied by a chill, adding ten drops of lavender and five drops of cinnamon oil to a warm bath at night can be helpful. Ten drops each of more stimulating oils such as eucalyptus or tea tree can be used in baths earlier in the day. All of the above oils can also be used for inhalations, and a mixture often works better than a single oil.

Naturopathy

Eat lots of fresh fruit because fruit is a great source of natural vitamins A, B and C. Add plenty of raw garlic to food. Cut out foods that contain sugar, starch or dairy. A short term cleansing diet consisting of just fresh fruit and salads, and plenty of liquids such as warm fruit juices or herbal teas, will help the body to fight off the cold more effectively.

Coughs

Coughing is an important way of keeping your throat and air passages clear. However, too much coughing may mean you have a disease or disorder.

A cough is a natural reflex reaction. It can occur in response to any irritation, blockage or inflammation that occurs in the airways. A cough often accompanies an infection such as a cold or bronchitis, but it can also come about through nervousness, with no direct irritation at all. Coughing can be vital as it keeps the bronchial tubes clear, therefore the goal of the treatment should be to make the cough more effective rather than just to suppress it.

Aromatherapy

A useful way of helping a cough perform its function more effectively is by using oils in a steam inhalation. Oils can soothe the lining of the air passages, fight infection and loosen mucus thus making it easier to remove. Soothing oils include benzoin and lavender. Many essential oils are antiseptic, especially thyme and eucalyptus. To increase expectoration, use frankincense or marjoram. All the above oils are helpful for dealing with coughs. Choose a blend that you like the smell of. Remember that if the cough persists after a few days, you should seek professional help.

Naturopathy

Initially, coughs can often be quite dry and painful. Taking a spoonful of honey can help soothe these initial effects. To make the honey more powerful, try mashing a small quantity of chopped raw onion or garlic into it. Cut out all dairy products from your diet. Either steam inhalation or a hot compress will encourage expectoration and help the lungs to work better. Once the coughing decreases, try not to slip back into eating patterns that include a lot of sugar or dairy, as these can lower the body's resistance to infection and cause the cough to linger or even to return in full force. If the cough persists, it is important to seek professional medical advice. Similarly, bright green or yellow mucus indicates the presence of an infection, and professional medical advice should be sought.

Asthma

Asthma is a chronic disease involving the airways in the lungs. These airways, or bronchial tubes, allow air to travel in and out of the lungs.

The airways of people with asthma are always inflamed. Their airways become even more swollen when something triggers their symptoms. This makes it difficult for air to move in and out of the lungs, which causes symptoms such as coughing, wheezing, shortness of breath and chest tightness.

Asthma is not generally a problem that should simply be tackled at home. Professional medical treatment is necessary. Childhood asthma tends to be associated with an allergic response. There may also be hay fever or eczema present in the family. When trying to identify the responsible allergens, it is valuable to consider external and internal factors, as well as conventional skin testing.

Aromatherapy

During an asthma attack, sniffing the aroma of a couple of drops of essential oil on a paper tissue can offer relief from the spasm of the airways. Choose from lavender, bergamot, frankincense or chamomile. In between attacks, massaging the chest with a choice of the above oils, in a diluted mixture, can assist with preventing the spasms and build-up of thick mucus, which causes the wheezing symptoms.

Naturopathy

For childhood asthma, or asthma with large quantities of thick mucus, it is worth trying a change in diet. Exclude dairy products, reduce sugar intake, and increase consumption of fresh vegetables and fruit. Breathing exercises may help, especially in cases with later onset of asthma or in cases where exercise aggravates symptoms. A simple way to deepen the breathing pattern is to blow up balloons. For best effects, blow them up until they burst. Regular back massages can also aid with releasing muscle tensions and improving circulation. Additionally, using hot and cold compresses on the upper back or chest will stimulate circulation through the lungs and help remove mucus.

Breathing Exercise

Put hands just below the breastbone and take a slow, deep breath. As you breathe in, push out the stomach. This should make the hands move apart a little in tandem with the movement of the diaphragm.

As you breathe out, pull the stomach in. The diaphragm will move back up and the hands will come together again. Repeat three or four times and then breathe normally.

Sore Throat

Sore throats are becoming increasingly common due to an increase in airborne pollution, the smoky, dry atmospheres that are commonplace in air-conditioned buildings, and so forth. Throat irritation can vary in intensity and may be related to other infections. When throat inflammation, or pharyngitis, reaches the larynx, the voice may also be adversely affected.

Aromatherapy

Use steam inhalations with oils such as benzoin, lavender or thyme. One drop of essential oil and lemon with half a teaspoon of honey can act as a powerful local antiseptic and have soothing effects.

Naturopathy

For adults and older children, the diet can be restricted to fruit juices for a maximum of one or two days. Younger children and infants will find it difficult to cope with just a fruit juice diet, so simply reduce their food intake and have them drink plenty of fruit juices. If the throat is swollen and hot, try a cold compress around it. Rest the voice, and stay exposed to a warm atmosphere. In modern offices where the dry air can lead to frequent sore throats try to make the air as moist ass possible by adding indoor plants to the work place.

Sinusitis

Sinusitus is an inflammation of the tissue that lines the sinuses. In normal conditions, sinuses are filled with nothing but air. When sinuses are blocked by fluids, germs can proliferate and cause infection.

The sinus cavities are air spaces in the bones of the skull located behind, above and below the eyes. They act as a sound box, allowing the voice to resonate. Like the nasal passages, sinus cavities are lined with mucus membranes. Nose and throat infections can spread to the sinuses. Acute sinusitis can be very painful and requires prompt treatment. Chronic sinusitis may be related to allergic reactions such as hay fever.

Aromatherapy

Steam inhalations are the best way to work directly on the membranes. They help loosen mucus and fight infection. You can use chamomile, eucalyptus, lavender, peppermint, pine, thyme or tea tree. Either use a combination of these oils, or use a single oil at a time. In cases of acute sinusitis, the inhalations can be taken four times a day to ease pain and relieve the congestion. As the symptoms ease, reduce to once daily until the sinuses fully clear up.

Naturopathy

Immediately cut out all dairy products and restrict intake of sugar and starches. Eat plenty of fresh fruit and vegetables. Avoid smoky atmospheres and air travel when nasal passages are acutely inflamed or blocked, as the abrupt changes in air pressure can cause severe pain and damage to the eardrum. Use alternating hot and cold light compresses or splash water around the nose. Begin with hot water for about three minutes and then switch to cold for no more than a minute. Repeat two to three times. These methods will reduce congestion and inflammation, which will help ease the pain. Using an inhalator can be a helpful supplementary method.

THE DIGESTIVE SYSTEM

The digestive system is composed of a group of organs that work together to convert food into energy and basic nutrients, and are responsible for feeding the entire body. Food passes through a large tube inside the body known as the alimentary canal or the gastrointestinal tract. The alimentary canal consists of the oral cavity, pharynx, esophagus, stomach, small intestines and large intestines

The digestive system is one of the most important set of organs in the body. This system allows us to absorb all the nutrients we need in order for all our cells to function properly.

The old adage 'we are what we eat' is valid, because poor nutrition can not only lead to problems such as constipation, flatulence or diarrhea, but also to more common ailments like headaches, chronic fatigue and poor concentration. The digestive system is also a key part of our immune defenses. It recognizes potentially toxic substances and either breaks them down into safer compounds or eliminates them. Western dietary and lifestyle habits have caused a whole host of disorders, from gastric ulcers to constipation and irritable bowel syndrome. Irritable bowel syndrome (IBS) has become a 'waste basket diagnosis' — if nothing else shows up, individuals will often be diagnosed with IBS. Treatment must be individualized, as stress, diet, posture and exercise all play a part in individual symptoms.

Indigestion

Indigestion is a general term used to describe discomfort in the upper belly or abdomen, which is often accompanied by symptoms such as bloating, acidity, heartburn, nausea or bowel disturbances. Typically, indigestion is a temporary problem caused by too much food, bad food, excess alcohol or stress. Digestive pains lasting for a longer duration may be a result of aspirin related drugs, heavy smoking or other digestive ailments.

Aromatherapy

A warm compress with chamomile or lavender oils may offer relief. Alternatively, try gently massaging a two per cent dilution of one of these oils into the abdomen if indigestion is milder.

Naturopathy

If indigestion symptoms are really strong, cut out solid food for twenty-four hours if possible, consuming only herbal teas or fruit juices. Pineapple juice is a particularly good choice because it contains digestive enzymes. Reintroduce foods to your diet gently, beginning with something light such as soup or pureed apple. Avoid drinking too many fluids with meals, as doing so will dilute your natural digestive juices.

Constipation

Anyone who has suffered from constipation knows it can be both painful and frustrating. Almost everyone gets constipated at some point during his or her life.

Constipation is a problem that is largely a result of our diet and lifestyle. Inadequate amounts of dietary fiber, and perhaps a lack of exercise, can lead to the slow passage of faeces through the bowel. This in turn allows water to be reabsorbed, leaving hardened, rabbit-like stools. The frequency of bowel movements is less important than the hardened consistency of the stools. Straining can result in piles, and it is thus important to address it before further complications arise.

Aromatherapy

One of the most effective methods of self-help is massaging the lower abdomen daily. A clockwise massage can be performed using two drops of lavender, marjoram or rosemary oils in one teaspoon of base oil. Lavender and marjoram are more relaxing oils, while rosemary has a more tonic effect.

Naturopathy

Increase dietary fiber intake by eating more fresh vegetables and fruit, whole grains and beans or pulses. Bran is a somewhat excessive form of fiber when taken on its own rather than as part of a meal, so eat only small amounts of bran if you choose to include it in your diet. Do more exercise, particularly for the abdominal muscles, and regularly practice deep breathing exercises. These will stimulate the diaphragm to move up and down, which internally massages part of the colon and aids with peristalsis. A little bit of plain yogurt daily can also help with constipation.

Acidity and Heartburn

When acid from the stomach leaks up into the gullet (oesophagus), a condition known as acid reflux results. Acid reflux may cause heartburn and other symptoms.

Many people occasionally suffer from acid dyspepsia, which is usually because of temporary issues. These issues include recent consumption of rich, spicy foods or a meal that was eaten too quickly during times of haste and stress. If the symptoms occur very regularly, you may need to carefully assess the food you eat and how quickly you eat. If you experience ongoing discomfort, seek professional medical treatment.

Aromatherapy

Applying hot or warm compresses to the abdomen, with a maximum of ten drops of chamomile or lavender oils in a bowl of water, can offer relief from the inflammation and spasms because of excess acidity. If the discomfort is not too much, you can gently massage these oils on the abdomen if you dilute them at two per cent in a base oil.

Naturopathy

A glass of milk is often suggested as a temporary measure because it has the ability to neutralize the acid. However, milk is not the best method, as dairy products can cause other digestive problems. The best method is to avoid solids for up to twenty-four hours after experiencing acid heartburn. Using a hot compress over the abdomen can aid with pain relief. Avoid coffee, alcohol, tobacco, sugar and spicy food for at least a couple of days, and if possible, cut them out completely.

Indigestion

Indigestion is a general term for discomfort, which includes bloating, acidity, heartburn, nausea or bowel disturbances. Usually it is a temporary issue, brought about by eating too much food, bad food, excessive alcohol consumption or stress. Long-term digestive pain may be brought about by aspirin related drugs, heavy smoking or other digestive issues.

Aromatherapy

A warm compress with chamomile or lavender oils can offer some relief. Additionally, you can try gently massaging a two per cent dilution of one of these oils into the abdomen if the indigestion symptoms are milder.

Naturopathy

If indigestion symptoms are really bad, cut out solid foods for twenty-four hours if possible. Drink only herbal teas or fruit juices. Pineapple juice is an especially good choice because it contains digestive enzymes. Reintroduce solid foods into your diet slowly and gently. Start with something light such as soup or pureed apple. Avoid drinking lots of fluids with meals, as they will dilute your natural digestive juices.

Diarrhea

Loose, frequent bowel movements can occur due to inflammation, infection or food poisoning and can have cleansing effects. A common experience is diarrhea during travel, which is a result of exposure to unfamiliar bacteria.

Aromatherapy

Massaging the abdomen with antiseptic and relaxing oils such as chamomile, lavender and neroli can help with diarrhea caused by minor issues. Eucalyptus can be used in the same way as the aforementioned oils. Add fennel or ginger if the diarrhea is accompanied by acute pain. When using any of these oils, dilute them to three per cent in a base oil.

Naturopathy

Drink plenty of fluids, especially mineral water or herbal teas. Consume easily digestible foods such as soups, fruit or vegetable juices. These food items can help replace lost nutrients, speed up recovery and allow the inflamed bowel to settle. Plain boiled rice and dry toast are some of the best first solids to consume. Additionally, you may want to consider a multi-mineral supplement if the diarrhea is intense. The supplement will help you replenish the lost materials. Fruit and vegetables can quickly be reincorporated into the diet as well.

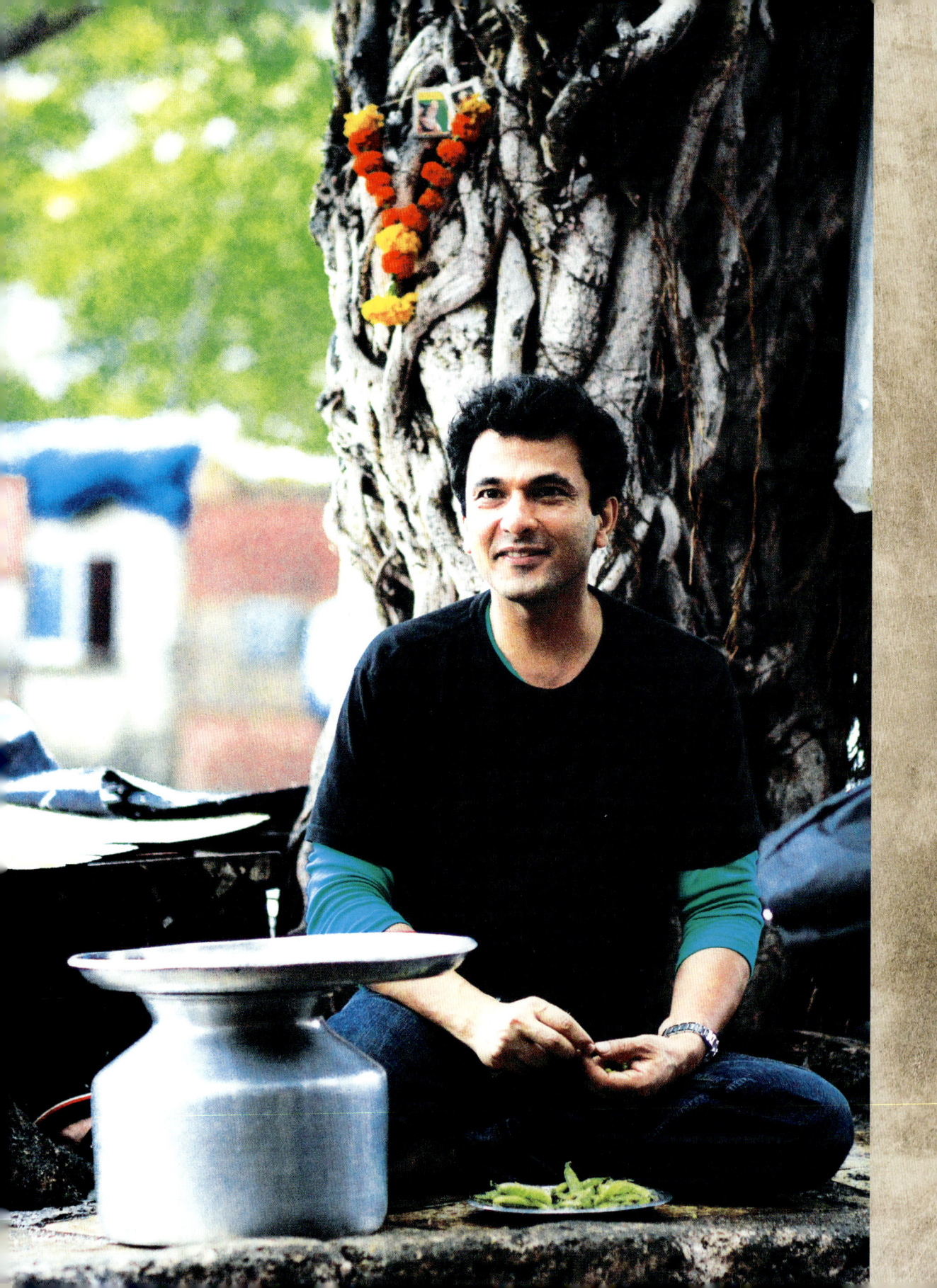

Yogic Food

by

Master Chef Vikas Khanna

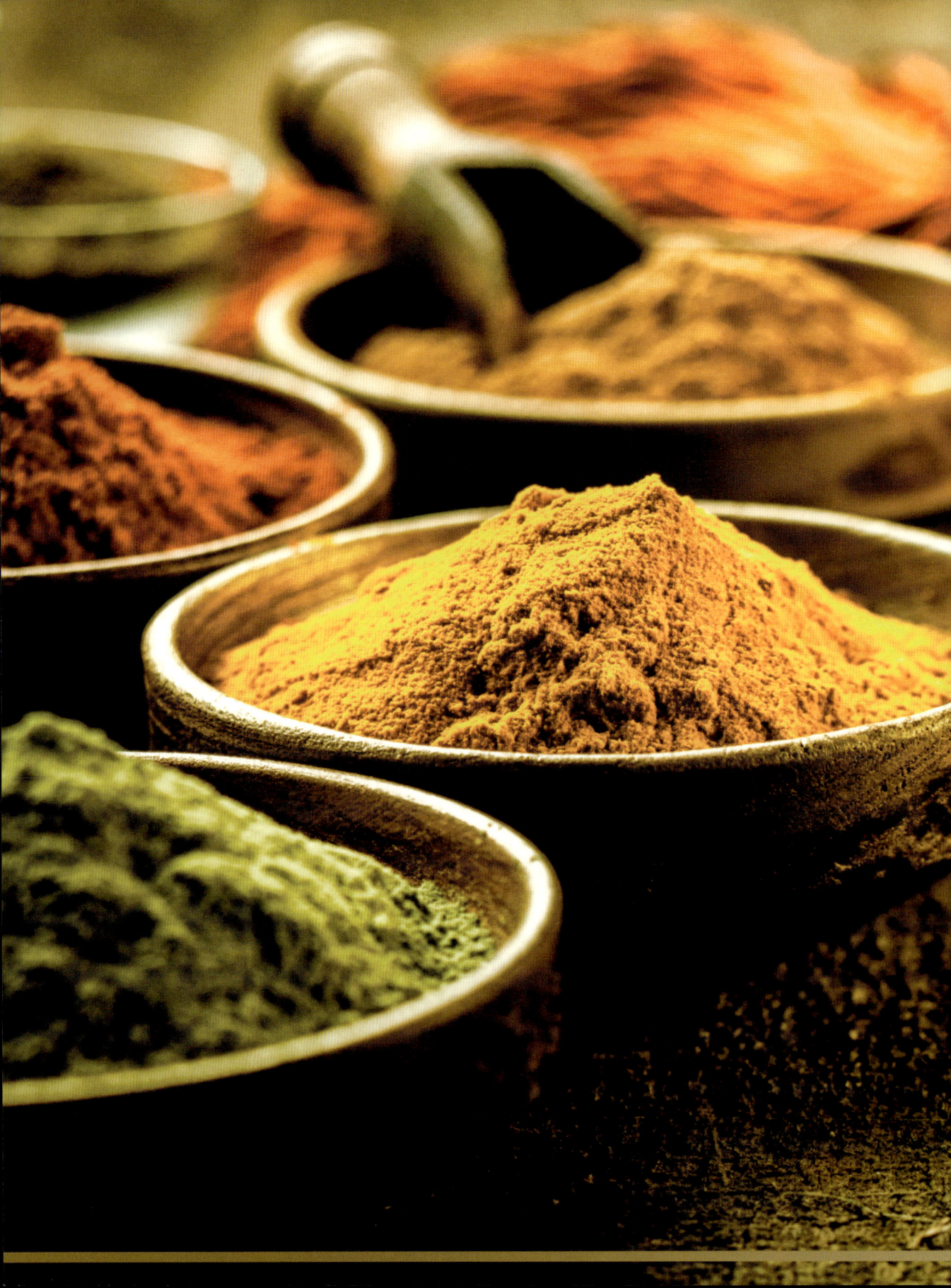

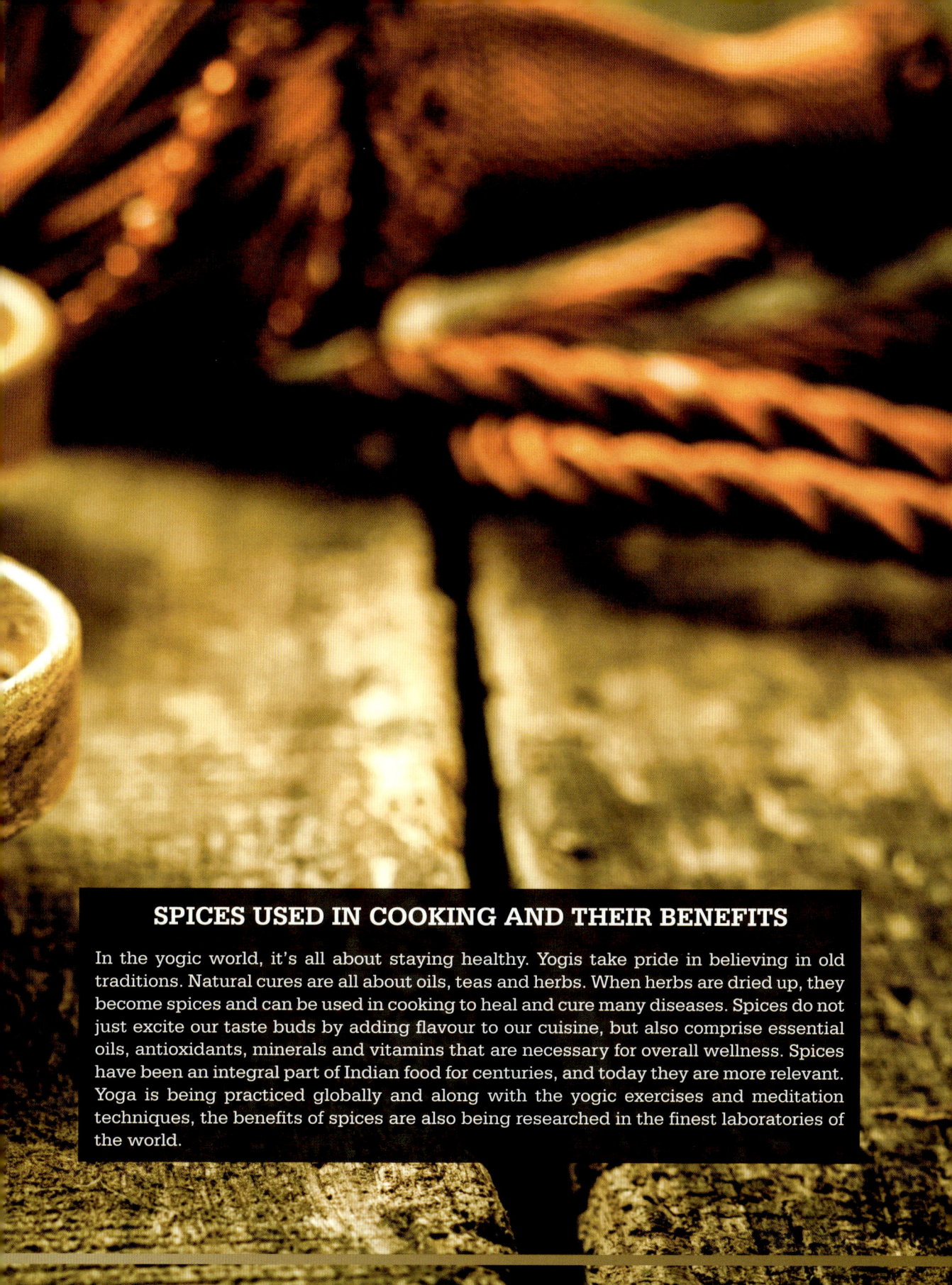

SPICES USED IN COOKING AND THEIR BENEFITS

In the yogic world, it's all about staying healthy. Yogis take pride in believing in old traditions. Natural cures are all about oils, teas and herbs. When herbs are dried up, they become spices and can be used in cooking to heal and cure many diseases. Spices do not just excite our taste buds by adding flavour to our cuisine, but also comprise essential oils, antioxidants, minerals and vitamins that are necessary for overall wellness. Spices have been an integral part of Indian food for centuries, and today they are more relevant. Yoga is being practiced globally and along with the yogic exercises and meditation techniques, the benefits of spices are also being researched in the finest laboratories of the world.

Here are a few spices and their benefits:

Asafetida

This is the dried resin from a rhizome of a giant fennel-like plant. It is sold in both lump and ground forms and used in very small quantities because of its strong and pungent flavour. It alleviates depression by acting as a nerve stimulant. I use and recommend the ground version because it comes mixed with rice flour and turmeric powder, which helps to mellow the flavour.

Used generally in Indian vegetarian cooking, even a small quantity of this strongly-smelling pungent spice adds a deep garlic-like flavour to the recipes. Small quantities soaked in water should be added while cooking. Asafetida must be stored in airtight containers.

Basil

Known across South Asia as a medicinal plant called *tulsi*, basil has an important role within many traditions of Hinduism, in which devotees perform worship involving tulsi plants or leaves. The subtle sweet flavour is not widely used in South Asian cuisine, except in some teas.

Basil powder is an anti-ageing blood purifier and an antiseptic.

Basil Seeds

These black seeds are known as *takmaria* in India. When soaked in water they become very gelatinous. They are used in drinks and desserts as they add a sweet taste and a wonderful texture. They are used for their medicinal properties in Ayurveda, the traditional medicinal system of India.

Bay Leaves

These are long, oval, pointed and smooth leaves of a hardy evergreen shrub. The leaves are dark green when fresh and turn olive green when dry. They are often used dry, whole or ground in curries and rice dishes. Filled with vitamins, for instance niacin and riboflavin, they help in balancing metabolism. Bay leaves are an important ingredient of garam masala, which you'll learn how to make in this section.

Black Cardamom

The robust aroma of black cardamom can improve nearly any curry or meat dish. It is excellent in *biryanis* (a rice dish). Black cardamom pods can be used in soups, chowders, casseroles and marinades for smoky flavour. It is highly valued for its therapeutic properties. It is one of the ingredients in the recipe for garam masala, a very extensively used spice blend in India.

Black Cumin Seeds

These tiny, oblong, aromatic seeds with herbal flavour are used to delicately flavour lentils and curries. The seeds are believed to increase heat in the body, making metabolism more efficient. Interestingly they were even found in King Tut's tomb, suggesting that even centuries ago, great respect existed for the beneficial health effects of black cumin seeds.

Black Salt

Black salt is an unrefined mineral salt. It is salmon pink to gray in colour and is available in lump or powder form. It helps in relieving heartburn. It adds an earthy, sulfurous flavour to our favourite street snacks, savoury drinks and fruit. First time users should know that this flavour won't appeal to all western palates.

Cardamom

These pods come in three different colours: mellow black, white and pale green. The pale green variety is the most common and flavourful. The black seeds inside the pod hold the fragrance, and are used in almost every part of Indian cuisine, ranging from savoury dishes to curries and desserts. The sharp and bitter taste mellows to a warm, sweet taste as it cooks. They are also known as the grains of heaven for their exceptional flavour.

Carom Seeds

These tiny black seeds of the carom plant, which resemble poppy seeds, are also known as lovage, omum, or bishop's weed. They are pungent in aroma and have a sharp taste. The thymol present in carom has antibacterial effects. I particularly use this spice in small quantities, as it gives the dish a very strong and distinctive flavour.

Cayenne Pepper

This is a red powder that is made from grinding the dried red skins of several types of chilli peppers. In India, it is simply called chilli powder. But I use the word cayenne pepper in all my recipes, as there are many different chili powders available in the United States. It adds a spicy flavour to dishes. It contains vitamins A and C and serves as an antioxidant due to the beta carotene.

Chaat Masala

This sweet, spicy and tangy combination of spices and seasonings is used in a variety of ways in Indian cooking.

Dried Chillies

These are whole dried red hot chillies that are usually infused with hot oil to give it a strong flavour. This process enhances and intensifies the flavour of the skins.

Cilantro

In India, street vendors generally give a bunch of cilantro and a handful of green chillies free when you buy produce. This shows how much we use them and how important they are to our cuisine. We use it fresh and add it to a dish at the last minute to preserve its fresh flavour. It keeps best refrigerated and wrapped in moist paper towels.

Cinnamon

This is a classic ingredient for curries and desserts. It is a great spice to ease stress, improve attention span and memory. The whole sticks are used in curry powders, garam masala, in marinades, meats, biryanis and curries. It is also available in powder which is rarely used in Indian cuisine. I have used ground cinnamon in some recipes for its convenience. As with everything, I encourage you to grind your own as you need it.

Clarified Butter

This is butter that has been rendered to separate the milk solids and water from the butterfat. Melting butter, and allowing the different components to sit and separate by density, produces clarified butter. The water evaporates, some solids float to the surface and are skimmed off, and the remainder of the heavier milk solids sink to the bottom and are left behind when the butterfat, which is clear and yellow is poured off the top. The milk solids are then discarded.

Cloves

These are the dried unopened buds of a tropical tree. Deep reddish brown cloves add a strong fragrance to rice and grain recipes. It is also an important ingredient in garam masala. They are lightly fried in hot oil, which perfumes the dish.

Coriander Leaves

Also known as cilantro leaves, these are one of the most commonly used herbs in Indian cuisine. It is generally used for garnishes, marinades and chutneys. The best way to store it is to keep it refrigerated, wrapped in a moist kitchen towel.

Coriander Seeds

Coriander seeds are ribbed peppercorn sized spherical pale green to beige-brown seeds of an annual fern-like plant of the parsley family. They are extremely aromatic, with a hint of spice. I always keep them in little quantities in airtight containers, as they lose their flavour with exposure and age.

When dry-roasted, the seeds impart a warm lemony aroma and flavour, which can then be ground before adding to the recipe. While preparing garam masala, the quantity of coriander seeds used is more in comparison to other spices because of its mild flavour.

Cumin Seeds

Varying in colour from beige to nearly black, cumin seeds are an essential flavouring in Indian cooking. Cumin has a strong earthy taste and warm aroma and should be used sparingly in recipes. It is commonly fried in oil to infuse the dish with the flavour of cumin and give it a deeper, woody flavour. It is one of the scents in a kitchen that most reminds me of my grandmother as she started many dishes by this method.

Curry Leaves

Curry leaves originate from the Kari tree of Southwest Asia. They are mainly used as an aromatic flavouring for most curries and soups. When starting a curry or soup dish, put the curry leaves into the oil to fry until crisp. For extended use, air dry them completely, and store in an airtight container. Their fresh citrus aroma is an integral ingredient of South Indian cooking. It is not a substitute for curry powder. Dried curry leaves are utilised much like bay leaves but all the recipes here call for fresh curry leaves.

Curry Powder

Curry powder is a mixture of spices, varying in composition. This was developed by the British during their colonial rule of India.

The word 'khari' from which 'curry' is derived, comes from southern India and refers to a sauce of any kind. The British, who wished to take the taste of Indian food home, developed curry powder. As a result, curry powder in the western world has a fairly standardised taste, but there are many varieties of curry flavours in South Asia.

Dill Leaves

Dill has a very distinctive flavour and is often paired with fish, cucumbers, potatoes, or is added to dips, salad dressings, or cream sauces. Dill loses flavour when it is heated, so always add it to cooked dishes at the last minute.

Dill Seeds

These seeds of the dill plant are straight to slightly curved, with a longitudinally ridged surface. The seeds have a much more potent flavour, similar to a combination of anise and celery.

Fennel Seeds

These are oval pale greenish yellow seeds of the common fennel plant. They are sweetly aromatic and have an anise-like flavour. They are used in both sweet and savoury dishes. Roasted fennel seeds are often chewed as a digestive and mouth freshener after Indian meals.

For most Indians, fennel seed means *mukhwas*, the tiny oblong licorice-like, candy-coated seeds that they chew after a meal. In cooking, the seeds have a more intense flavour than the leaves and are an important component of spice blends. Like cumin and many other spices, they are first fried to bring out the flavour before being added to various dishes.

Fenugreek Leaves – Dried

Called *kasoori methi* in India, this leaf lends a rich and pleasantly bitter flavour to curries. Fresh leaves are available in season and can also be found frozen but I use them dried in all of these recipes.

Fenugreek Seeds

These are dried rectangular yellow brown seeds of a strongly scented annual herb of the legume family. They are used in small quantities because of their strong flavour. The greens of the plant are very frequently used for their aromatic and somewhat bitter flavour.

These small yellow brownish seeds have a powerful, bitter taste. A small amount is enough to add substantial flavour. It is a key ingredient of some spice blends, especially the *paanch phoron* mix used to flavour curries. While frying or dry roasting these seeds, care should be taken not to overcook them as that will make the fenugreek excessively bitter and inedible.

Five Spice Mix

Also known as paanch phoran, this is a traditional Bengali spice mix and quintessential spice in the east Indian cuisines. It lends a lovely aroma when fried in oil. Fennel seeds, nigella seeds, fenugreek seeds, mustard seeds and cumin seeds are combined in equal portions for this spice mix.

Garam Masala

This is the most important spice blend in north Indian cuisine. Adding a little pinch of this mixture at the end of cooking or right before serving adds more flavour to the dish.

Garlic

Garlic is a close relative of onion, shallot and leek. It has been used throughout recorded history for both culinary and medicinal purposes. It has a characteristic pungent, spicy flavour that mellows and sweetens considerably with cooking.

Ginger

A paste of puréed ginger and garlic is one of the first ingredients that goes into the hot oil for many dishes. We use ginger everywhere for its rich, pungent aroma and peppery bite. It instantly arouses the taste buds and is considered beneficial for health. It promotes general wellness and energy enhancement. Fresh ginger is best when the roots are firm and the knobs snap when broken. Dried ground ginger should have an intense characteristically gingery aroma or it is old.

Goan Curry Powder

This distinctive spice mix from the coastal regions of Goa is a combination of dry-roasted coconut with spices. Though you can reduce the level of spice, this blend has a wonderful deep flavour.

Green Chillies

Chillies are one of the most important ingredients for pungency and heat in Indian cuisine. In most of the regions, they are even served raw on the side with the meal. I often remove the seeds and only use the skin to reduce the heat.

Himalayan Salt

Salt is the world's oldest food additive known to man. Crystals of Himalayan salt have been a part of my pantry ever since I lived in Nepal. These crystals add a wonderful aroma and earthy taste to food and can be found at many specialty stores.

Kaffir Lime Leaf – Dried

Kaffir lime leaves add a memorable taste to a variety of foods, and are highly popular in south east Asian cuisine. Used in a selection of soups and curries, kaffir lime leaf is an important ingredient in many foods from Thailand and other South East Asian countries as well.

Kewra

This is an extract that is distilled from the pandanus flowers and is used to flavour meats, drinks and desserts in India and South East Asia. These flowers have a sweet, perfumed odour with a pleasant quality similar to rose flowers, but are significantly kewra is fruitier.

Kokum

This is the sun-dried, dark purple to black, sticky, and curly-edged fruit of a mangosteen tree. It has a citrus-like, refreshingly sour taste, and a sweet aroma. It is native to the south Indian coastal regions.

Long Black Pepper

Known as pippali in India, this is a close relative of the black pepper plant, and has a similar, though generally hotter, taste.

Mace

Mace is the deep amber-coloured covering of the nutmeg kernel. Its flavour is similar to nutmeg, only more intense. I always buy it in flakes or blades rather than ground because its flavour is best preserved that way.

Mango Powder

The dried pulp of unripe mangoes is ground to make mango or amchoor powder. It is beige in colour, slightly fibrous in appearance, and sweet and sour in taste. Mango powder contains phenol compounds and is high in antioxidants. It is used particularly to add sourness to a dish such as a salad or a chaat, but the ingredients need to be kept dry.

Mint

Mints are aromatic, almost exclusively perennial, rarely annual, herbs. They are used in marinades, chutneys, drinks and desserts because of their refreshing taste. I also use dried mint to make breads in my kitchens.

Mustard Seeds

Of all the varieties of mustard that are available in the world, it is the black seeds that are commonly used in Indian cuisine. They are also the source of the commonly used mustard oil. We use black mustard whole for the most part and briefly fry them in oil when starting a dish. Note that mustards prepared elsewhere and yellow mustard seeds cannot be used as substitutes in these recipes.

Nutmeg

The rich brown seed of the fruit of a tropical evergreen, nutmeg has a warm, spicy flavour with hints of sweetness and is used to season both savoury and sweet dishes. It is available in whole and ground forms. For best results, I always prefer buying it whole and then preparing a freshly ground batch according to the recipe. Nutmeg helps reduce stress and stimulate the brain. It has been highly regarded as a brain tonic since the ancient times.

Paprika

It is a red powder made from dry, mild chillies. It is mainly used for adding a rich red colour to curries or marinades. It is sometimes called Kashmiri mirch in Indian stores but I have found that Hungarian mild paprika works very well in my recipes.

Parsley

There are two common varieties of parsley in the market. The feathery flat-leaf parsley adds a great flavour to sauces and chutneys. The curly parsley has less flavour than the flat-leaf parsley, but it works as a terrific garnish.

Peppercorns

Peppercorns, salt and sugar - it seems like much of history through the Renaissance was centered on the search for these precious ingredients. In our cuisine, we rarely use white pepper as we like the deeper, mellower flavour of black pepper. The favourite variety of most chefs is the Tellicherry peppercorn which comes from the Malabar coast of Kerala in South -west India. We make chutneys out of pickled green peppercorns which have a lighter and more ethereal taste than the powerful black pepper.

Pomegranate Seeds – Dried

These sun-dried, kernel-like seeds of the wild Indian pomegranate are ground to give a sour and tangy flavour to dishes. They impart a dark brown colour to curries when cooked in hot oil. The fresh pomegranate seeds are not the substitute of the dried ones because of their totally different character.

Rose Buds – Dried

Rose buds have been used for centuries in Indian and Middle Eastern cuisines for the aromatic and fruity flavour they add to food. They have a very soft texture and swell up in curries.

Rose Spread – Gulukand

In Ayurveda, rose is known for its soothing and cooling effect on the body, mind and emotions. It is used as a sweetener in *paan* – beetel leaf wrap – a traditional Indian palate cleanser.

Rosewater

This is a hydrosol portion of the distillate of rose petals. It imparts an intoxicating scent of roses to rice dishes, desserts and drinks. Considered very auspicious for its aroma, it is also diluted with water and sprinkled at various religious and cultural ceremonies.

When using rosewater for the first time, use it with a light hand until you get used to the floral flavour. I recommend making your own rosewater as store-bought flowers nearly always have pesticides on it.

Rosemary

This pungent herb with its needle-like leaves is often used to flavour meats and tomato sauces. Rosemary stems, stripped off their leaves, can also be used as skewers for *kebabs*. Dried rosemary is an excellent substitute for the fresh herb.

Saffron

These intense yellow threads are the dried orange to deep red stigmas of a small purple crocus, a member of the iris family. It is the world's most expensive spice, as it takes almost seventy-five thousand handpicked blossoms to make one pound of saffron. It is painstakingly harvested by hand from the *crocus sativa* only in the early morning hours.

It has a distinctly warm, rich, powerful and intense flavour, with no substitute. It can be purchased in strands or ground. I recommend the strands for the sake of quality.

The most highly regarded saffron in India is the deep maroon coloured variety from Kashmir. It is the darkest one there is and has an aroma that will make you dizzy.

Sage

The velvet leaves of sage are often combined with other strong herbs to flavour meat dishes and poultry stuffing. Dried sage is an excellent substitute for the fresh herb.

Star Anise

Star anise is a dried star-shaped dark brown pod containing flavourful seeds in each section, and is a fruit of the evergreen tree of the magnolia family. These licorice-like seeds are used to flavour both sweet and savoury dishes.

Star anise has a more pronounced licorice flavour than fennel or anise seed. Dropping one piece of it into a curry dish adds a powerful dimension. I sometimes use fennel seed and star anise ground together for a really intense flavour.

Tamarind

The curved brown bean pod of the tamarind tree contains a sticky pulp enclosing one to twelve shiny black seeds. It is the pulp that is used as a flavouring for its sweet, sour, fruity aroma and taste. It is used to make chutneys, preserves and curries and is available as a pressed fibrous slab or as a jam-like bottled concentrate. I have used the jam-like bottled concentrate in all my recipes for convenience.

The tartness of tamarind is a gift from the south of India. The sticky, sour pulp from the tamarind bean pod adds its essence to chutneys and assorted preserves of all kinds. It is a power house of anti-oxidants, vitamins and minerals. In the restaurant we boil a slab of tamarind, which still has seeds in it and then strain it to make a sauce but for home use it's easier to use the paste version that comes in jars.

Turmeric

This is a dried rhizome of a tropical plant of the ginger family. Intensely yellow ground turmeric is used to colour many curries. It is actually boiled, peeled, sun-dried and ground into a bright yellow-orange powder. The deep, astringent flavour is indispensible, somewhat reminiscent of ginger. It has a warm, peppery aroma and a strong bitter taste, which mellows upon cooking. Its antiseptic and antibacterial properties add to its popularity.

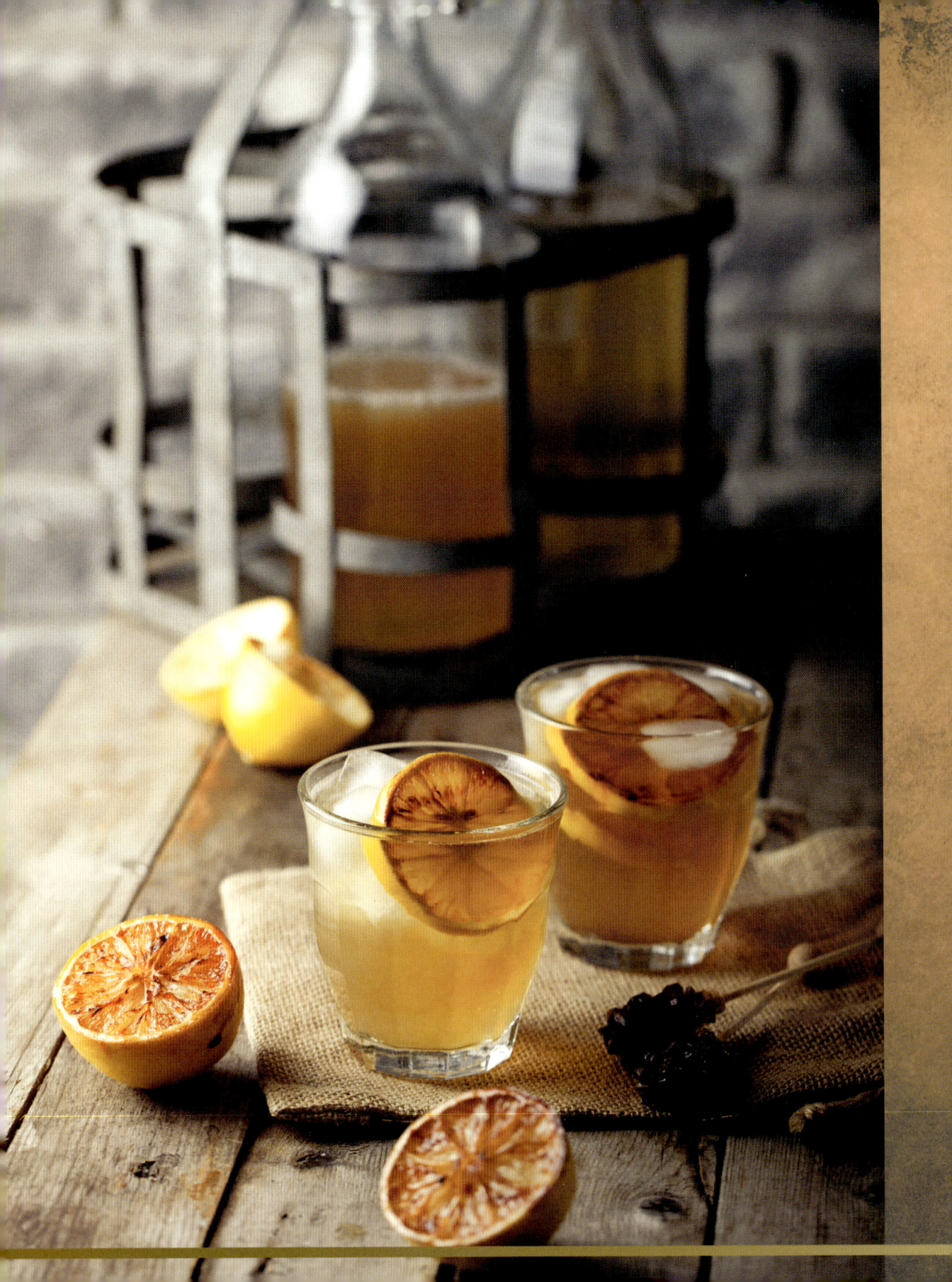

Healthy Recipies

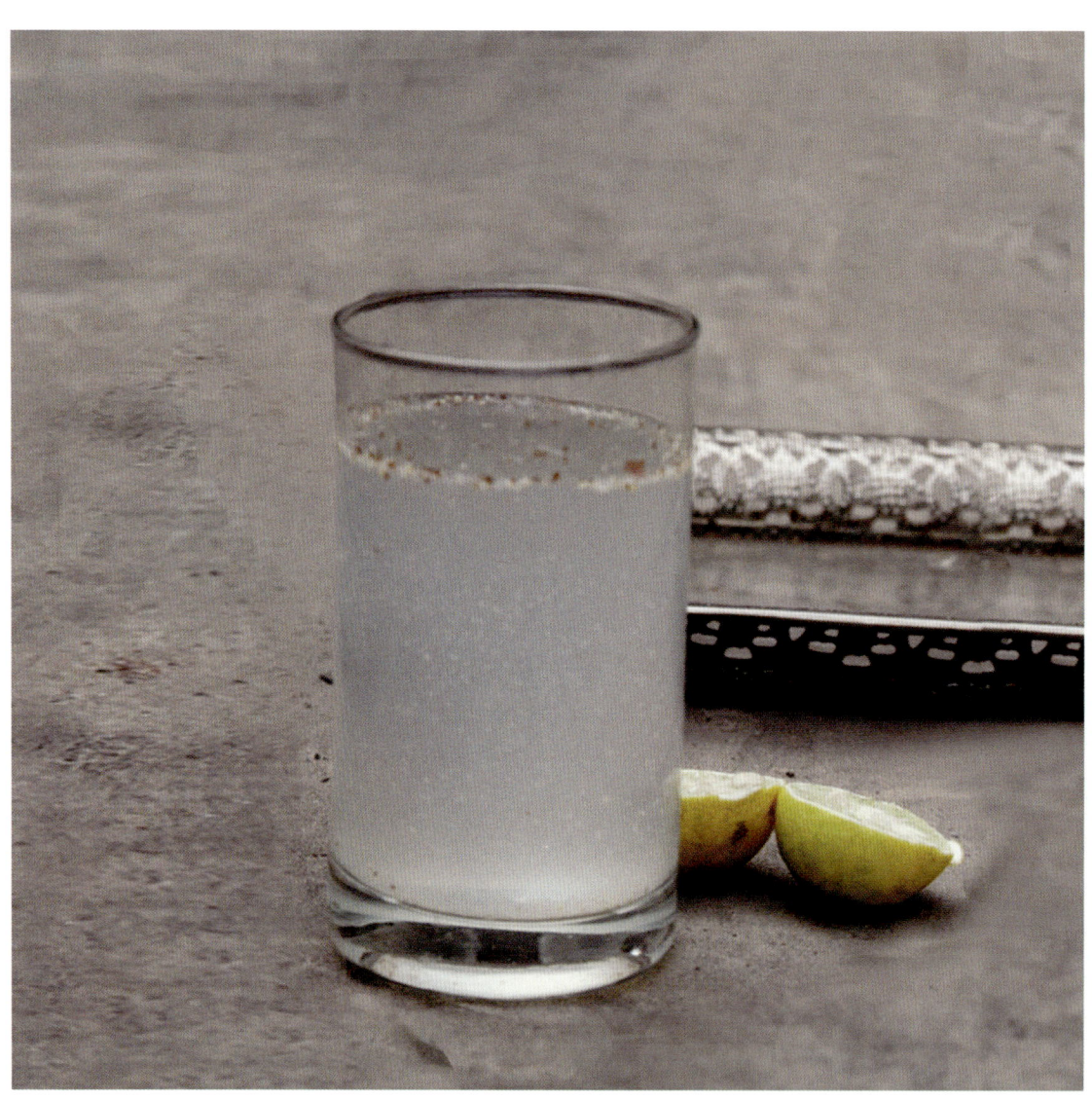

MORNING GLORY SPICY LEMON DRINK

Juice of ½ lime

1 cup boiling water

Pinch of cayenne pepper (optional)

Sugar syrup to taste (or honey) (optional)

Method

Combine all ingredients in a cup and stir to mix well.

Makes 1 serving.

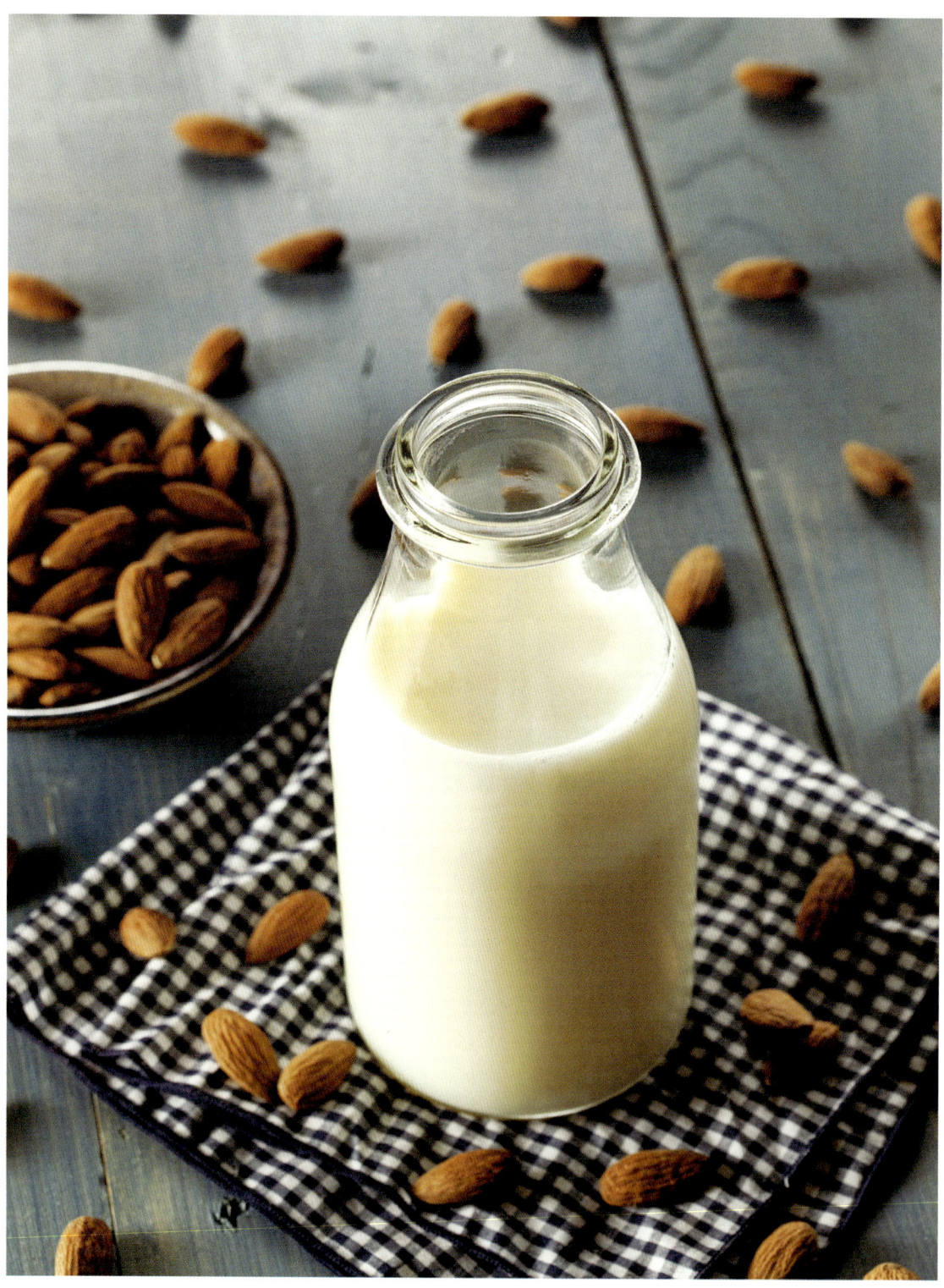

CREAMY ALMOND AGAVE SMOOTHIE

1 cup almonds

2 cups water (for soaking)

3 cups water (for blending)

Agave syrup to taste (or honey) (optional)

Method

Soak almonds overnight in a bowl with two cups of water. Drain and remove skin.

Transfer the almonds to a blender or food processor, and blend until very smooth. Add three cups of water and blend for another two to three minutes.

Strain the almond mixture through cheesecloth to collect the liquid into a pitcher.

Add agave or honey to liquid in pitcher and mix.

Remaining almond mixture can be saved for future use in recipes that require nuts.

Makes 3 cups.

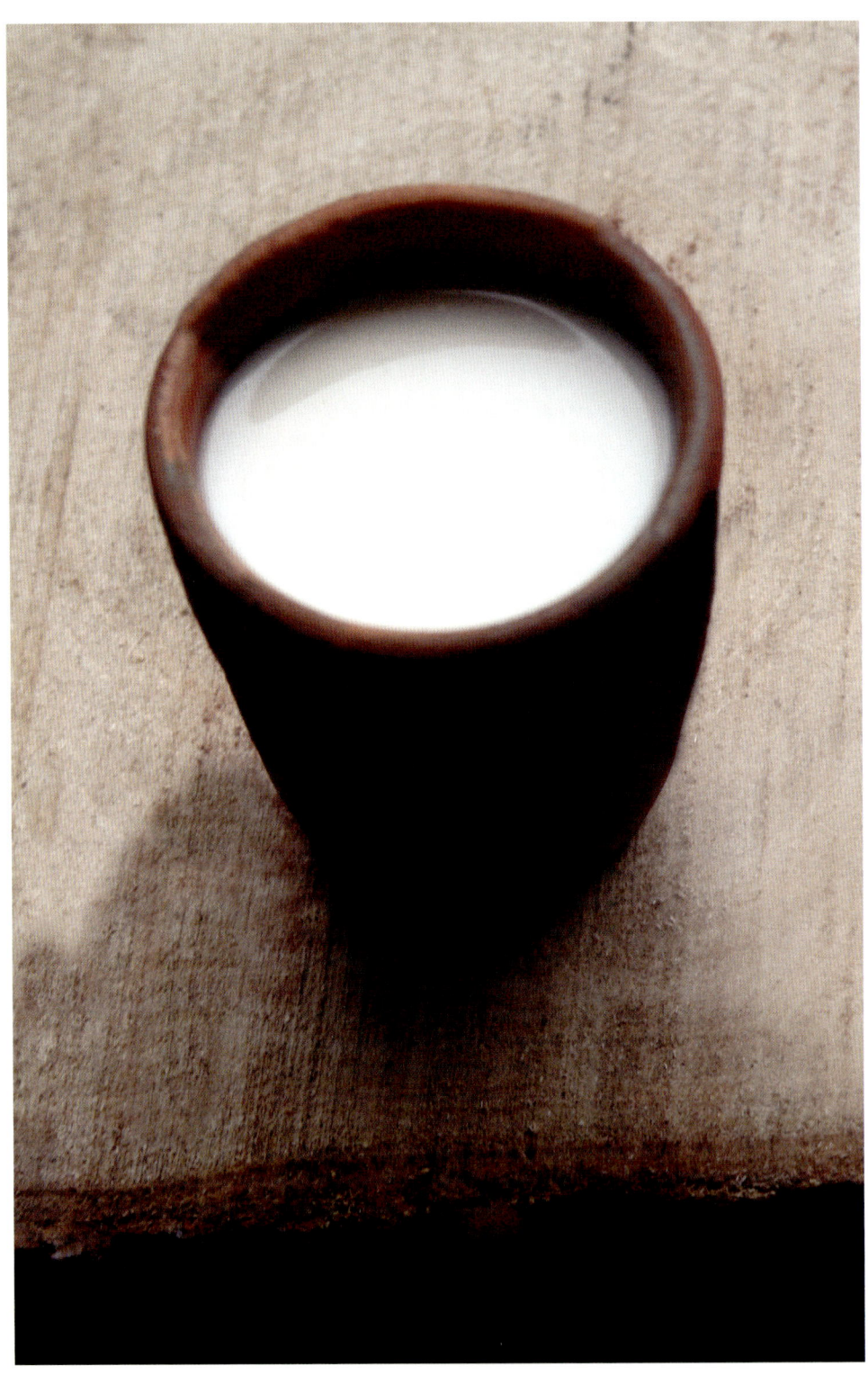

BROWN RICEY ICY MILK

½ cup short-grain organic brown rice, uncooked

8 cups water

½ tsp salt

Honey to taste

Method

Place rice, water, salt, and honey in a large pot and bring to a boil over high heat. Reduce heat to low and simmer covered. Cook for about an hour and a half.

Remove from heat, and transfer to a food processor or blender. Purée until smooth and serve.

This milk can be stored in refrigerator for upto seven days.

Makes about 6 cups.

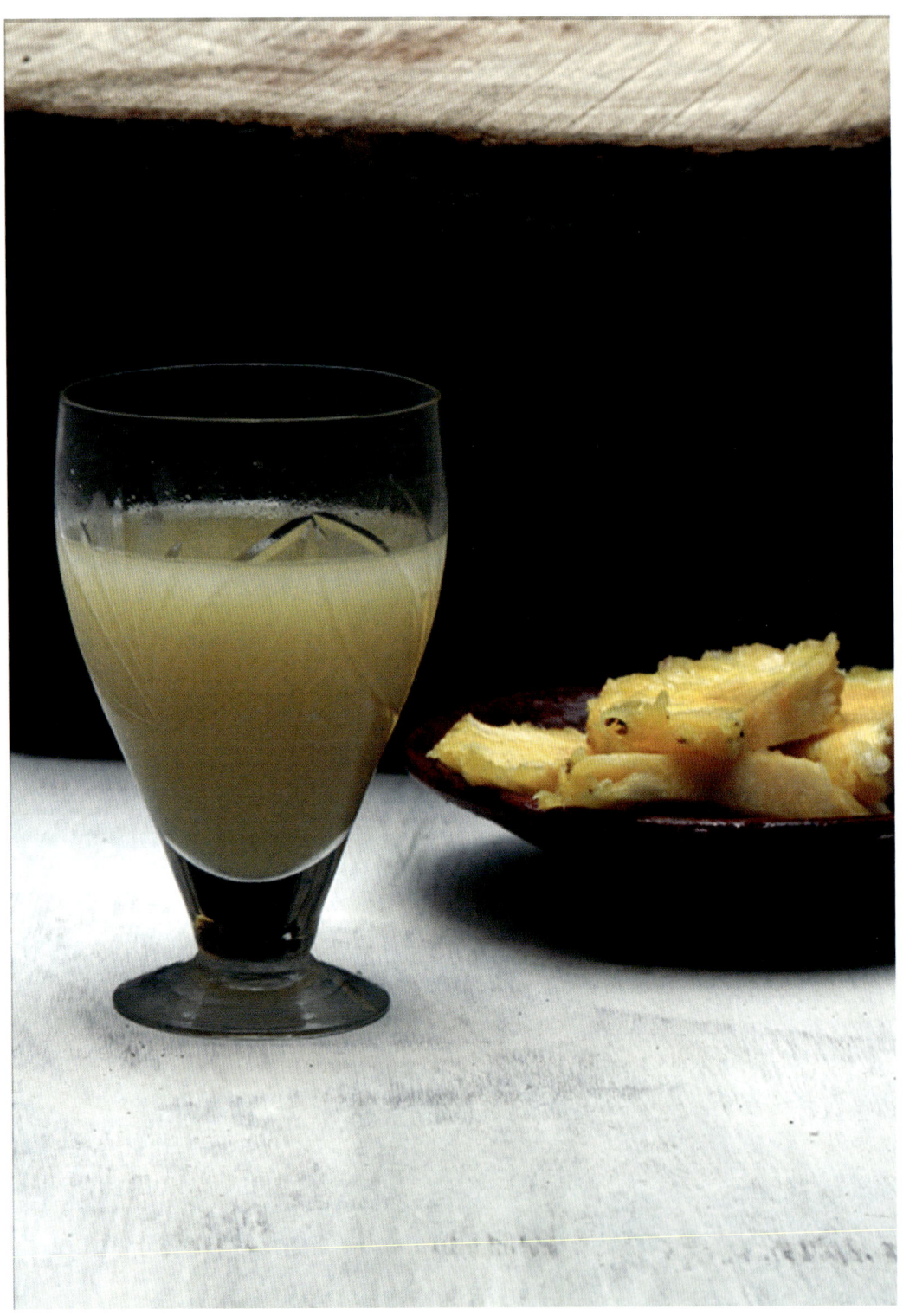

HOMEMADE PIÑA COLADA

3 cups pineapple juice

1 cup coconut milk

2 tsp sugar syrup (optional)

½ tsp lime juice

4 raspberries (for garnish)

4 mint leaves (for garnish)

Method

In a pitcher, mix together pineapple juice, coconut milk, sugar syrup and lime juice. Chill in the refrigerator for at least two hours or overnight.

Pour evenly into four glasses. Garnish with raspberries and mint leaves.

Makes 4 servings.

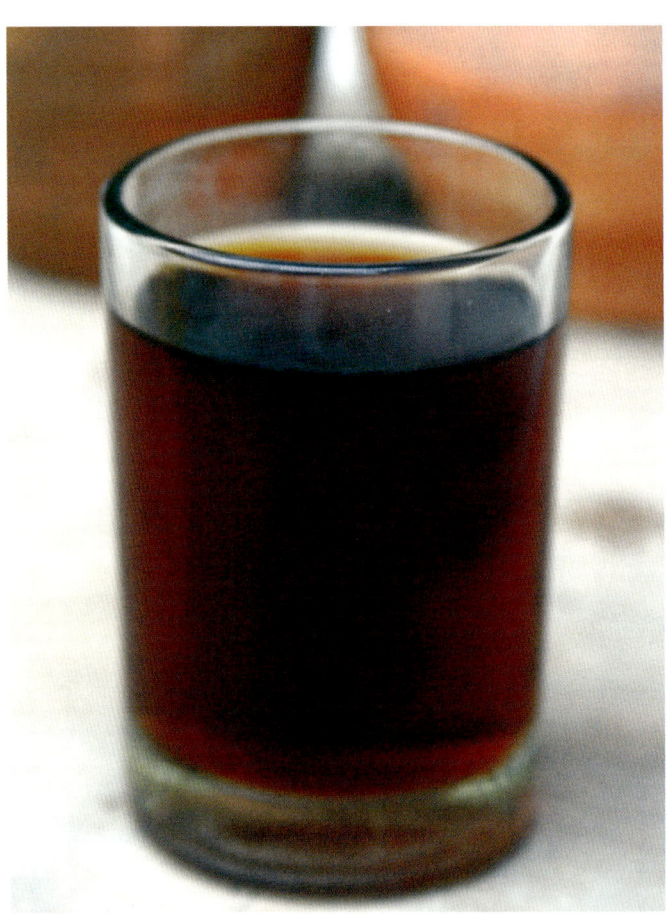

CLOVE-SCENTED MASALA CHAI MIX

1 tsp cloves

1 tsp freshly ground black pepper

1 tsp cardamom seeds

½ tsp nutmeg, grated

1 5-cm piece cinnamon bark (or 1 tsp ground cinnamon)

1 tsp ground ginger

Method

Combine all ingredients in a dry frying pan over medium and toast for three to four minutes, stirring constantly. Remove from heat.

Place in a spice or coffee grinder and working in batches, grind the spice mixture. Store in an non-reactive airtight container.

Makes about ¼ cup.

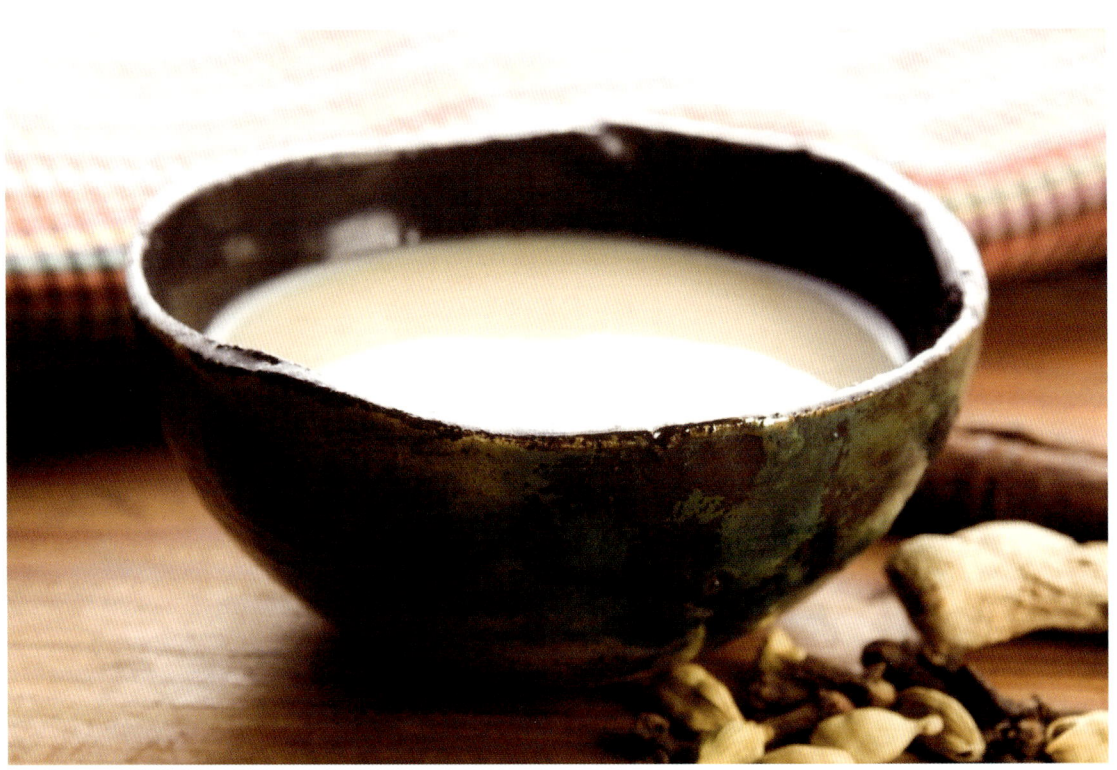

MILKY JAGGERY MASALA CHAI

3 cups water

1 cup milk (or soy milk)

½ - ¾ tsp masala chai mix

1-2 tsp loose leaf black tea (or 1-2 tea bags)

2 tbsp grated jaggery, or to taste

Method

Heat a large pot on high heat. Add water, milk, chai mix, tea and jaggery.

Bring to a boil, stirring frequently to make sure that the milk does not burn. Reduce heat to low and simmer for about five minutes. Strain into cup and add sweetener to taste, and serve.

Makes 4 servings.

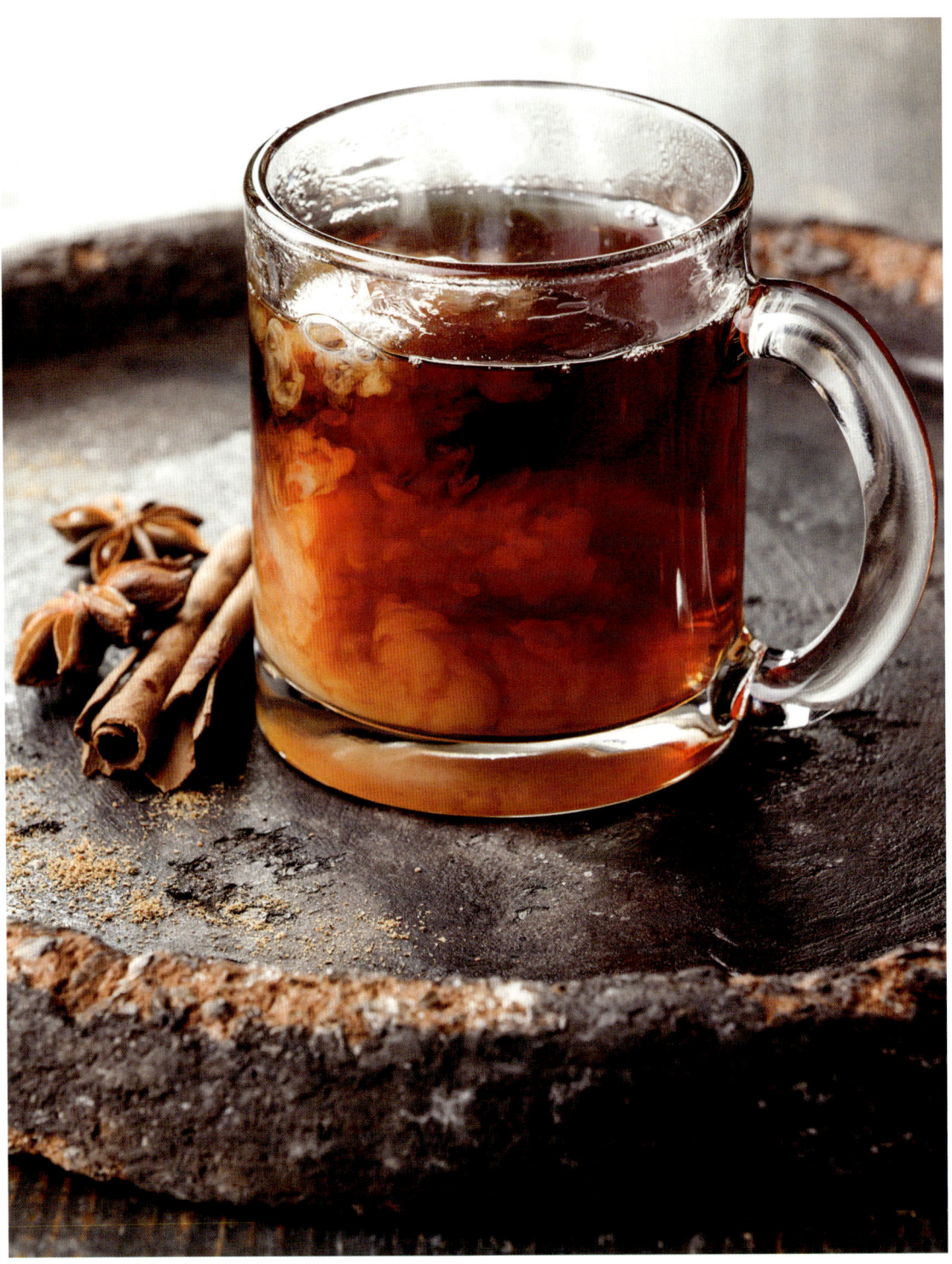

WARM HEART YOGI TEA

6 small pieces cinnamon bark

1 tsp whole fenugreek seeds

1 tsp cardamom pods

1 tsp cloves

1 tsp whole peppercorns

2 tsp fennel seeds

2 tsp ginger, chopped

Method

Combine all the ingredients with 4 cups water in a pot over medium heat, and bring to a boil.

Remove from heat and let the flavours infuse for three to four minutes. Strain and serve hot.

Makes 4-5 servings.

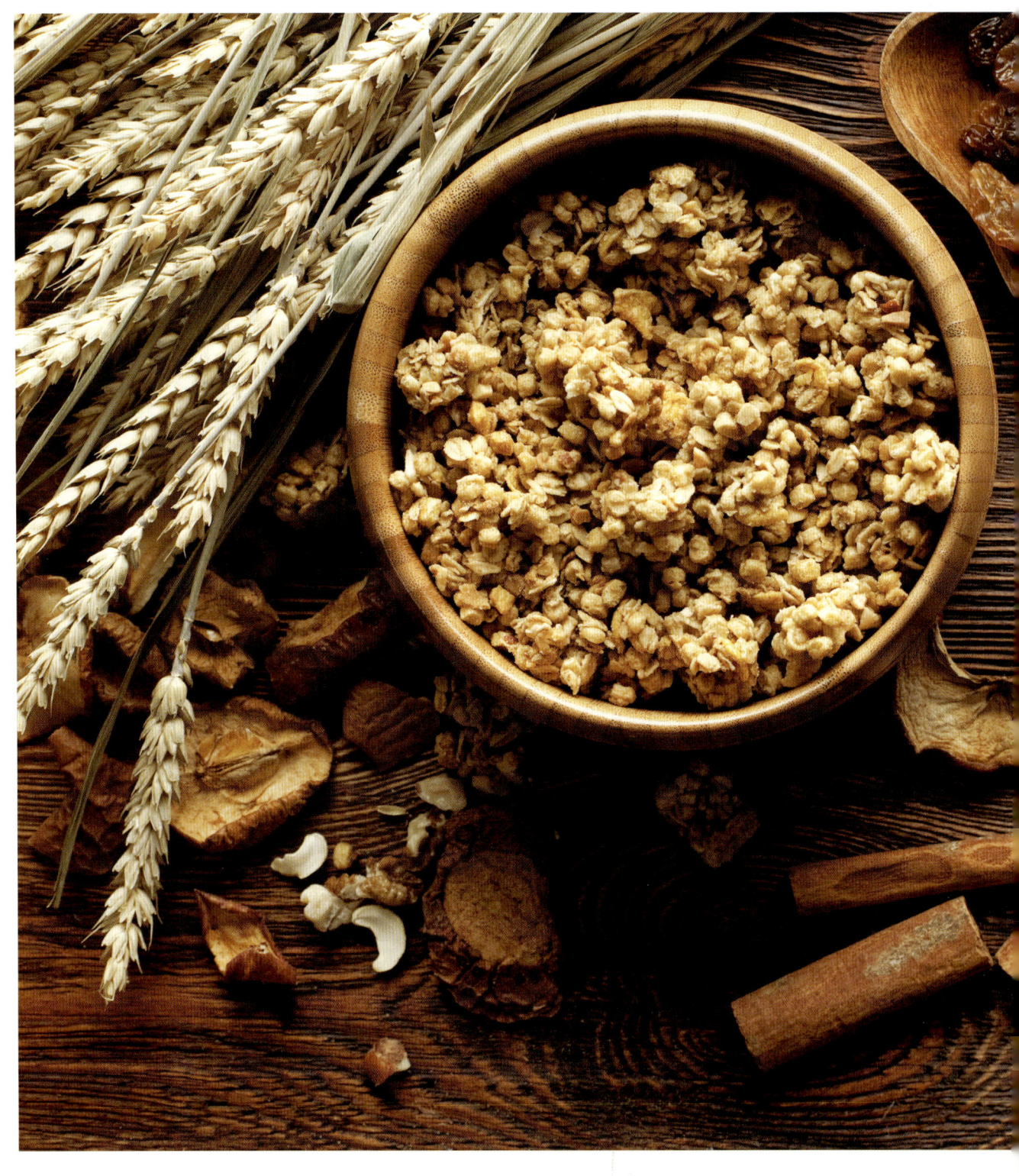

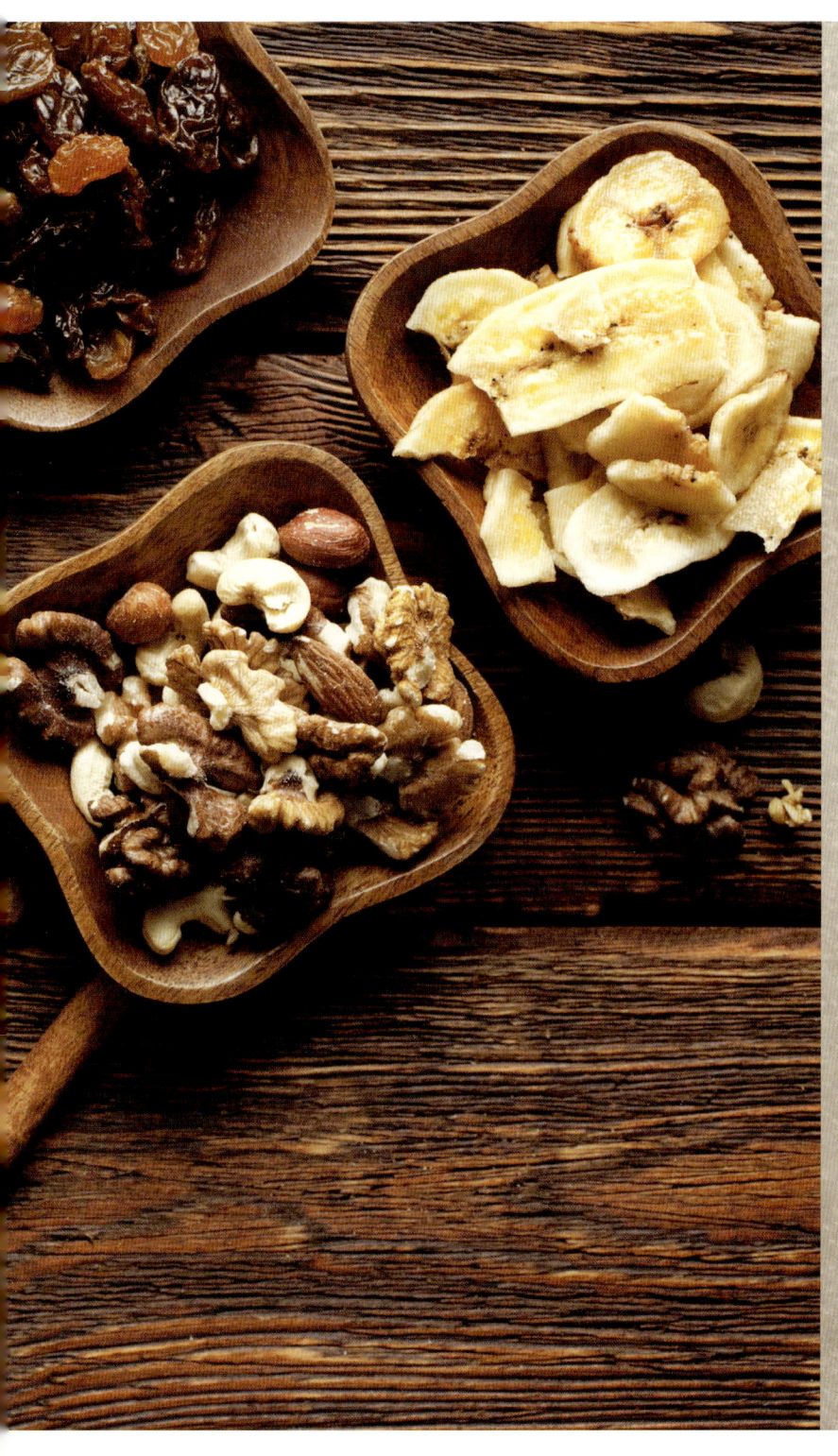

Breakfast

Following your morning yoga routine, try one of these delicious and healthy breakfast recipes that can balance the *doshas*. A promising start to a great day!

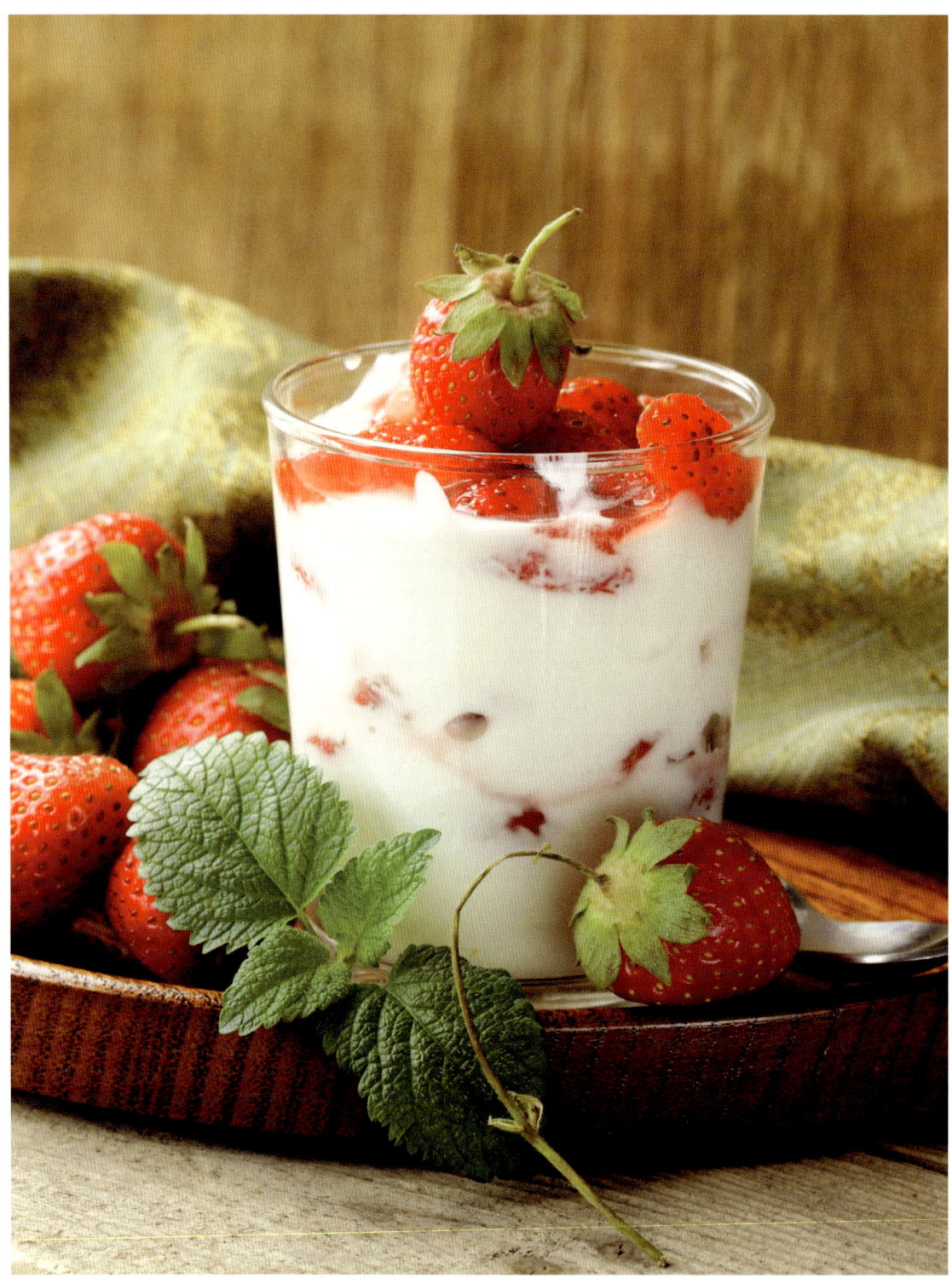

UNION SQUARE FARMERS MARKET FRUIT SALAD

2 cups strawberries, hulled and sliced

1 cup blueberries

2 bananas, sliced

2 tbsp flax seeds, ground

2 cups plain low fat yoghurt (may use vanilla-flavoured yogurt)

Mint leaves (for garnish)

Method

In a large mixing bowl, combine strawberries, blueberries, bananas, flax seeds, and yogurt. Serve fresh with a garnish of mint leaves.

Makes 4 servings.

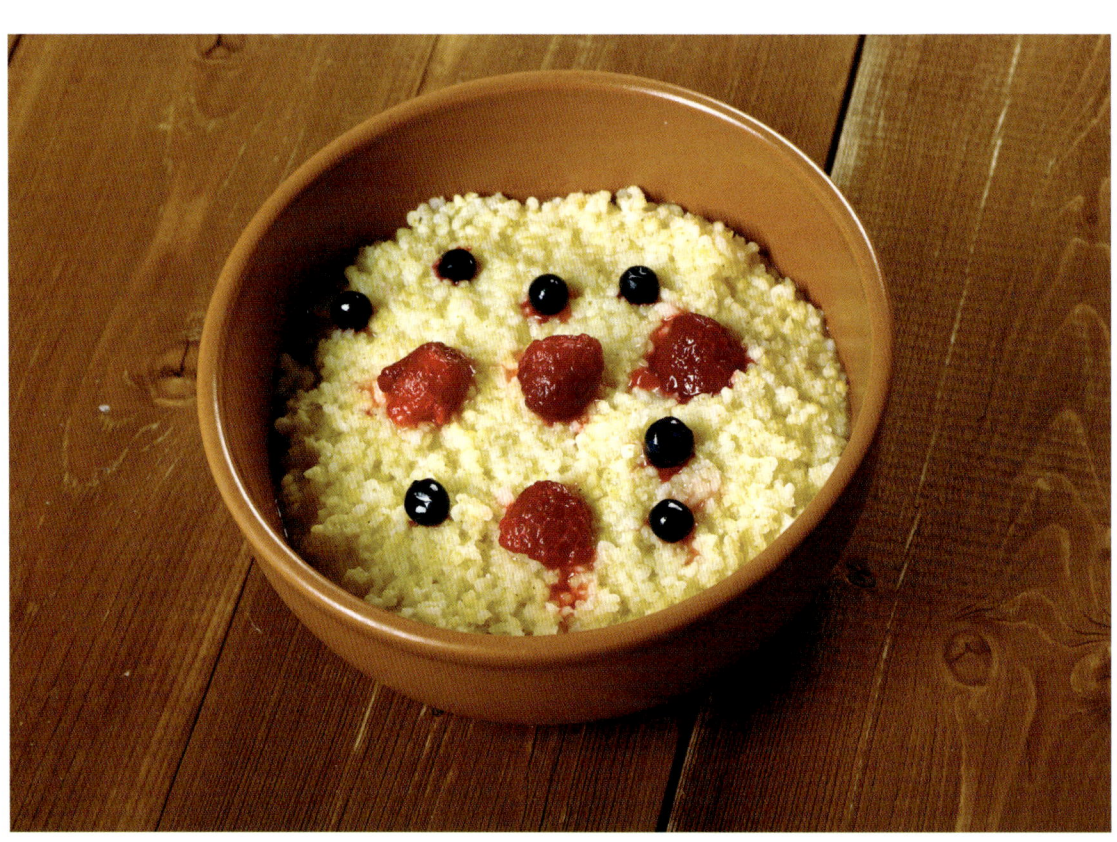

VINTAGE PORRIDGE WITH STEWED BERRIES

1 cup porridge oats

1 cup water

1 cup soy milk

¼ tsp salt

¾ cup mixed berries

1 tsp honey

1 tbsp flax seeds

Method

Heat a pot over medium heat. Add porridge oats, water, milk and salt. Increase heat to high and bring to a boil. Reduce heat to low and simmer. Add in mixed berries and cook for about 10 minutes, until the oats are cooked.

Remove from heat, add honey and flax seeds. Serve hot and fresh.

Makes 1-2 servings.

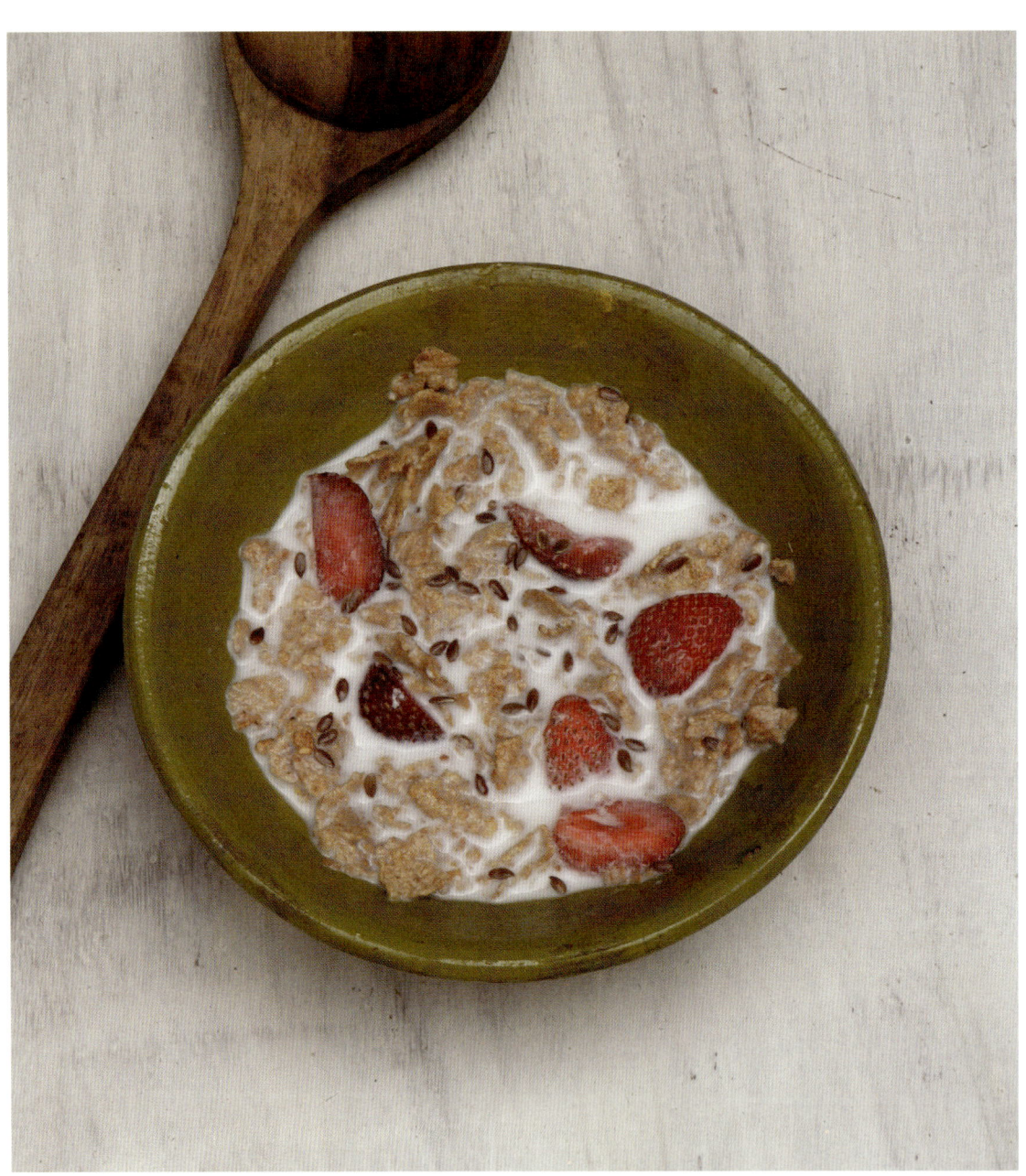

MULTI GRAIN WALNUT CEREAL

1 cup multi-grain cereal

2 tbsp bran

1 tbsp flax seeds, ground

1 tbsp walnuts, lightly roasted and roughly crushed

2 cups milk

½ cup fresh berries

Method

In a mixing bowl, combine cereal, bran, flax seeds, walnuts and milk and let it rest for 20-30 minutes. Add berries and serve immediately.

Makes 1-2 servings.

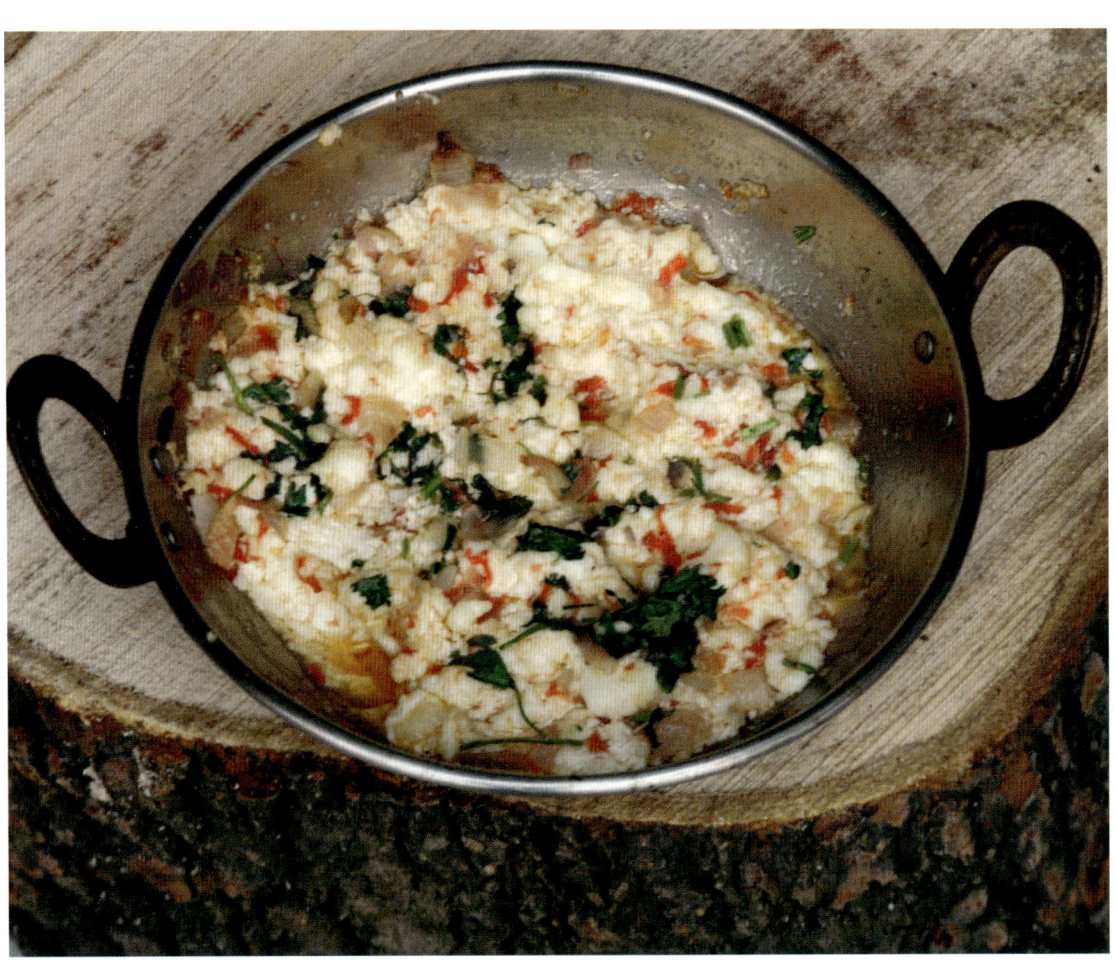

FRESH TURMERIC SCRAMBLED TOFU

3 tbsp milk or water

½ tsp salt

¼ tsp freshly ground pepper

1 tbsp oil

1 tbsp onions, minced

1 tsp fresh ginger, minced

2 tbsp turmeric, freshly grated

1 ½ tsp fresh green chillies, minced

5 cups crumbled tofu

2 tbsp coriander leaves, chopped

Method

In a medium mixing bowl, add milk, salt, and pepper, and mix to combine well. Reserve.

Heat oil in a frying pan over medium-high heat. Add onions and ginger, and cook for a minute. Add turmeric and green chillies, and mix to combine well.

Reduce heat to low and add tofu and cook for three to four minutes.

Serve hot topped with coriander leaves.

Makes 3-4 servings.

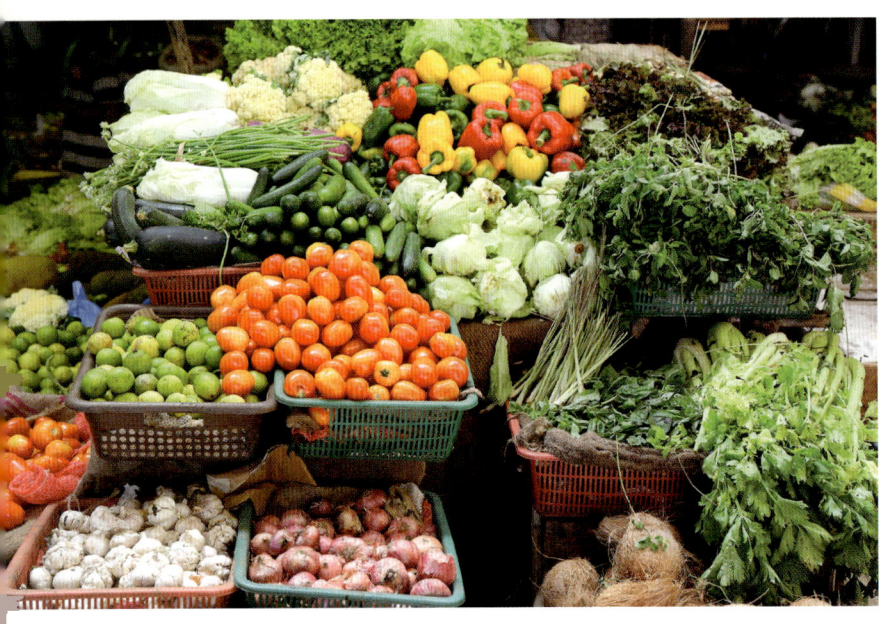

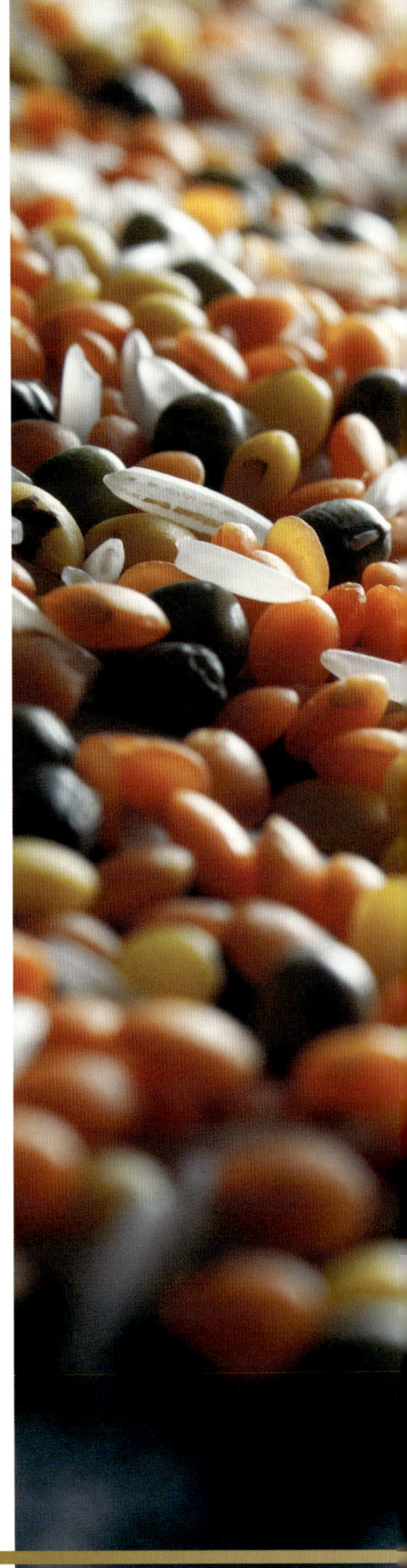

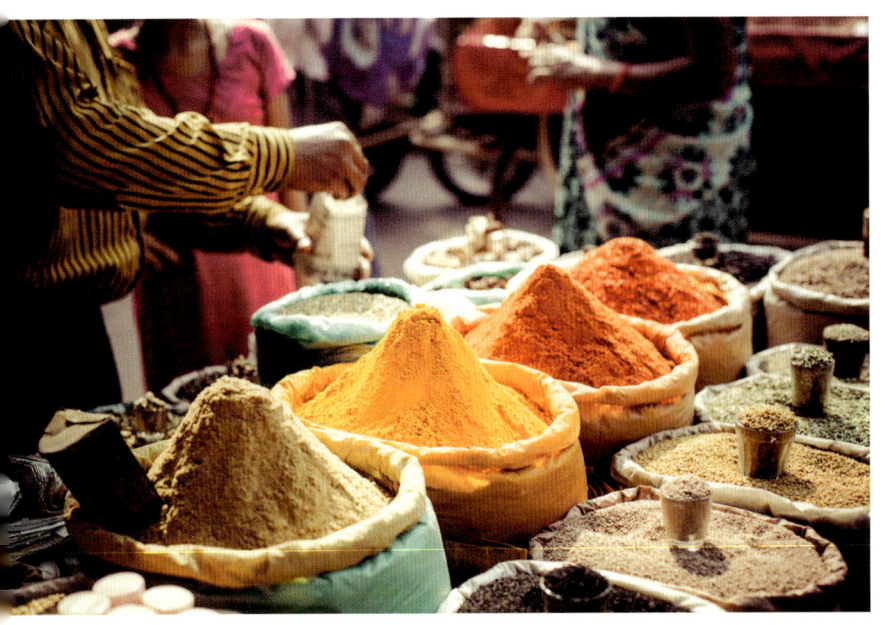

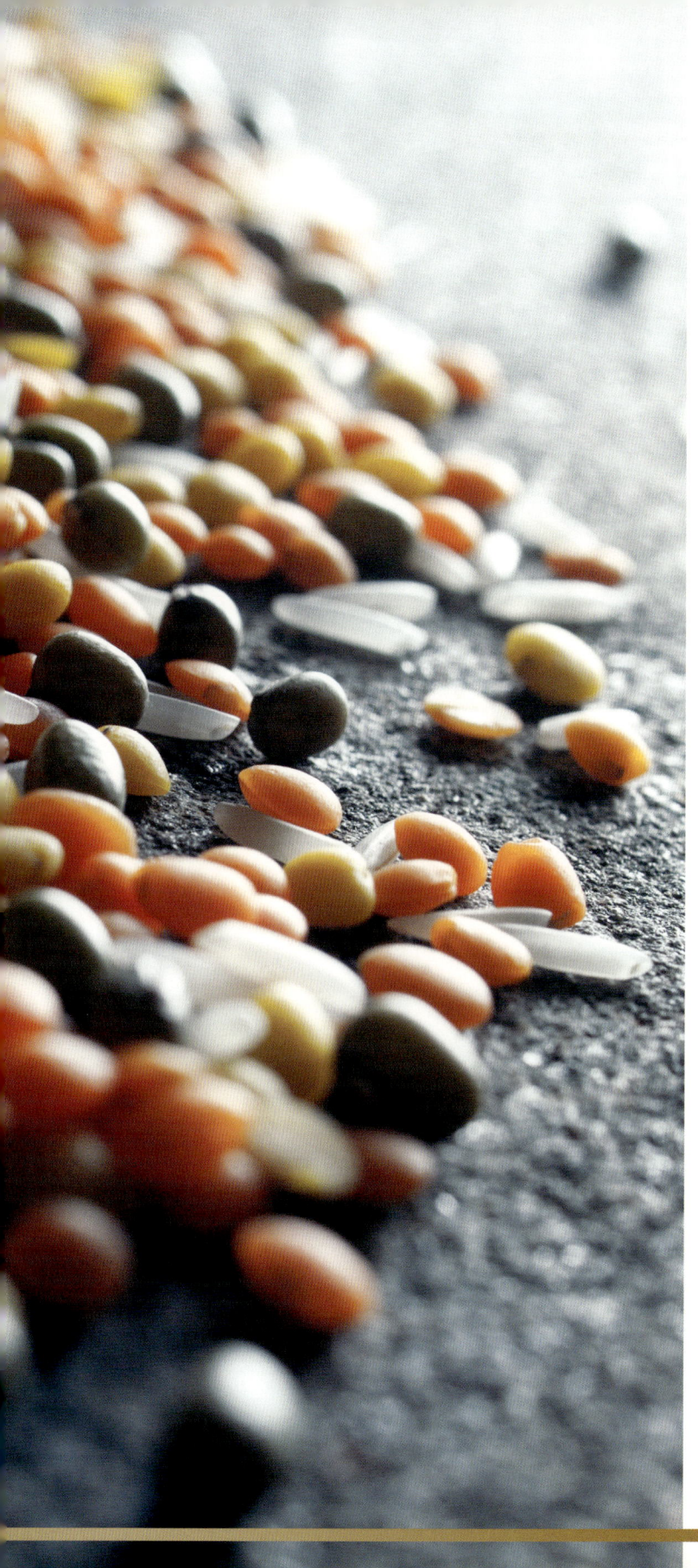

Light Meals

Salads

Soups

Lentils

Desserts

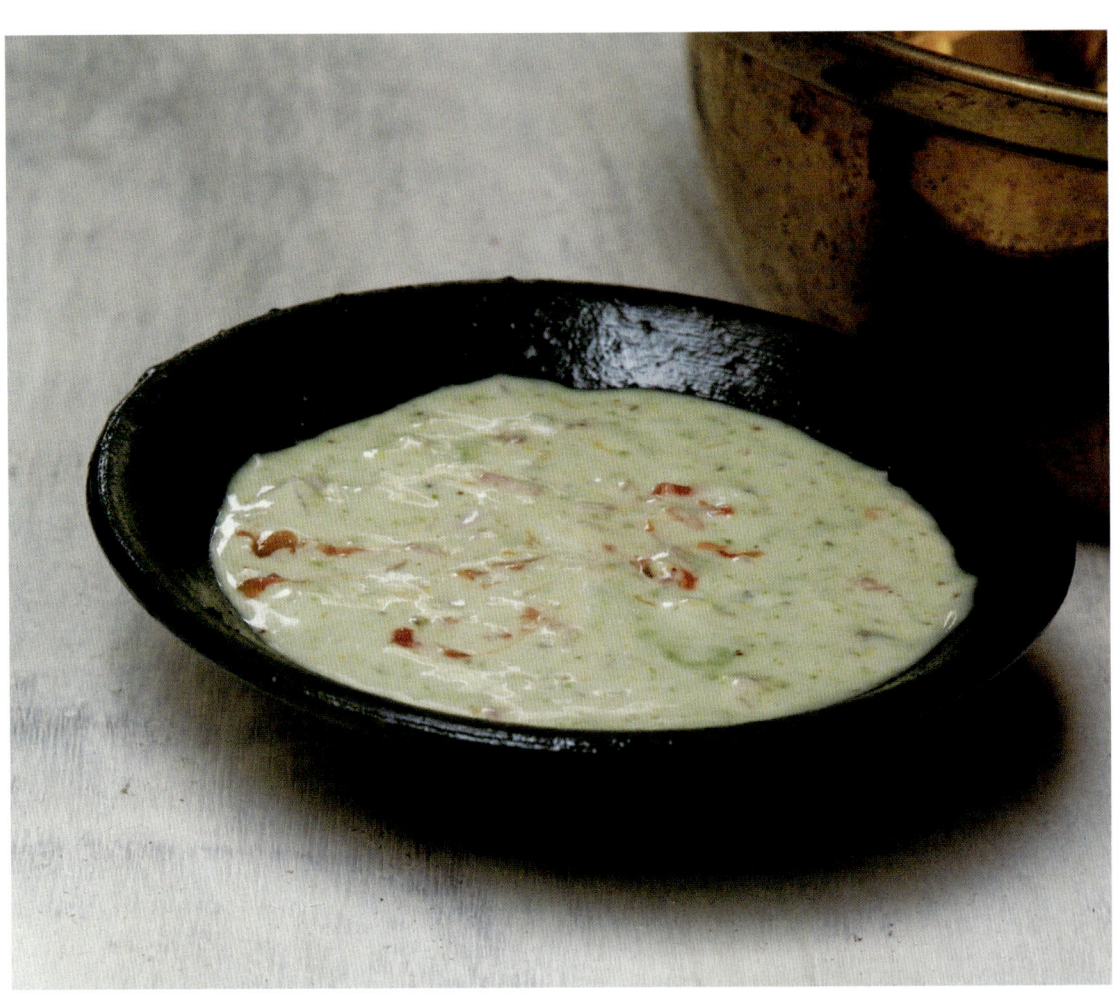

AVOCADO MULTI-LAYER BEAN SPREAD

2 cups avocados, mashed

1 tbsp lemon juice

½ tsp salt

¼ tsp freshly ground pepper

1 cup sour cream

2 tbsp honey

½ cup spring onions, chopped

2 cups tomatoes, chopped

½ cup black olives, pitted and chopped

2 cups cheddar cheese, grated

1 ½ cups boiled and mashed beans

Method

In a mixing bowl, add avocados, lemon juice, salt and pepper, and mix well to combine. Reserve.

In a small bowl, mix together sour cream and honey. Reserve

In a medium bowl, mix together onions, tomatoes, olives and cheese.

Stir together, and then set aside.

Spread mashed beans evenly in the bottom of a pan. Cover with a layer of avocado mixture, followed by a layer of sour cream mixture, and finally top with the olive and cheese mixture.

Makes 8 servings.

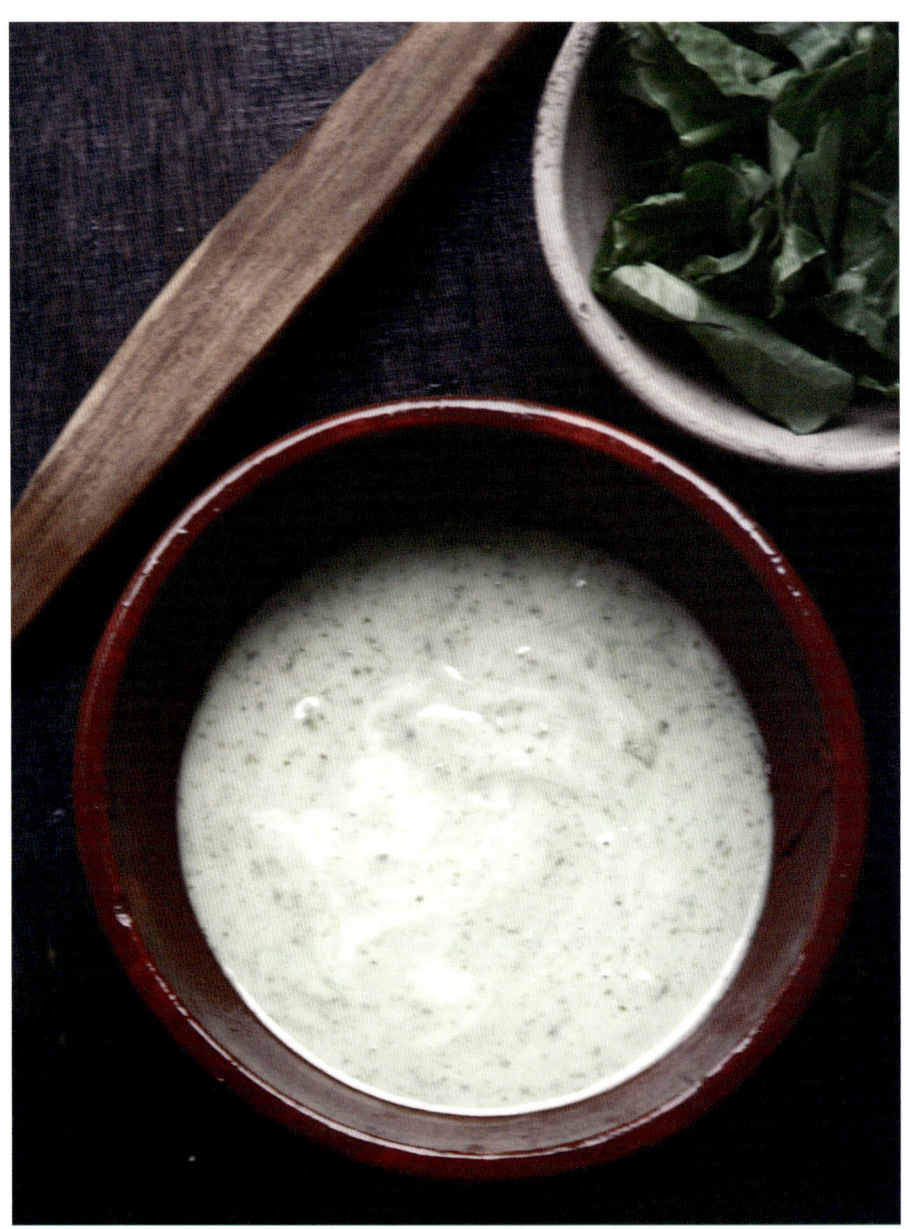

MUSTARD GARLICKY DIP

5 cups mustard greens, stemmed and roughly chopped

4 cloves garlic

2 tbsp green onions, chopped

½ green chili, or to taste

¼ cup basil leaves

¼ cup coriander leaves

1 tbsp lemon juice

Salt and freshly ground pepper to taste

2 cups light sour cream

¼ cup Greek yoghurt

Method

Bring water to boil in a medium pot over high heat. Add mustard greens and cover with lid. Blanch for two to three minutes, until the mustard is wilted. Drain and transfer to a bowl of iced water for three to four minutes.

Drain and reserve.

Pulse garlic, green onions, and chili in a food processor until smooth.

Add basil and coriander, and pulse for few more seconds. Add mustard, and then pulse again. Add lemon, salt, pepper, sour cream and yoghurt, and blend until mixed.

Makes 2½ cups.

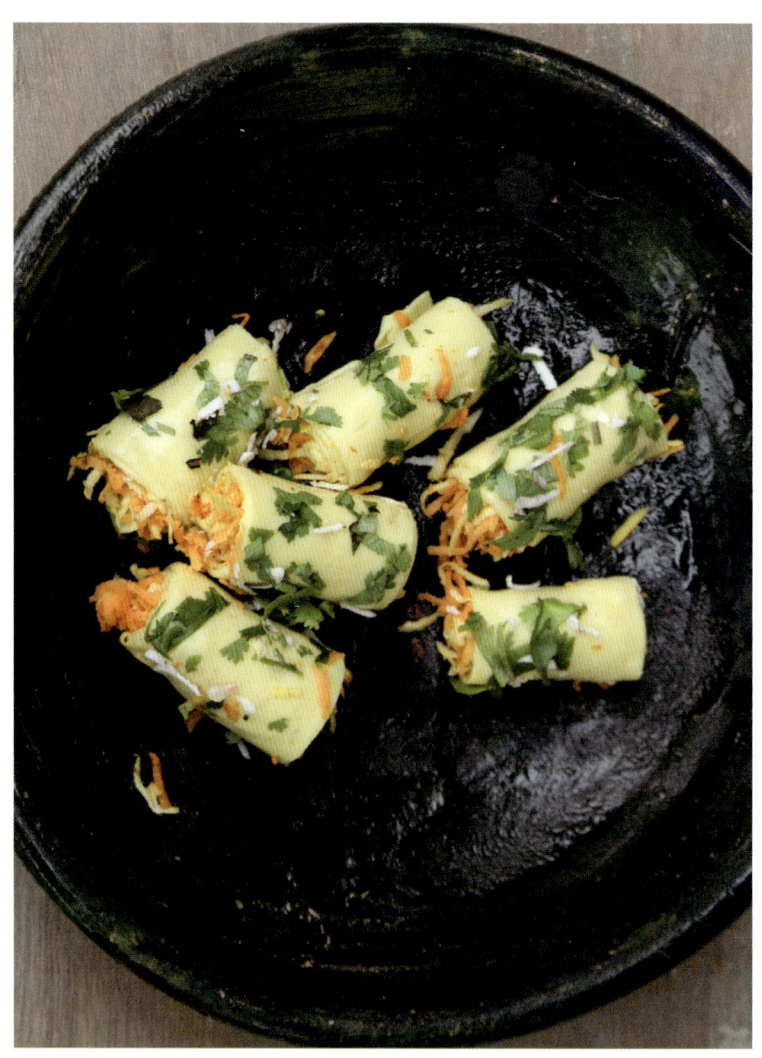

CHICKPEA ROLLS STUFFED WITH KALAMATA OLIVES

1 cup plain yoghurt

½ cup water

1 cup gram flour

Salt to taste

¼ tsp turmeric

3 tbsp lemon juice

¼ cup pitted kalamata olives, finely chopped

1 tbsp vegetable oil

1 tsp mustard seeds

1 tsp white sesame seeds

1 green chili, split

¼ cup coriander leaves, chopped (for garnish)

Method

In a large bowl, add yoghurt, water and flour, and mix until smooth. Add salt, turmeric and lemon juice.

Heat a pot on high heat, add mixture and bring to a boil. Reduce heat to low and simmer, whisking continuously. Continue to cook until mixture is thick and coats the back of a spoon.

Remove from heat and immediately spread on a greased baking sheet. Let it cool and dry for about fifteen minutes. Once cooled, cut into one to one-and-a-half inch wide strips. Gently spread the olives and roll lengthwise.

Repeat the process with all the sheets.

Heat oil in a small pot over medium heat. Add mustard seeds and cook for about 30 seconds until they sputter. Add sesame seeds and chilli and cook for a minute.

Sprinkle rolls with sesame seed chilli mixture. Garnish with the mixture and fresh coriander.

Makes 8-12 rolls.

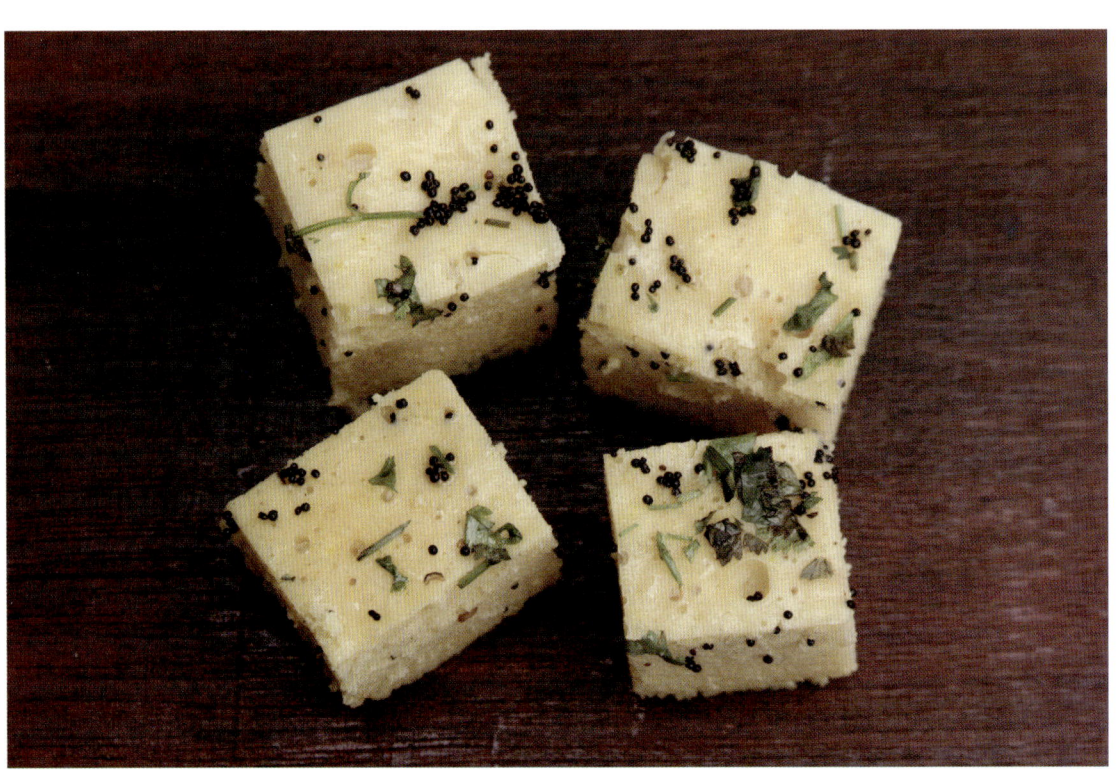

CITRUSY DHOKLA

1 cup cream of wheat

Salt to taste

1 tsp canola oil

¼ tsp turmeric

½ tsp whole cumin seeds, crushed

1-2 tbsp coriander leaves, chopped

1½ tsp lemon juice

1 cup plain yogurt

Juice of 1 orange

Juice of 1 grapefruit

1 tsp Eno Fruit salt

Method

Combine all ingredients except Eno in a large bowl and mix well. The batter should have the consistency of a pancake batter, add a little water if required.

Pour batter into a microwavable dish. Add the Eno and stir quickly, as it will activate immediately.

Cover and steam in a steamer until cooked through.

Serve hot or at room temperature.

Makes 12-16 squares.

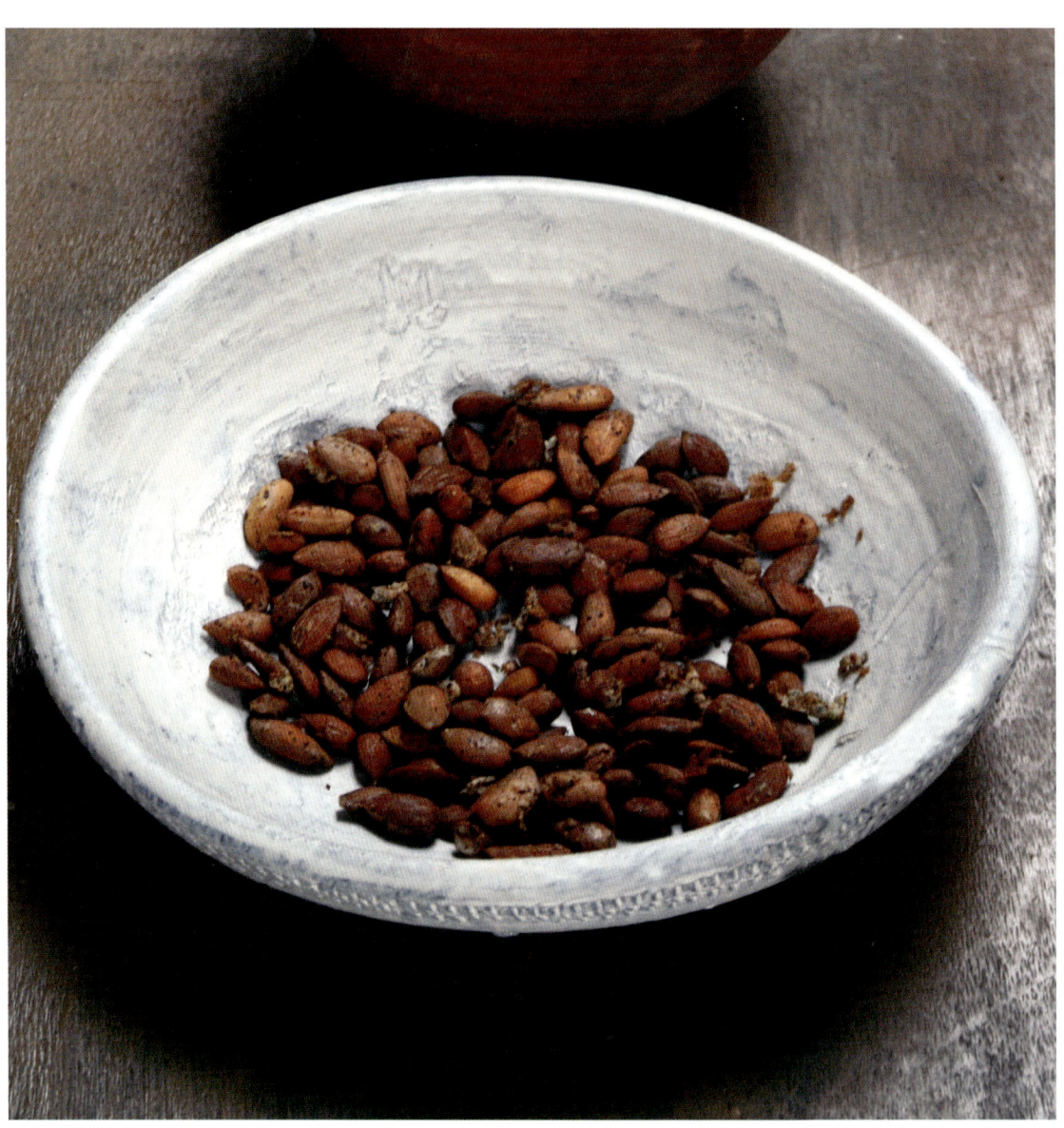

HONEY-SPICED ALMONDS

1 large egg, white only

1 ½ tsp cumin, light roasted and ground

Salt to taste

¼ tsp smoked paprika, or more to taste

2 ½ cups almonds, blanched

2 tbsp honey

Olive oil spray

Method

Preheat oven to 150°C.

Beat egg white in a small bowl until frothy. Add cumin, salt and paprika. Whisk well until combined.

Add the almonds and honey, and toss to combine.

Lightly grease a baking sheet with olive oil spray.

Place almonds in a single layer on the baking sheet and bake for about twenty-five to thirty minutes, turning once or twice.

Remove from oven and let cool. Serve hot or at room temperature.

Makes 2½ cups.

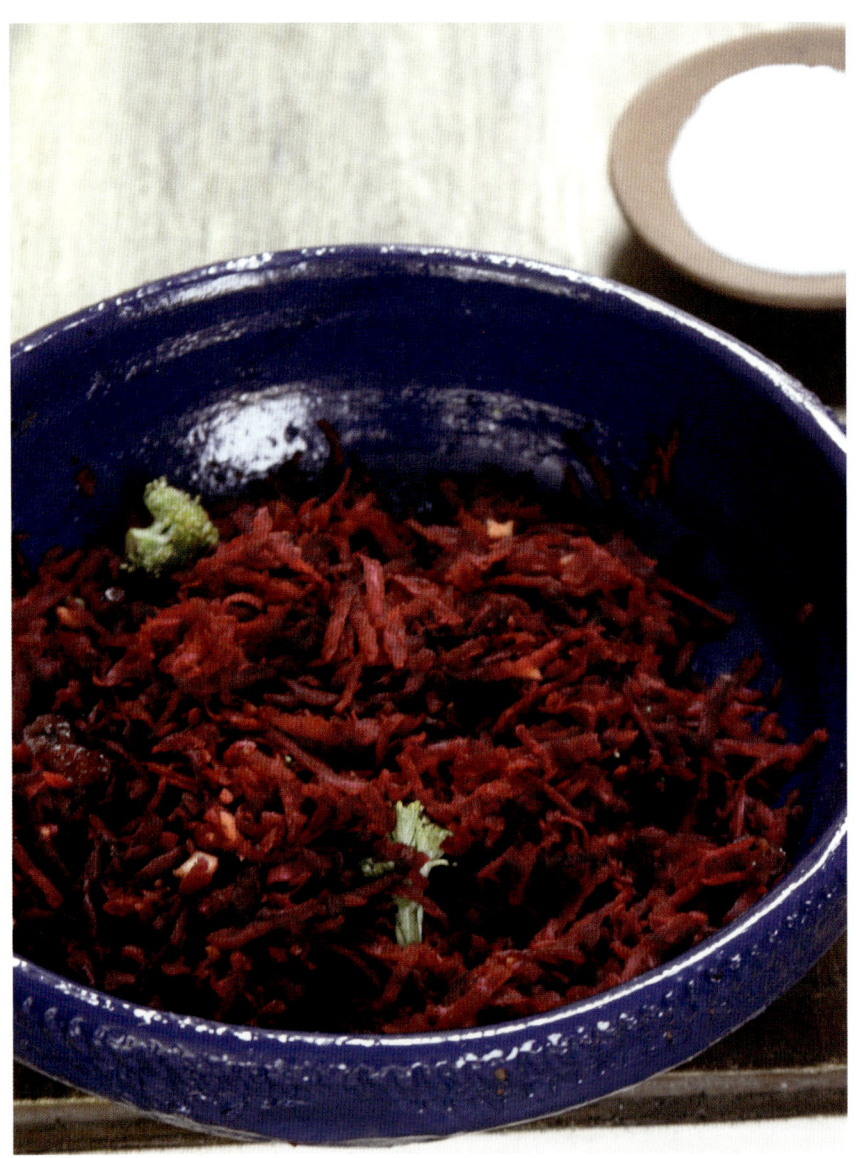

SALAD WITH LEMONY DRESSING

2 cups mixed greens

1 cup sunflower seed sprouts, loosely packed

1 medium carrot, peeled and grated

1 medium beet, peeled and grated

¼ cup finely chopped broccoli

1 tbsp dried cranberries

1 tbsp raw pumpkin seeds

¼ cup mint leaves, chopped

Dressing:

Juice of 1 lemon

4 tbsp hemp seed oil or olive oil

1 clove garlic, crushed

Salt and freshly ground pepper

Method

In a large mixing bowl, add all salad ingredients. Toss to combine

Combine all dressing ingredients in a jar and shake well.

Right before serving, pour the dressing and gently toss to evenly coat the salad.

Makes 4-6 servings.

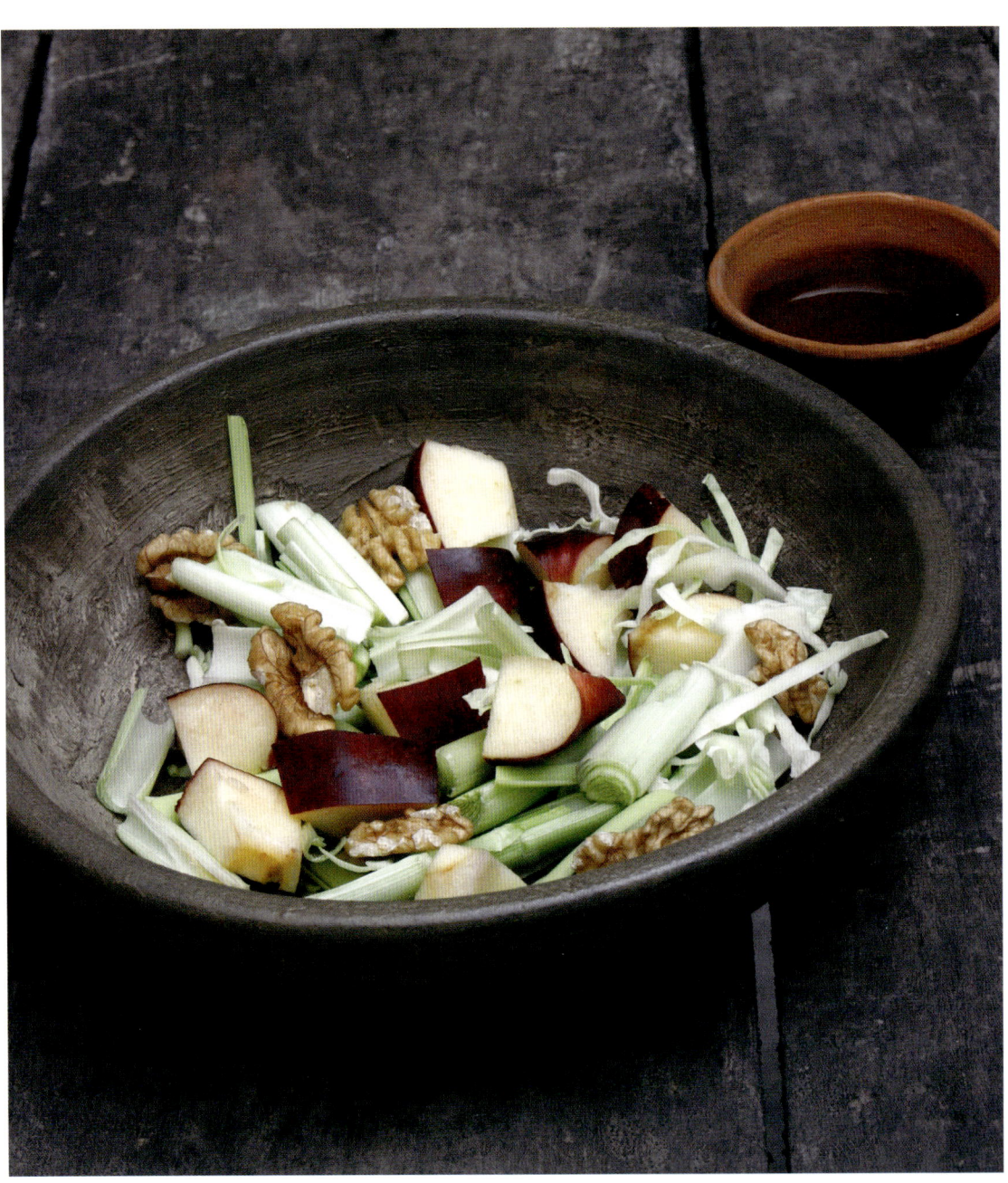

LETTUCE EAT SALAD

6 cups red leaf lettuce, shredded

2 unpeeled red apples, cored and diced

2 stalks celery, thinly sliced

½ cup walnuts, chopped

Dressing:

Juice of 1 lemon

2 tbsp extra virgin olive oil

Pinch of white pepper

Method

In a medium mixing bowl, combine all salad ingredients and toss. Drizzle with lemon juice and olive oil over the salad, and toss to combine. Serve fresh, sprinkled with white pepper.

Makes 4-6 servings.

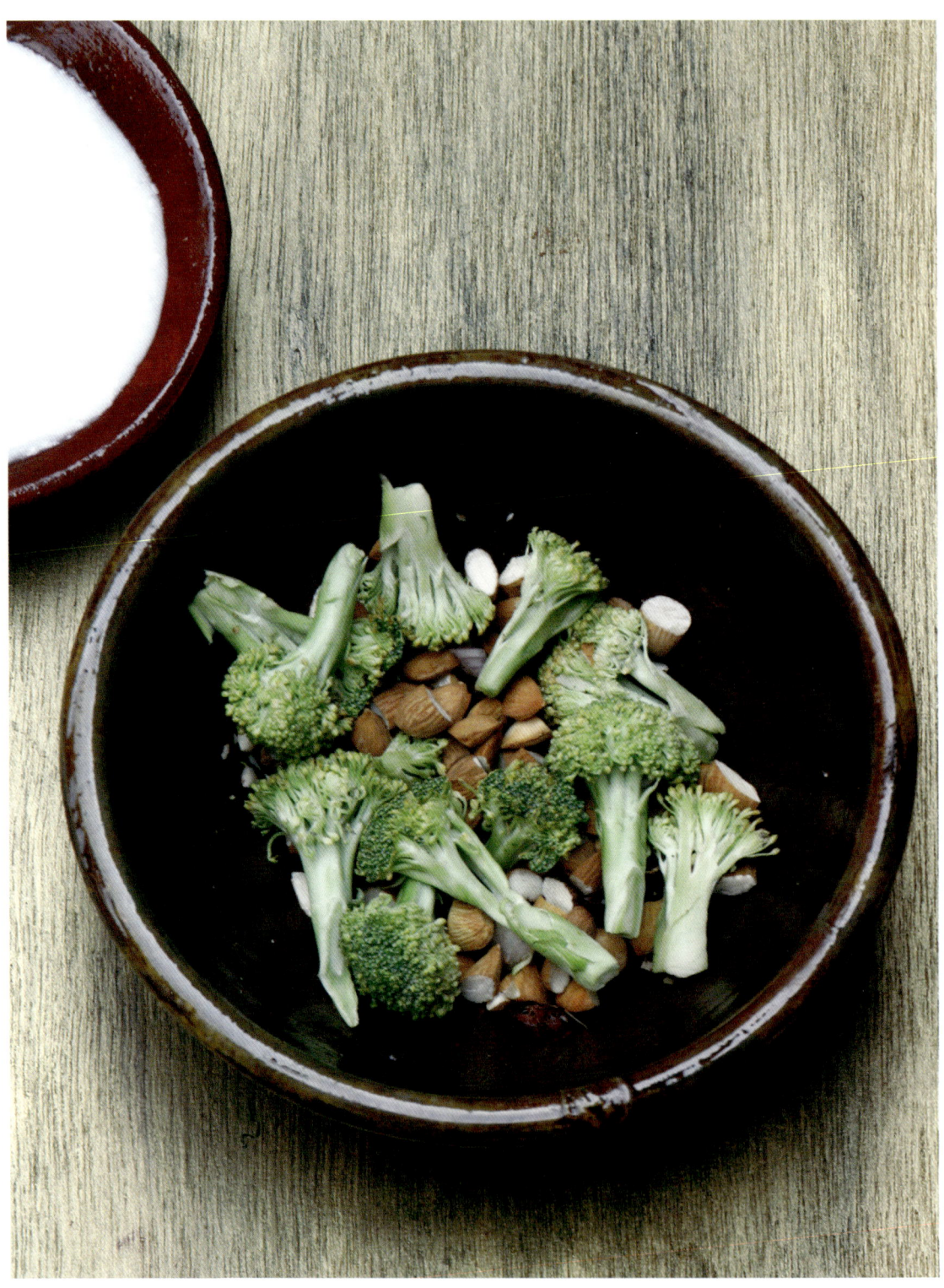

ROASTED ALMOND AND CURRANT SALAD

3 cups broccoli florets

½ cup red onions, chopped

¼ cup almonds, lightly roasted and chopped

½ cup black currants

Dressing:

½ cup plain light yoghurt

2 tbsp fresh ginger juice

2 tbsp honey

1 tbsp rice wine vinegar

Salt and freshly ground pepper

Method

In a large mixing bowl, add all salad ingredients and toss to combine.

Combine all dressing ingredients in a jar and shake well. Pour the dressing over the salad as per taste, toss to combine and serve.

Serve fresh.

Makes 4 servings.

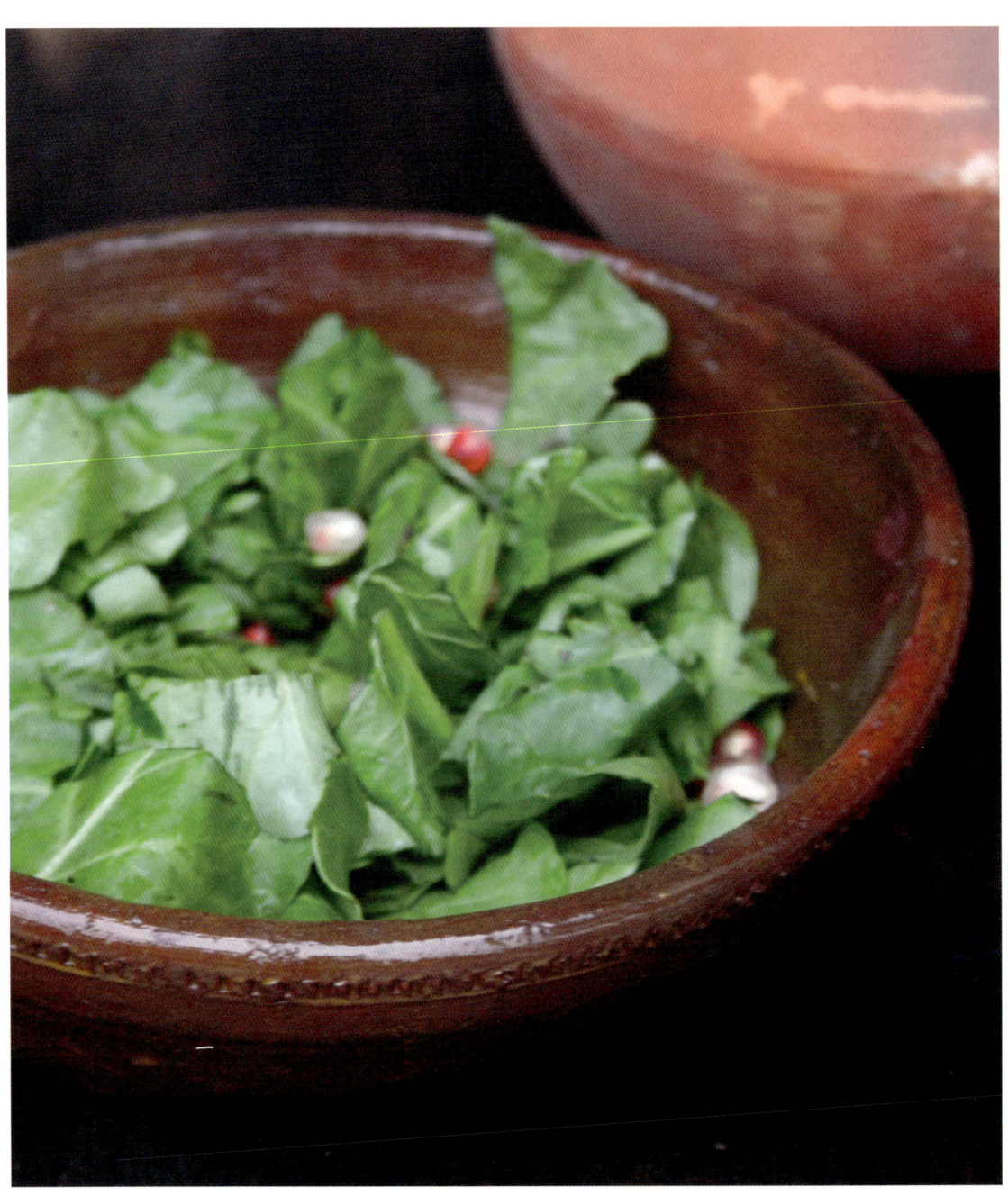

POMEGRANATE AND SPINACH SALAD
WITH GINGER-SCENTED DRESSING

5-6 cups baby spinach leaves, trimmed and coarsely chopped

$\frac{1}{3}$ up coriander leaves, chopped

1 cup fresh pomegranate seeds

$\frac{1}{3}$ cup pine nuts, toasted

$\frac{1}{4}$ cup red onions, sliced

Dressing:

4 tbsp olive oil

4 tbsp apple cider vinegar

2 tsp honey

1 tsp dry mango powder

Salt and freshly ground pepper to taste

Method

In a large mixing bowl, add all salad ingredients and toss to combine.

Combine all dressing ingredients in a jar and shake well. Pour the dressing over the salad as per taste, toss to combine and serve.

Makes 4-5 servings.

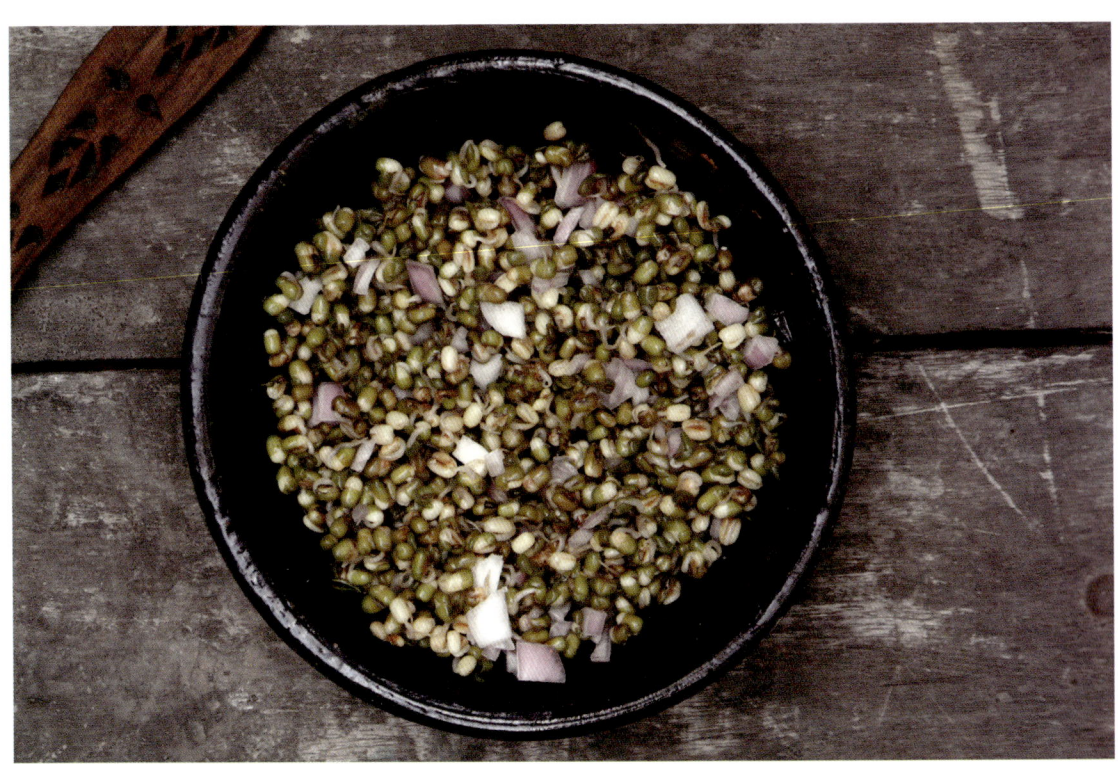

SPROUTS AND GRAPE SALAD

2 cups mixed beans sprouts

1 cup red bell peppers, chopped

1 cup celery, chopped

1 medium red onions, finely chopped

10-12 grapes, cut into half

Dressing:

$1/3$ cup rice vinegar

$1/3$ cup olive oil

1 tsp mustard

1 tsp garlic, minced

1 tsp honey

Salt and ground pepper to taste

Method

In a medium mixing bowl, combine all salad ingredients and toss.

In a jar, combine all dressing ingredients and shake well.

Pour over salad and toss again. Serve fresh.

Makes 4-5 servings.

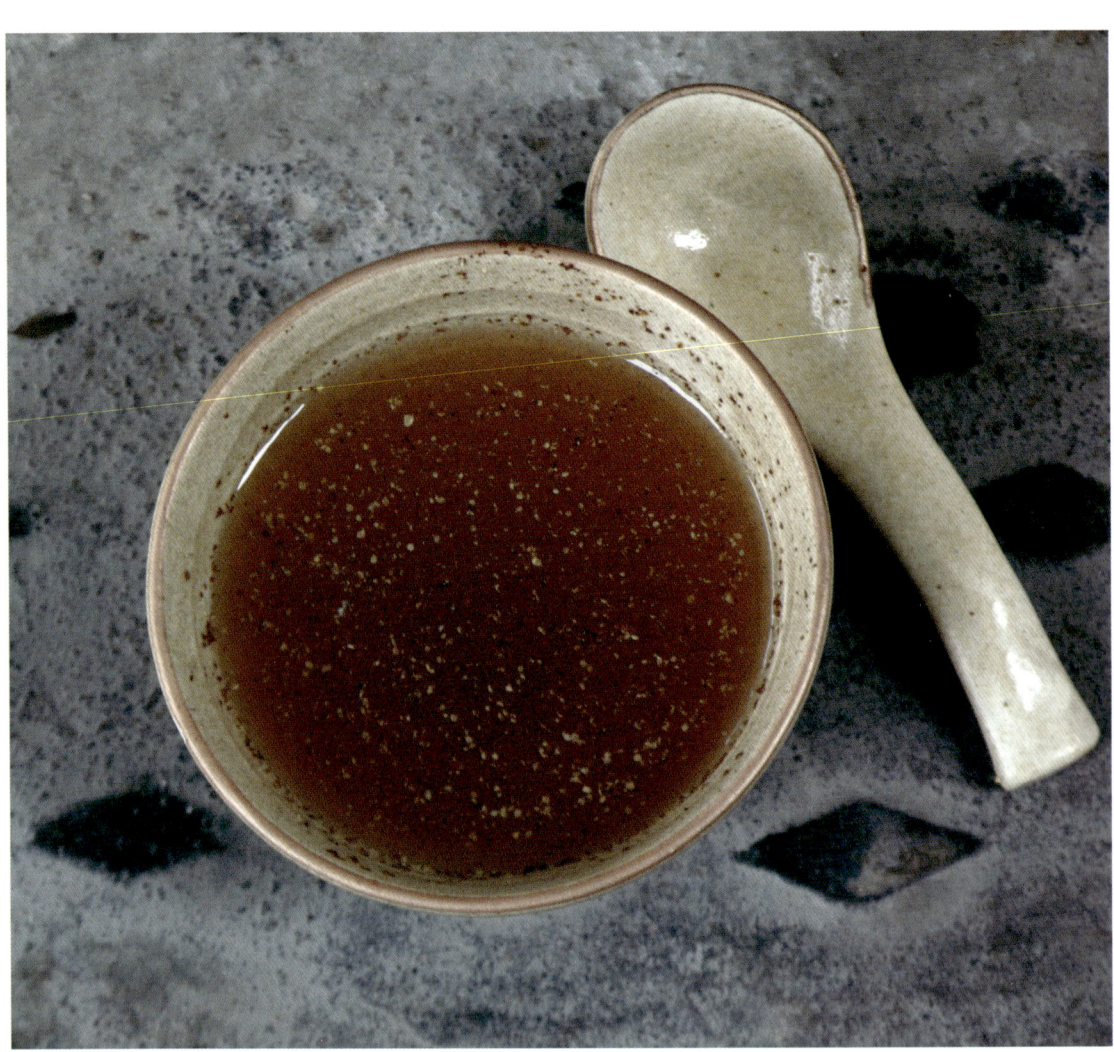

WARM COMFORTING APPLE AND VEGETABLE SOUP

1 red onion, roughly chopped

2 medium carrots, peeled and roughly chopped

2 red apples, cored and roughly chopped

2 tbsp grated ginger

2 bay leaves

8-10 whole peppercorns

2 cloves

Salt to taste

1 tsp turmeric

Method

Heat a large heavy bottom pot on high heat. Add all ingredients with four to five cups of water and bring to a boil.

Reduce heat to a low and simmer covered for thirty-five to forty-five minutes, until flavours have combined well, adding a little water if required.

Transfer the mixture to a blender and process until smooth and strain before serving.

Serve hot.

Makes 8-10 cups.

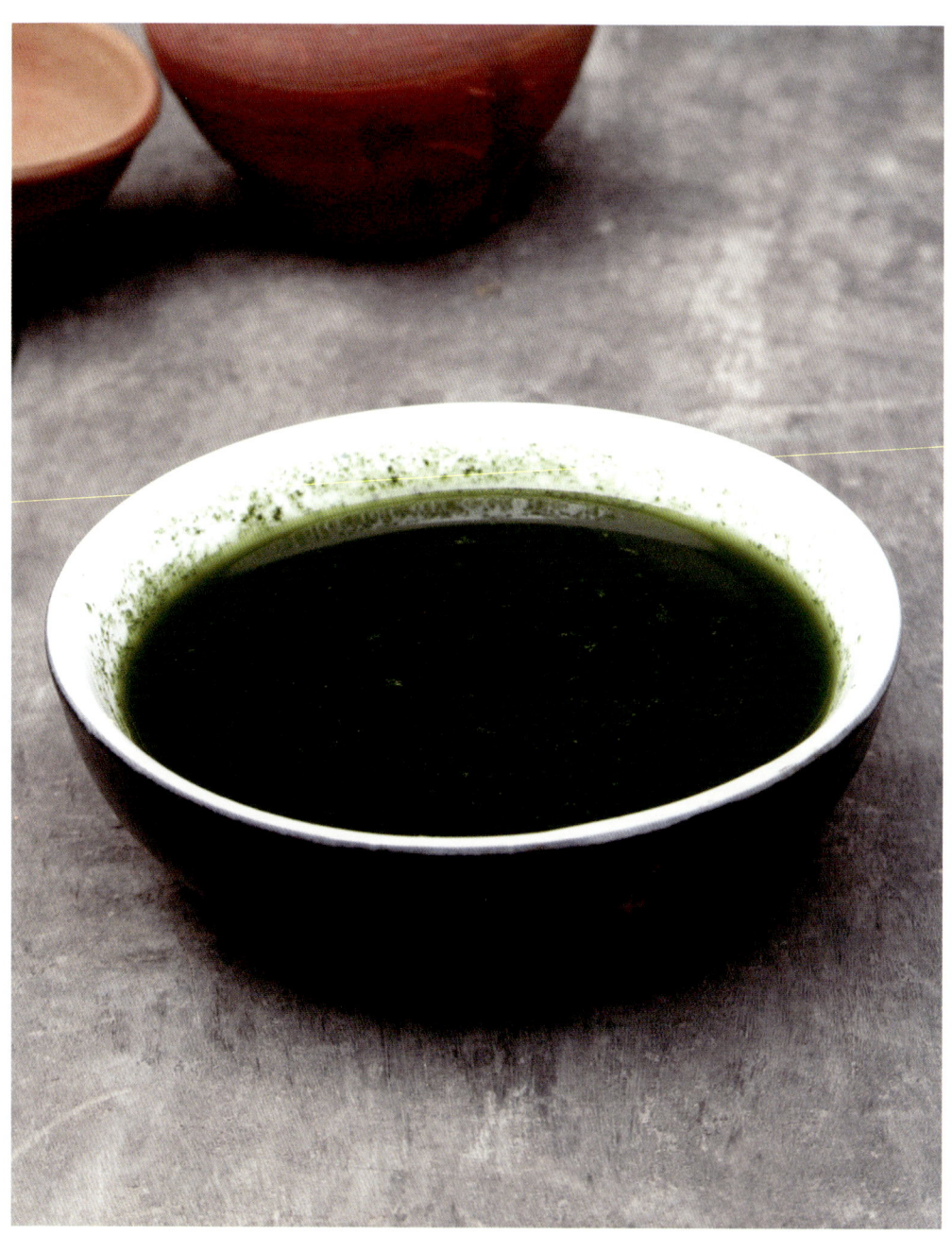

ONCE A DAY GREEN MACHINE SOUP

1 tbsp olive oil

1 red onion, thinly sliced

½ tsp minced ginger

1 tsp cumin

Pinch of asafetida

4 cups of vegetable stock

1 cup broccoli florets

5-6 cups spinach, chopped

¼ cup green peas

Salt and freshly ground pepper to taste

Method

Heat oil in a large heavy bottom pot on medium-high. Add onions and ginger. Sauté for about five minutes, until onions begin to caramelize. Add cumin, asafetida and sauté for another minute.

Add vegetable stock, broccoli, spinach and peas, and cook for about ten minutes, until all flavours have combined well. Season with salt and pepper to taste and serve hot.

Makes 4-6 cups.

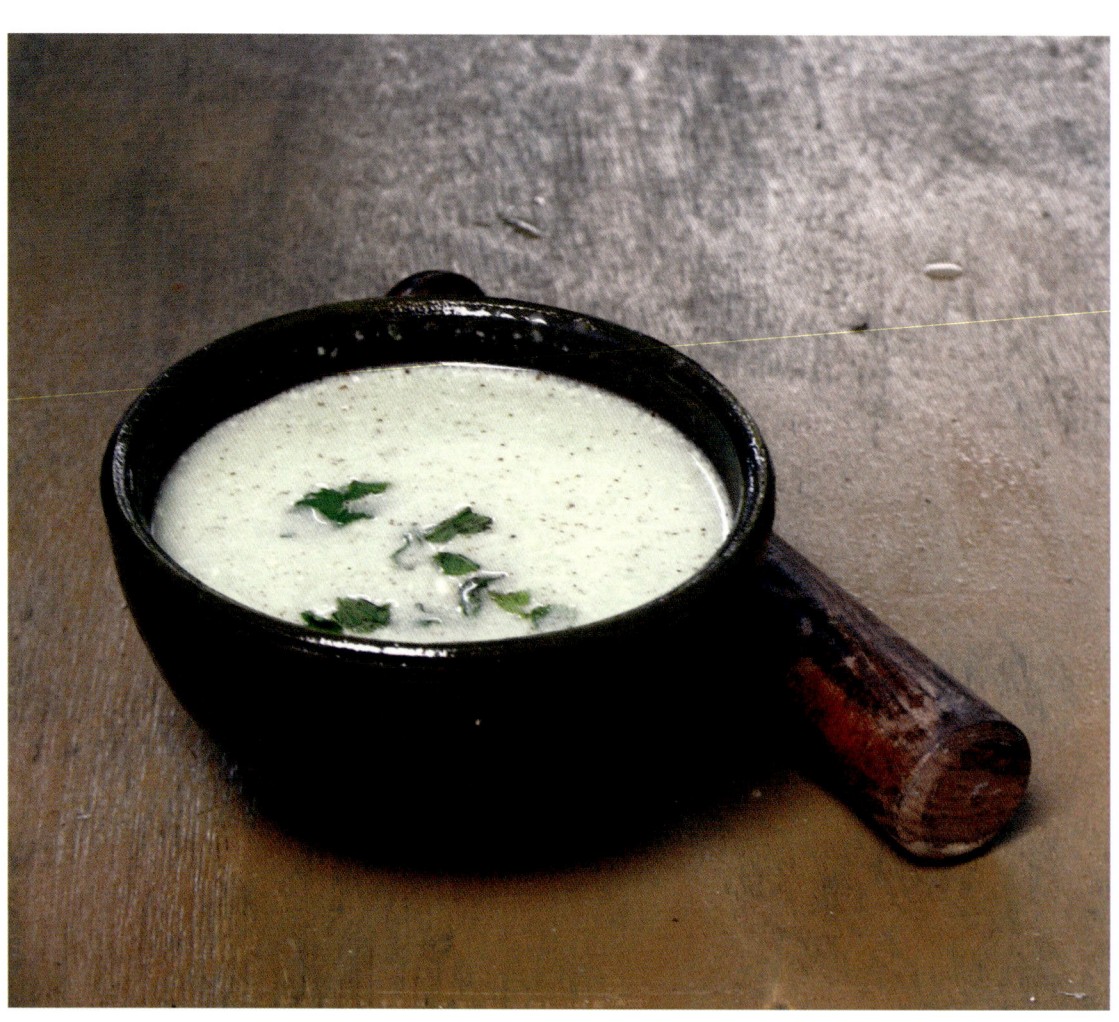

CHILLED CUCUMBER AND ORANGE SOUP

2 English cucumbers, chopped

Salt to taste

2 cloves garlic

¼ cup mint leaves, chopped

Juice of 1 lime

¼ tsp ground cumin

1 cup fresh orange juice

2 cups plain low fat yoghurt

¼ cup coriander leaves, (for garnish)

1 tsp green chilies, minced (optional)

Method

Combine all the ingredients in a medium non-reactive mixing bowl.

Refrigerate overnight, covered.

Garnish with coriander leaves, sprinkle green chilies, and serve.

Makes 4 cups.

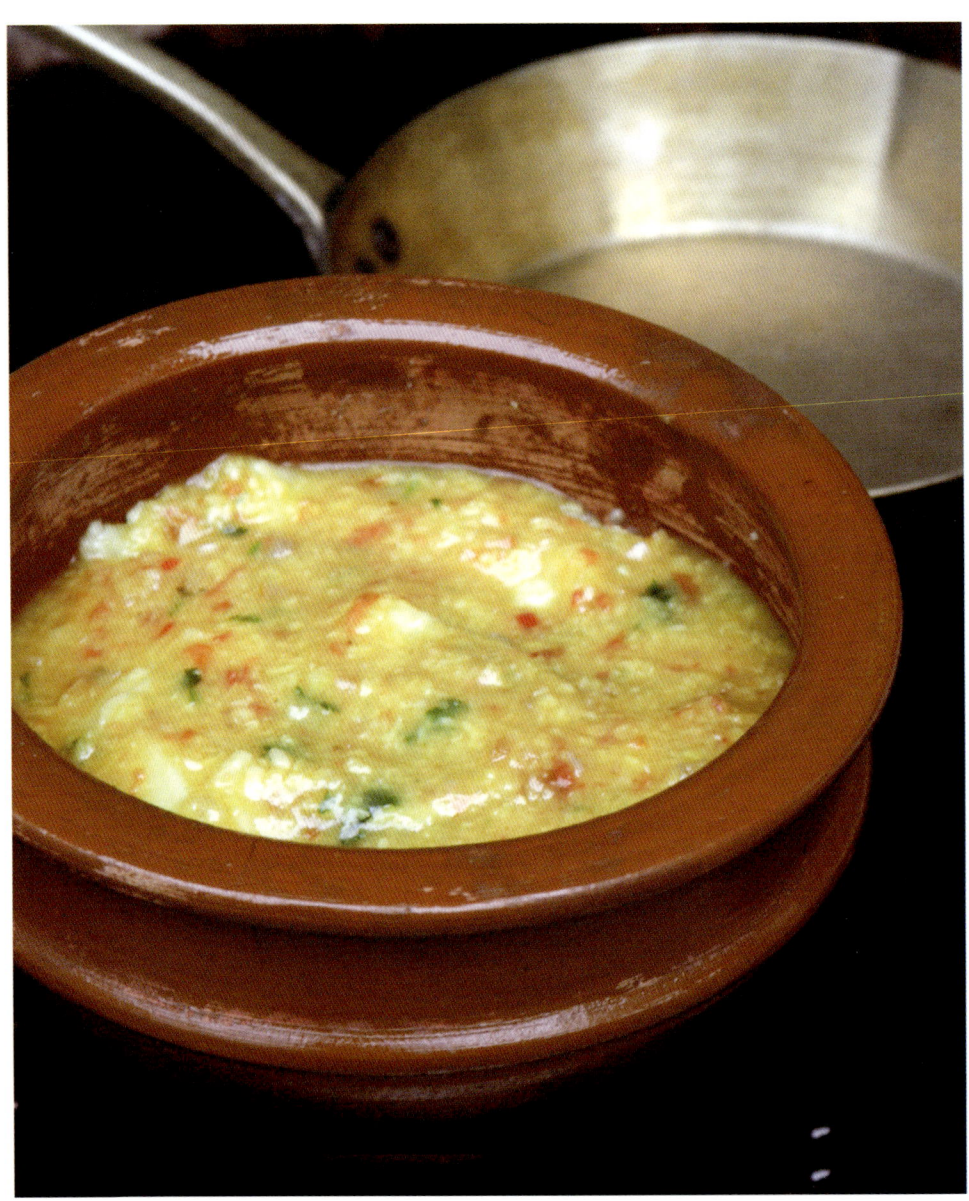

EVERYDAY COMFORT MUNG DAL

Dal:

2 cups split yellow mung dal

5-6 cups water

1 medium red onion, finely chopped

1 green chili, slit at end

Salt to taste

¼ tsp turmeric

1 tsp olive oil

Tadka:

1 tbsp olive oil

1 tsp whole cumin seeds

Pinch of asafetida

1 green chili, minced

1 medium tomato, sliced

¼ cup coriander leaves, chopped (for garnish)

Method

Heat a large pot on high heat. Add all dal ingredients and bring to a boil.

Reduce heat to low and simmer, while covered until done, which should take about twenty minutes. Using a slotted spoon, skim off the white foam and discard frequently.

In a frying pan on medium-high, heat oil. Add cumin and asafetida, and cook for 10 seconds until they sizzle. Add chilli and tomato, and cook, stirring for another three to four minutes.

Transfer the mixture to the cooked dal and stir to combine flavours.

Serve hot, garnished with coriander leaves.

Makes 4-6 servings.

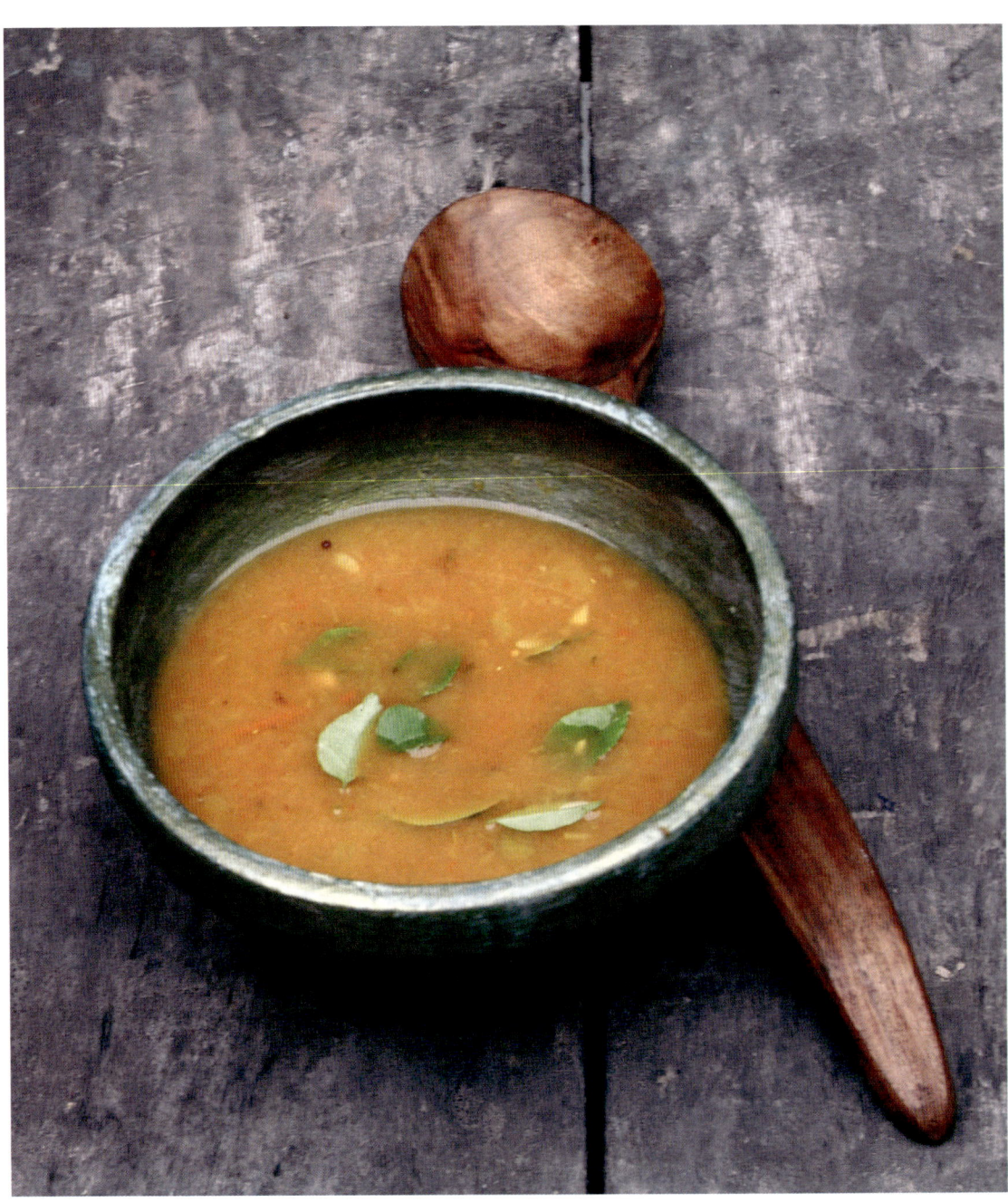

WHOLESOME TUR DAL

Dal:

2 cups tur dal or pigeon peas

5-6 cups water

1 medium carrot, finely chopped

1 green chili, slit at end

Salt to taste

¼ tsp turmeric

1 tsp olive oil

Tadka:

1 tbsp olive oil

1 tsp mustard seeds

10 curry leaves

1 green chili, minced

1 medium tomato, sliced

¼ cup coriander leaves, chopped (for garnish)

Juice of 1 lemon

Method

In a large pot, combine all dal ingredients and bring to a boil on high heat.

Reduce heat to low and simmer while covered until done, which should take about twenty minutes. Using a slotted spoon, skim off the white foam and discard frequently.

Heat oil in a frying pan over medium-high heat. Add mustard seeds and curry leaves, and cook for about ten seconds until they sizzle. Add chilli and tomato, and cook, stirring for another three to four minutes.

Transfer the mixture to the cooked dal and stir to combine flavours.

Garnish with coriander leaves and drizzle with lemon juice. Serve hot.

Makes 2-4 servings.

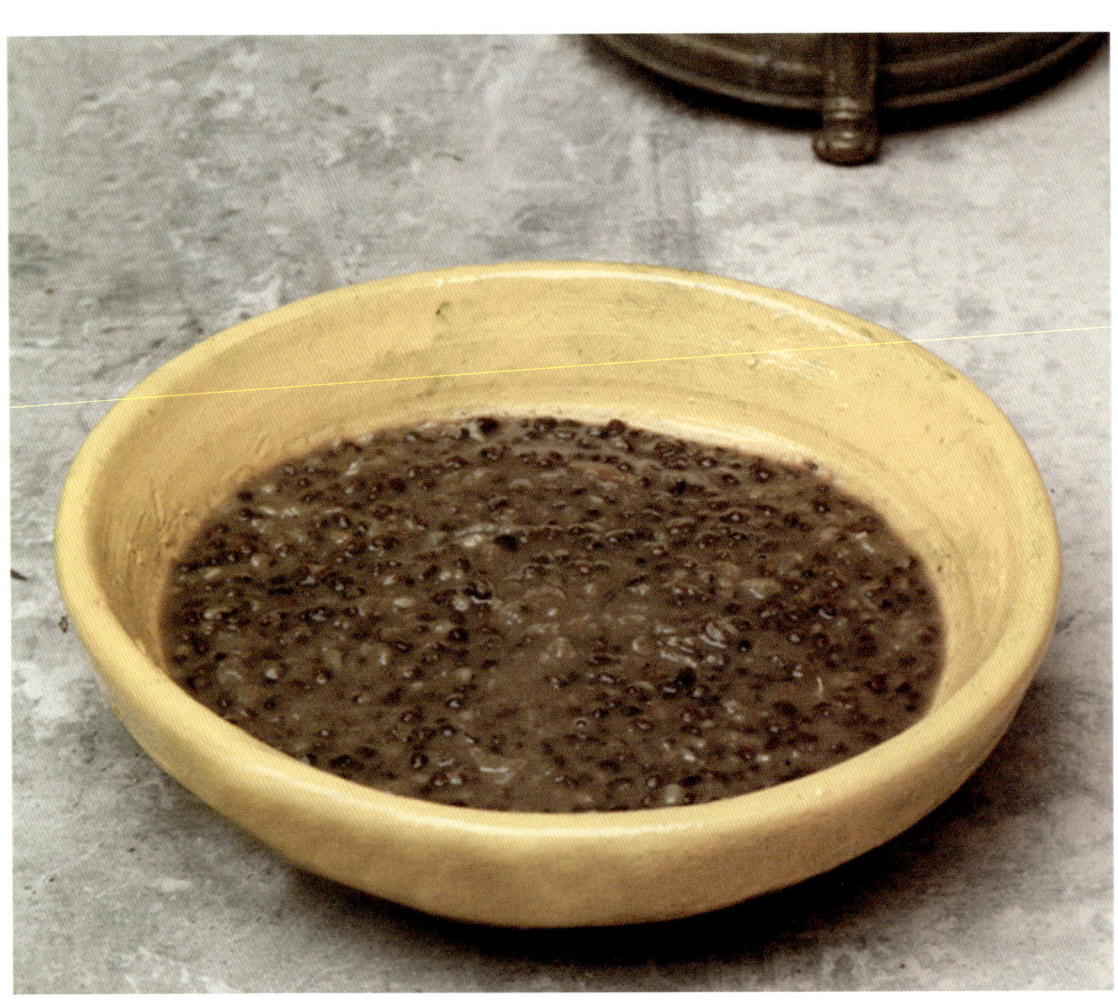

GRANDMA'S HEALING MINTY DAL

Dal:

2 cups whole urad dal

5-6 cups water

1 medium red onion, finely chopped

1 green chili, slit at end

2 cloves garlic, chopped

2 tbsp grated ginger

Salt to taste

¼ tsp turmeric

1 tsp olive oil

Tadka:

1 tbsp olive oil

1 tsp whole cumin seeds

Pinch of asafetida

1 green chili, minced

1 medium tomato, sliced

¼ cup mint leaves, chopped (for garnish)

Method

In a large pot, combine all dal ingredients and bring to a boil on high heat.

Reduce heat to low and simmer covered until done, which should take about twenty minutes. Using a slotted spoon, skim off the white foam and discard frequently.

Heat oil in a frying pan over medium-high. Add cumin, asafetida and cook for ten seconds until they sizzle. Add chili, tomato and cook, stirring for another three to four minutes.

Transfer the mixture to the cooked dal and stir to combine flavours.

Garnish with mint leaves and serve hot.

Makes 6-8 servings.

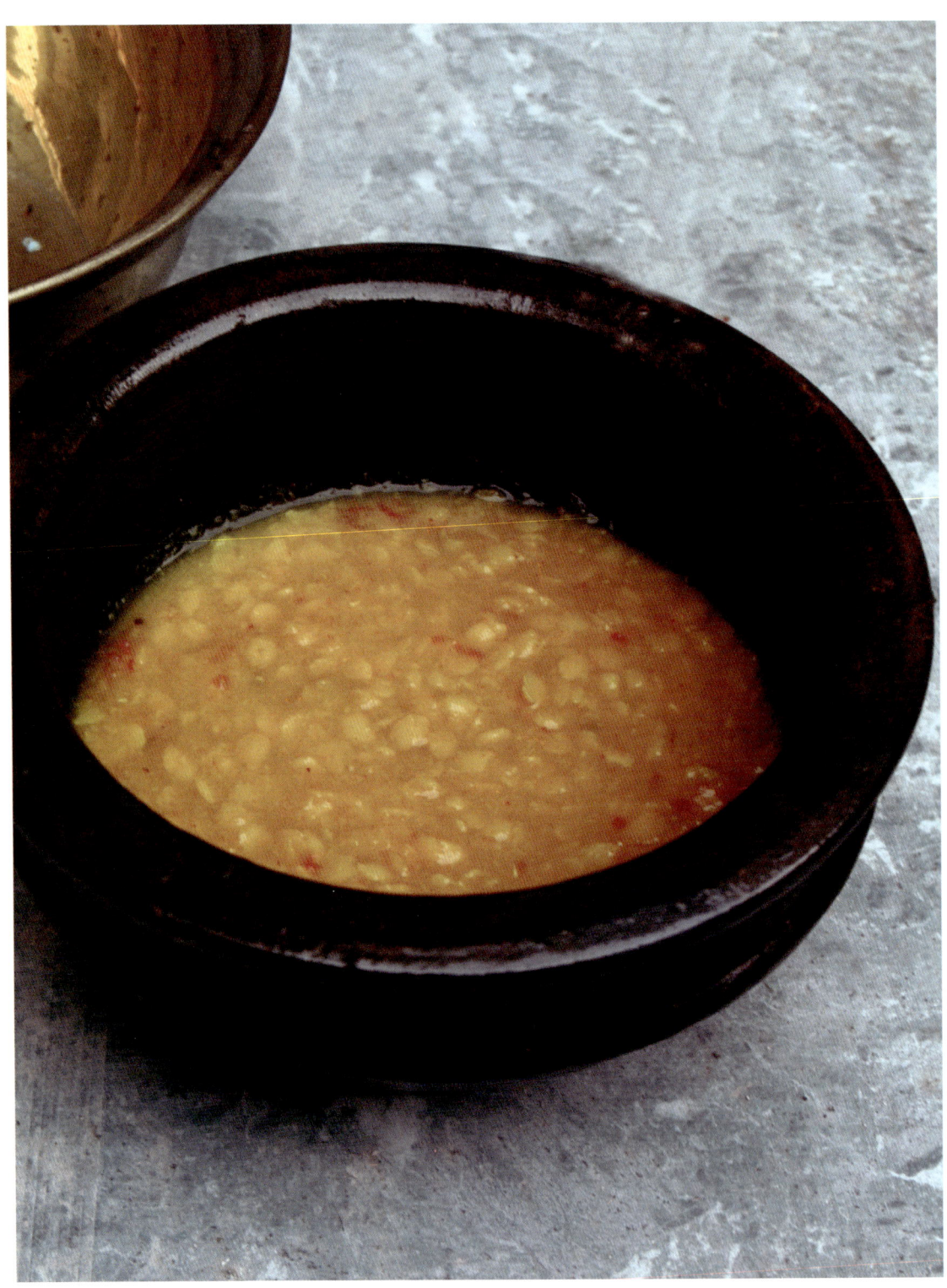

SWEET AND SOUR CHANA DAL

Dal:

1 ½ cups channa dal

1 medium red onion, finely chopped

1 green chilli, slit at end

Salt to taste

¼ tsp turmeric

1 tsp olive oil

Tadka:

1 tbsp olive oil

1 tsp whole cumin seeds

Pinch of asafetida

1 green chilli, minced

2 tbsp grated jaggery

2 tbsp tamarind paste

Method

Soak the dal in enough water overnight. Drain and reserve the dal.

Combine all dal ingredients with four cups of water in a large pot. Bring to a boil on high heat.

Reduce heat to low and simmer while covered until done, which should take about twenty minutes. Using a slotted spoon, skim off the white foam and discard frequently.

In a frying pan on medium-high, heat oil. Add cumin, asafetida and chilli, and cook for ten seconds until they sizzle.

Transfer the mixture to the cooked dal, jaggery and tamarind, and stir to combine flavors. Continue to cook for the right consistency.

Serve hot.

Makes 6-8 servings.

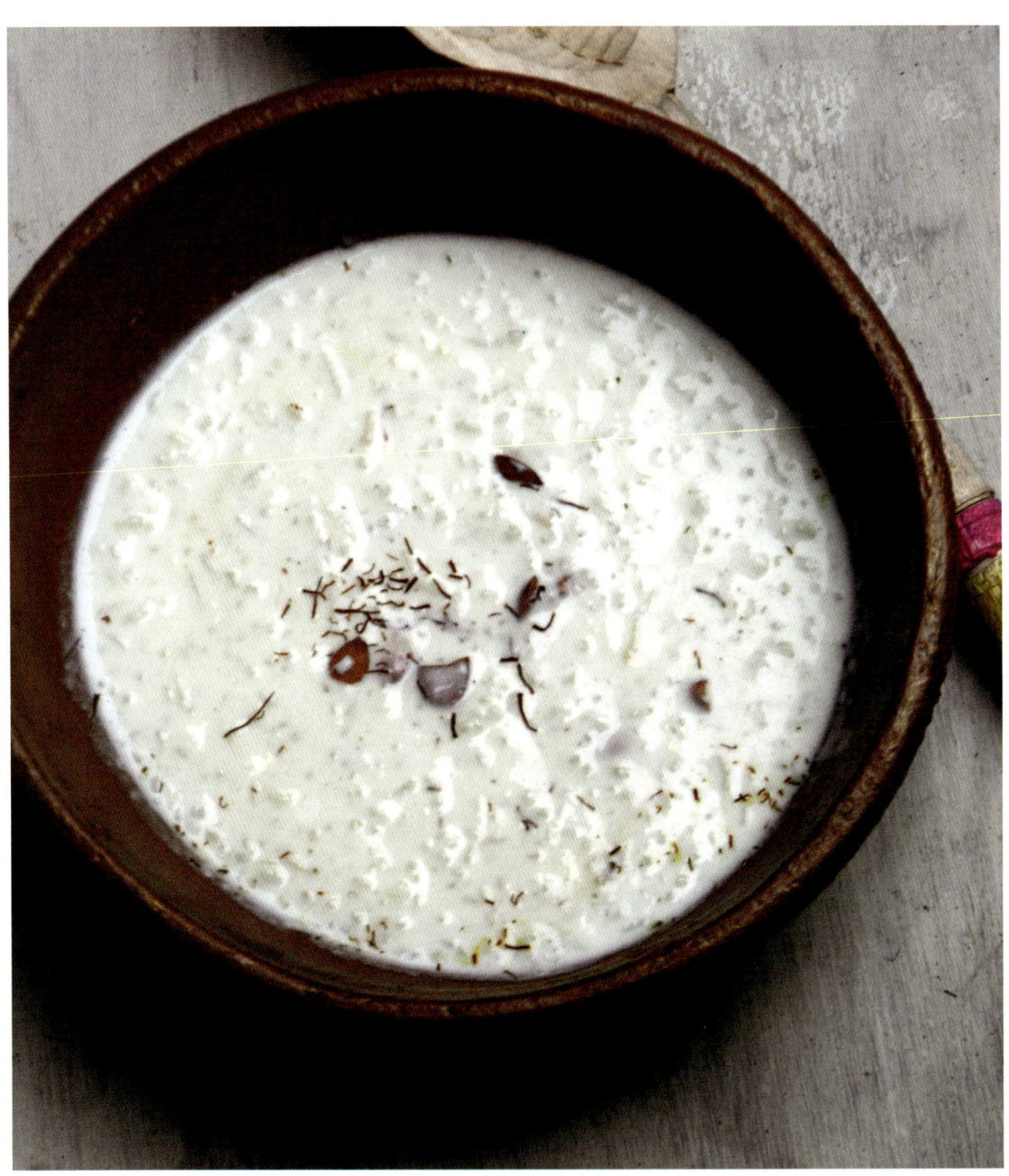

ON-THE-GO NUTTY RICE PUDDING

1 cup basmati rice, cooked and coarsely mashed

4 cups whole milk

¼ tsp ground cinnamon

4 tbsp jaggery or brown sugar, or to taste

3 tbsp raisins

1 tsp pistachios, coarsely chopped

1 tsp almond slivers

Method

Heat a large pot on high heat. Add rice, milk, cinnamon, jaggery and raisins, and bring to a boil.

Reduce heat and simmer while covered, for about twenty minutes, stirring occasionally. Garnish with pistachios and almonds. Serve hot or cold.

Makes 4 servings.

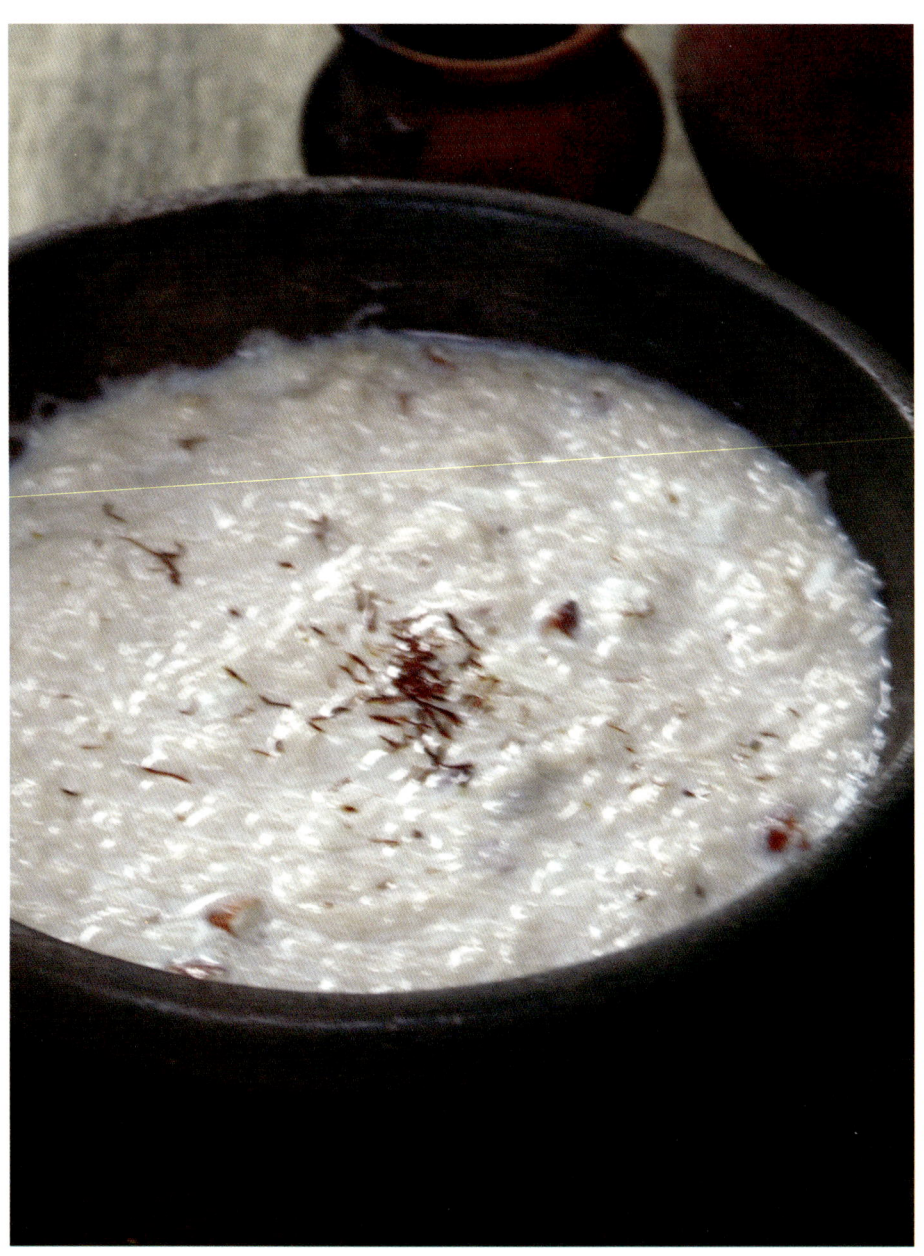

genera Elettaria and Amomum in the family Zingiberaceae.

Caste – Each of the hereditary classes of Hindu society, distinguished by relative degrees of ritual purity or pollution and of social status.

Cayenne – A hot, pungent powder made from various tropical chillies.

Cerebrospinal – Of or relating to the brain and spinal cord or to these together with the cranial and spinal nerves that innervate voluntary muscles.

Chakra – an energy point or node in the subtle body.

Chakrasana – Wheel pose.

Chariot – a type of carriage using animals to provide rapid motive power. Chariots were used for war as 'battle taxis'.

Charioteer – A chariot driver.

Chaturanga – An ancient Indian strategy game which is the common ancestor of the board games chess.

Cinnamon – A spice obtained from the inner bark of several trees from the genus Cinnamomum that is used in both sweet and savoury foods.

Coccyx – Commonly referred to as the tailbone, is the final segment of the vertebral column in humans.

Concentric – Denoting circles, arcs, or other shapes that share the same center, the larger often completely surrounding the smaller.

*D*andasana – Staff pose.

Deity – A God or Goddess.

Deltoids – In human anatomy, the muscle forming the rounded contour of the shoulder.

Dendrites – A short-branched extension of a nerve cell, along which impulses received from other cells at synapses are transmitted to the cell body.

Dhanurasana – Bow pose.

Dharana – Concentration, the process of holding or fixing the attention of mind onto one object or place.

Dharma – In Hinduism, the religious and moral law governing individual conduct and is one of the four ends of life.

Dhyana – Meditation or concentration.

Dorsal – The back of an animal or human being.

Dorsiflexion – Flexion or bending toward the extensor aspect of a limb, as of the hand or foot.

Doshas – According to Ayurveda, one of three bodily humors that make up one's constitution.

Drishti – Focused gaze, a means for developing concentrated intention.

Dualism – In philosophy of mind, a view about the relationship between mind and matter which claims that mind and matter are two ontologically separate categories.

*E*ndocrine – The major endocrine glands include the pineal gland, pituitary gland, pancreas, ovaries, testes, thyroid gland, parathyroid gland, hypothalamus, gastrointestinal tract and adrenal glands.

Epic – A long poem, typically one derived from ancient oral tradition, narrating the deeds and adventures of heroic or legendary figures or the history of a nation.

Equidistant – At equal distances.

*F*akir – A religious ascetic who lives solely on alms.

Fascia – A sheet of connective tissue covering or binding together body structures.

Femoris – The rectus femoris muscle is one of the four quadriceps muscles of the human body.

Fennel – The fruit is a dry seed from 4–10 mm long, half as wide or less, and grooved. Dried fennel seed is aromatic.

Flexion – The action of bending or the condition of being bent, especially the bending of a limb or joint.

Flexor muscles – Flexion is typically instigated by muscle contraction. A muscle that flexes a joint is called a flexor.

Fontanel – Soft spot of the skull.

Fulcrum – The support about which a lever pivots.

*G*arudasana – Eagle pose.

Gastrocnemius – a muscle located on the back of the lower leg, being one of the two major muscles that make up the calf.

Glutei – Any of three muscles in each buttock that move the thigh, the largest of which is the gluteus maximus.

Gomukhasana – Cow face pose.

Gracilis – one of the muscles found in the groin.

Groin – The area between the abdomen and the thigh on either side of the body.

Gunas – In Vedanta, any of the three interdependent modes or qualities of nature.

Guruvaar – Thursday.
Gyan – Knowledge.

*H*alasana – Plow pose.
Hatha – denotes a system of physical techniques supplementary to a broad conception of yoga.
Hiranyagarbhaya – Form of prayer.
Humerus – a long bone in the arm or forelimb that runs from the shoulder to the elbow.

*I*liacus – muscle found in the lower portion of the trunk, covered in a thick fascia (connective tissue).
Iliopsoas – the combination of the psoas major and the iliacus at their inferior ends.
Infraspinatus – In human anatomy, is a thick triangular muscle, which occupies the chief part of the infraspinatous fossa.
Isometric – *isometrics* are a type of strength training in which the joint angle and muscle length do not change during contraction.
Isotonic – a type of muscle contraction;

*J*nana – Knowledge.

*K*akasana – Crow pose.
Kapalbhati – a Pranayama, the yogic system of body cleansing techniques.
Kapha – In ayurveda, one of the three doshas, condensed from the elements, water and earth. It is the principle of stabilizing energy, governs growth in the body and mind, is concerned with structure, stability, lubrication, and fluid balance, and is eliminated from the body through the urine.
Kapotasana – Pigeon pose
Karma – Destiny or fate, following as effect from cause.
Kleshas – a term from Indian philosophy and yoga, meaning a 'poison'.
Kriya – Exercises and breathing techniques intended to purify and cleanse the body's energy channels.
Kundalini – Means 'coiled up' or 'coiling like a snake'.

*L*atissimus – Either of a pair of large, roughly triangular muscles covering the lower part of the back, extending from the sacral, lumbar, and lower thoracic vertebrae to the armpits.
Levator – A muscle that serves to raise a body part compare depressor.

Ligaments – A ligament is the tissue that connects two bones to form a joint.
Locomotive – The ability of cells or organisms to move and propel itself from place to place.

*M*ahabharata – One of the two major Sanskrit epics of ancient India.
Mangalvaar – Tuesday
Manipura – Solar plexus/navel chakra is the third primary chakra according to Hindu tradition.
Mantra – A word or sound repeated to aid concentration in meditation.
Masala – Blend of spices.
Matsyasana – Fish pose.
Matsyendrasana – Spinal twist.
Maya – that 'which is not' (i.e. illusion), refers to accepting the temporary as having lasting value, and looking for enduring happiness in this world.
Mayurasana – Peacock pose.
Medius – One of the three gluteal muscles, is a broad, thick, radiating muscle, situated on the outer surface of the pelvis.
Milieu – A person's social environment.
Mudra – Closure or seal. Mudra hand positions are physical gestures that have an effect on the energy flow of the body.
Muladhara – Root chakra is one of the seven primary chakras according to Hindu tantrism.

*N*adi – The channels through which, in traditional Indian medicine and spiritual science, the energies of the subtle body is said to flow. They connect at special points of intensity called chakras.
Namaskar – With all the depths and charms of my mind and all the love and cordiality of my heart, the divinity within me greets the divinity within you.
Natrajasana – Dancer's pose.
Neuro-Musculoskeletal – describing the inter-actions between nerves, muscles, and the skeleton.
Nidra – Sleep.
Nidrasana – Yogic sleep pose.

*O*m – Is a mystic syllable, considered the most sacred mantra. It appears at the beginning and end of most Sanskrit recitations, prayers, and texts.

*P*admanasana – Lotus pose.

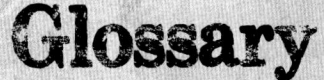

Glossary

Abdominal – The belly, that part of the body that contains all of the structures between the chest and the pelvis.

Abdominis – Long flat muscle on either side of the linea alba extending along the whole length of the front of the abdomen.

Abduction – The movement of a limb or other part away from the midline of the body, or from another part.

Abductor – A muscle whose contraction moves a limb or part away from the midline of the body, or from another part.

Adductor – A muscle whose contraction moves a limb or other part of the body toward the midline of the body or toward another part.

Adishesha – The king of all the serpent deities and one of the primal beings of creation.

Advaita – A Vedantic doctrine that identifies the individual self (atman) with the ground of reality (brahman).

Agnisar – Stimulating the digestive fire.

Agnostics – A person who claims neither faith nor disbelief in God.

Agonist – A substance that acts like another substance and therefore stimulates an action.

Ahimsa – Compassion and not to injure.

Ajna – The Ajna chakra is positioned in the stomata, directly behind the center of the forehead.

Anahata – It is associated with a calm, serene sound devoid of violence.

Anatomical – Of or relating to bodily structure.

Aarti – Religious ritual of worship.

Antagonist – A person who actively opposes or is hostile to someone or something.

Anterior – Situated in the front of the body or nearer to the head.

Anulom – With the grain or natural.

Aphorisms – A concise statement of a scientific principle, typically by an ancient classical author.

Appendicular – Consists of the bones or cartilage that support the appendages of vertebrates.

Ardha – Half.

Aryan – People speaking an Indo-European language who invaded northern India in the 2nd millennium BC, displacing the Dravidian and other aboriginal people.

Asana – A posture adopted in performing hatha yoga.

Asceticism – Severe self-discipline and avoidance of all forms of indulgence, typically for religious reasons.

Ashtanga – A type of yoga based on eight principles and consisting of a series of poses executed in swift succession, combined with deep, controlled breathing.

Ashva – Horse.

Atharva Veda – The fourth Veda in Hinduism.

Atheists – Atheism is not a disbelief in gods or a denial of gods; it is a lack of belief in gods.

Atma or Atman – The individual self, known after enlightenment to be identical with Brahman.

Aura – The distinctive atmosphere or quality that seems to surround and be generated by a person, thing, or place.

Axial – To an axial position or location of a group.

Axons – It is the elongated fiber that extends from the cell body to the terminal endings and transmits the neural signal.

Ayurveda – Is a system of Hindu traditional medicine.

Balasana – Child's pose.

Bandha – Body locks.

Bhagavad Gita – Referred to as simply the Gita, is a 700 – verse Hindu scripture in Sanskrit that is part of the Hindu epic *Mahabharta*.

Bhagavate – Lord.

Bhakti – Within Hinduism it is the love felt by the worshipper towards their personal God.

Bhujangasana – Cobra Pose.

Biceps – Two-headed muscle that lies in the upper arm.

Bija – Seed.

Bipedal – Walking on two feet.

Brachialis – muscle in the upper arm that flexes the elbow joint. It lies deeper than the biceps brachii, and is a synergist that assists the biceps brachii in flexing at the elbow.

Brachii – Brachii muscle is the larger of the two muscle bodies that forms the entire biceps brachii muscle.

Brahma – the Hindu God of creation.

Brevis – Several muscles in the human body.

Budhvaar – Wednesday.

Camphor – A waxy, flammable, white or transparent solid with a strong aromatic odor.

Cardamom – sometimes called cardamon, spice made from the seeds of several plants in the

Paschimottasana – Seated forward bend.

Pashupati – an incarnation of the Hindu Lord Shiva as 'Lord of animals'.

Pineal gland – also known as the pineal body, conarium or epiphysis cerebri, is a small endocrine gland in the vertebrate brain.

Pitta – In ayurveda, one of the three doshas, condensed from the elements fire and water.

Pituitary – The main endocrine gland. It is a small structure in the head. It is called the master gland because it produces hormones that control other glands and many body functions including growth. The pituitary consists of the anterior and posterior pituitary.

Plantar – Of or relating to the sole of the foot.

Plexus – A network of nerves or vessels in the body.

Prakriti – Nature.

Prana – Life force.

Pranayama – The regulation of the breath through certain techniques and exercises.

Pratyahara – the fifth element among the Eight stages of Patanjali's Ashtanga Yoga.

Pronation – the inward movement of the foot as it rolls to distribute the force of impact of the ground as you run.

Psoas – Each of a pair of large muscles that run from the lumbar spine through the groin on either side and, with the iliacus, flex the hip. A second muscle, the psoas minor, has a similar action but is often absent.

Purusha – One's true self, regarded as eternal and unaffected by external happenings.

Putra – Son.

*Q*uadratus – Any of several roughly square or rectangular muscles, e.g., in the abdomen, thigh, and eye socket.

Quadriceps – The large muscle at the front of the thigh, which is divided into four distinct portions and acts to extend the leg.

*R*ajas – the force which promotes or upholds the activity of the other aspects of nature (prakriti) such as one or more of the following: action, change, mutation; passion, excitement; birth, creation, generation.

Ramayana – a Sanskrit epic poem ascribed to the Hindu sage and Sanskrit poet Valmiki. It is regarded as one of the two great works of Indian literature, along with the Mahabharata.

Ravivaar – Sunday.

Rectus – Each of a pair of long flat muscles at the front of the abdomen, joining the sternum to the pubis and acting to bend the whole body forward or sideways.

Reincarnation – the religious or philosophical concept that the soul or spirit, after biological death, can begin a new life in a new body.

Rig Veda – an ancient Indian sacred collection of Vedic Sanskrit hymns.

Rituals – A religious or solemn ceremony consisting of a series of actions performed according to a prescribed order.

*S*ahasrara – Crown chakra is the seventh primary chakra, according to Hindu tradition.

Sakti – The female principle or organ of reproduction and generative power in general.

Salabhasana – Locust pose.

Sama Veda – the third of the four Vedas, the ancient core Hindu scriptures. It ranks next in sanctity and liturgical importance to the Rigveda.

Samadhi – a spiritual state of consciousness.

Samkya – It is one of the six orthodox schools of Hindu philosophy. It is described as the rationalist school of Indian philosophy. It is most related to the Yoga school of Hinduism, and its rationalism was influential on other schools of Indian philosophies.

Samskara – The concept of imprints or impressions left on the mind by experience in Indian philosophies.

Sanchalasana – Low lunge pose.

Sartorius – a long, narrow muscle running obliquely across the front of each thigh from the hipbone to the inside of the leg below the knee.

Sarvangasana – Shoulder Stand.

Sattva – In Ayurveda, the element or mode of prakriti or nature associated with purity, wholesomeness, and virtue.

Scapular – Relating to the shoulder or shoulder blade.

Serratus – A muscle in the trunk (thorax).

Shanivaar – Saturday.

Shanti – Peace.

Shastras – commonly used to mean a treatise or text written in explanation of some idea, especially in matters involving religion.

Shavasana – Corpse pose.

Shukrvaar – Friday.

Siddhasana – Accomplished pose.

Sirsasana – Head stand.

Soleus – located in the superficial posterior compartment of the leg.

Somvaar – Monday.

Sruti – 'That which is heard', and refers to the body of most authoritative, ancient sacred texts comprising the central canon of Hinduism.

Supine – Lying face upward.

Supta – Fallen asleep.

Surya – Sun.

Sushumna – The movements indicate the flow of Prana through the central canal and in the process, the sushumna makes the way for the ascent of Kundalini.

Sutras – an aphorism or a collection of aphorisms in the form of a manual or, more broadly, a text in Hinduism or Buddhism.

*T*adasana – Tree pose.

Tamas – The element or mode of prakriti or nature associated with lethargy, darkness, and ignorance.

Tandava Nritya – a vigorous dance that is the source of the cycle of creation, preservation and dissolution.

Tantra – a divinely revealed body of teachings, explaining what is necessary and what is a hindrance in the practice of the worship of God; and also describing the specialized initiation and purification ceremonies that are the necessary prerequisites of Tantric practice.

Trimurti – The triad of gods consisting of Brahma the creator, Vishnu the preserver, and Shiva the destroyer as the three highest manifestations of the one ultimate reality.

*U*ddiyana – It involves, after having exhaled all the air out, pulling the abdomen under the rib cage by taking a false inhale while holding the breath and then release the abdomen after a pause.

Upanishads – a series of Hindu sacred treatises written in Sanskrit circa 800–200 BC, expounding the Vedas in predominantly mystical and monistic terms.

Upvaas – Fast.

Ustranasana – Camel pose.

Uttanasana – Standing forward bend.

*V*ata – In ayurveda, one of the three doshas, condensed from the elements air and space. It is the principle of kinetic energy in the body.

Vedanta – one of the world's most ancient religious philosophies and one of its broadest. Based on the Vedas, the sacred scriptures of India, Vedanta affirms the oneness of existence, the divinity of the soul, and the harmony of religions.

Vedas – a large body of texts originating in ancient India.

Vinyasa – a gradual progression or a step – by – step approach that connects one pose to another.

Virabhadrasana – War pose.

Vortex – A mass of whirling fluid or air, especially a whirlpool or whirlwind.

Vratas – a religious practice to carry out certain obligations with a view to achieve divine blessing for fulfillment of one or several desires. Etymologically, vrata, a Sanskrit word, means to vow or to promise.

Vyasa – a central and revered figure in most Hindu traditions.

*W*armonger – A person who advocates, endorses, or tries to precipitate war.

*Y*antra – A geometric diagram, or any object, used as an aid to meditation in tantric worship.

Yoga – To unite.

Yuj – To control.

FESTIVE SAFFRON VERMICELLI

2 tbsp ghee

2 cups roasted vermicelli, broken into pieces

6 cardamom pods, lightly crushed

2 cinnamon sticks

1 ½ cup milk

1 tsp saffron threads, soaked in 2 tbsp of warm milk

⅓ cup honey

1 ½ tbsp almonds, coarsely ground (for garnish)

Method

Preheat oven to 180°C.

Heat a pot on medium heat. Add ghee and vermicelli and sauté until it is evenly browned. Add cardamom and cinnamon and sauté until fragrant, about one minute.

Add milk, saffron and honey, and bring to a boil on high heat. Reduce the heat to low, simmer until the vermicelli is cooked and all the flavours have combined well. Add a little water if required.

Garnish with almonds and serve hot.

Makes 4 servings.